T0201233

Practical Procedures in
Aesthetic Dentistry

# Practical Procedures in Aesthetic Dentistry

**Edited by**

**Subir Banerji** *BDS MClinDent(Prostho) PhD MFGDP(UK) FICOI FICD*

*Private Dental Practitioner;*
*Senior Clinical Teacher,*
*Programme Director, Aesthetic Dentistry MSc*
*King's College London Dental Institute, UK;*
*Board Member of the Academy of Dental Excellence*

**and**

**Shamir B. Mehta** *BDS BSc MClinDent(Prostho)(Lond) MFGDP(UK)*

*Dental Practitioner;*
*Senior Clinical Teacher,*
*Deputy Programme Director, Aesthetic Dentistry MSc*
*King's College London Dental Institute, UK;*
*Faculty Member of the Academy of Dental Excellence*

**and**

**Christopher C.K. Ho** *BDS Hons(SYD) GradDipClinDent(Oral Implants) MClinDent(Prostho)(LON), FPFA*

*Prosthodontist, Sydney, Australia;*
*Visiting Clinical Teacher, King's College London Dental Institute, UK;*
*Faculty Member of the Global Institute for Dental Education;*
*Board Member of the Academy of Dental Excellence*

WILEY Blackwell

This edition first published 2017 © 2017 by John Wiley & Sons Ltd.

*Registered office:*  John Wiley & Sons, Ltd., The Atrium, Southern Gate, Chichester, West Sussex, PO19 8SQ, UK

*Editorial offices:*  9600 Garsington Road, Oxford, OX4 2DQ, UK
The Atrium, Southern Gate, Chichester, West Sussex, PO19 8SQ, UK
1606 Golden Aspen Drive, Suites 103 and 104, Ames, Iowa 50010, USA

For details of our global editorial offices, for customer services and for information about how to apply for permission to reuse the copyright material in this book please see our website at www.wiley.com/wiley-blackwell

The right of the author to be identified as the author of this work has been asserted in accordance with the UK Copyright, Designs and Patents Act 1988.

All rights reserved. No part of this publication may be reproduced, stored in a retrieval system, or transmitted, in any form or by any means, electronic, mechanical, photocopying, recording or otherwise, except as permitted by the UK Copyright, Designs and Patents Act 1988, without the prior permission of the publisher.

Designations used by companies to distinguish their products are often claimed as trademarks. All brand names and product names used in this book are trade names, service marks, trademarks or registered trademarks of their respective owners. The publisher is not associated with any product or vendor mentioned in this book. It is sold on the understanding that the publisher is not engaged in rendering professional services. If professional advice or other expert assistance is required, the services of a competent professional should be sought.

The contents of this work are intended to further general scientific research, understanding, and discussion only and are not intended and should not be relied upon as recommending or promoting a specific method, diagnosis, or treatment by health science practitioners for any particular patient. The publisher and the author make no representations or warranties with respect to the accuracy or completeness of the contents of this work and specifically disclaim all warranties, including without limitation any implied warranties of fitness for a particular purpose. In view of ongoing research, equipment modifications, changes in governmental regulations, and the constant flow of information relating to the use of medicines, equipment, and devices, the reader is urged to review and evaluate the information provided in the package insert or instructions for each medicine, equipment, or device for, among other things, any changes in the instructions or indication of usage and for added warnings and precautions. Readers should consult with a specialist where appropriate. The fact that an organization or Website is referred to in this work as a citation and/or a potential source of further information does not mean that the author or the publisher endorses the information the organization or Website may provide or recommendations it may make. Further, readers should be aware that Internet Websites listed in this work may have changed or disappeared between when this work was written and when it is read. No warranty may be created or extended by any promotional statements for this work. Neither the publisher nor the author shall be liable for any damages arising herefrom.

*Library of Congress Cataloging-in-Publication Data are available*

ISBN: 9781119032984

A catalogue record for this book is available from the British Library.

Wiley also publishes its books in a variety of electronic formats. Some content that appears in print may not be available in electronic books.

Cover image: Courtesy of Subir Banerji.

Set in 10/12pt Warnock Pro by Aptara Inc., New Delhi, India
Printed and bound by CPI Group (UK) Ltd, Croydon, CR0 4YY

C001221_091121

# Contents

# List of Contributors

**Subir Banerji** BDS MClinDent(Prostho) PhD MFGDP(UK) FICOI FICD. Programme Director, MSc Aesthetic Dentistry and Senior Clinical Teacher, King's College London Dental Institute. In private practice in London and Faculty and Board member, Academy of Dental Excellence.

**Jorge André Cardoso** DMD(Portugal) MClinDent(Prostho)(UK). Tutor, MSc Aesthetic Dentistry and Secretary, Portuguese Society of Esthetic Dentistry, In private practice in Espinho, Portugal and Faculty member Academy of Dental Excellence.

**Brian Chee** BDS MSc DClinDent(Perio) MFDSRCS(Eng). Greenhill Periodontics & Implants, Wayville, South Australia.

**Tom Giblin** BSc BDent(Hons) CertPros. In private practice in Sydney, Australia and Diplomate, ICOI.

**Christopher C.K. Ho** BDSHons(SYD) GradDipClinDent(Oral Implants), MClinDent(Prostho)(LON), FPFA. Visiting Clinical Lecturer, King's College London, Faculty member, Global Institute for Dental Education and Faculty and Board member, Academy of Dental Excellence.

**Kyle D. Hogg** DDS, MClinDent (Prostho). Visiting Clinical Teacher and Postgraduate Tutor, MSc Aesthetic Dentistry, King's College London. Previous Honorary Clinical Teacher, University of Florida College of Dentistry – Jacksonville. Faculty and Editorial Board member, Academy of Dental Excellence and in private practice, Dental Health Professionals, Cadillac, MI, USA.

**Russ Ladwa** BDS LDS FDSRCS MGDS DGDP FFGDP. Past Dean, Faculty of General Dental Practice (UK), at the Royal College of Surgeons of England and Past President, Odontology Section of the Royal Society of Medicine, London.

**Il Ki Ricky Lee** RDT. Sydney dental specialist.

**Shamir B. Mehta** BDS BSc MClinDent(Prostho)(LON) MFGDP(UK). Deputy Programme Director, MSc Aesthetic Dentistry; Senior Clinical Teacher, Department of Conservative and MI Dentistry, King's College London Dental Institute; in private practice in London and Faculty member Academy of Dental Excellence.

**Bill Sharpling** MBA, DipCDT RCS(Eng). Director of the London Dental Education Centre (LonDec) and Senior Clinical Teacher and Associate Dean (CPD) at King's College London Dental Institute.

**Andrea Shepperson** BDS(Otago). Member of the American Academy of Cosmetic Dentistry (AACD), Honorary Life Member of the New Zealand Academy of Cosmetic Dentistry (NZACD), Member of the American Academy of Oral and Systemic Health (AAOSH), Member of the New Zealand Dental Association. Digital Smile Design Instructor and Kois Center Mentor.

**Charles A.E. Slade** BDS LDS RCS MFGDP(UK) MClinDent(Prostho). Clinical Lecturer, London Deanery, Clinical Teacher, King's College London Dental Institute and Faculty member, Academy of Dental Excellence. Key opinion leader Biomet 3i. In private practice, Lister House, Wimpole Street, London and No45 Dental, Chichester, UK.

# Foreword

Dr Banerji is to be congratulated for assembling such an impressive, international array of co-authors, all of whom I know to be highly talented clinicians and teachers. Collectively, they bring together a wealth of clinical experience and knowledge.

This very practical work is clearly aimed at the senior dental undergraduate/newly qualified dental practitioner, but will also prove of value to more experienced clinicians. The ambition of the authors, set out in the Preface, is to supplement established standard textbooks and the many hands-on courses available to us. The combination in each chapter of concise text, practical clinical tips, high-quality illustrations, and particularly the many hours of 'live' video that accompany a majority of the chapters, ensures that this ambition will be achieved. A companion website is also available to complement this work.

The inclusion of high-quality 'live' video is a major strength and a huge advance on the static illustrations in most standard textbooks. Several of the videos show actual clinical procedures from start to finish and, along with narrated presentations from the authors, allow a level of understanding that cannot be achieved using static images alone. Their extensive clinical experience has also enabled the authors to compile a whole series of extremely helpful clinical tips. Every reader will find something to adopt here to enhance their own clinical practice.

Even today, there probably remains, in the minds of some people, a stigma associated with the terms 'aesthetic' or 'cosmetic' when applied to healthcare. The inclusion of a chapter on 'Ethics' is, therefore, entirely appropriate. It should also be noted that many of the procedures described are additive or minimally invasive, and fully accord with the principles of best practice.

This work covers a comprehensive range of aesthetic clinical procedures and will be a very useful addition to every library. For many clinicians, it will be a 'must have' book!

*Stephen M. Dunne BDS LDS FDS PhD*
*Professor of Primary Dental Care and Advanced General*
*Dental Practice, King's College London*
*Clinical Director, Genix Healthcare Ltd*
*Specialist in Restorative Dentistry*
*President of the European Federation of Conservative Dentistry*

# Preface

With changing trends associated with increased patient demands (often perpetuated by a growing wealth of ready-access, media-based and online digital information), it has become increasingly apparent that the attainment of a high-quality, predictable and desirable aesthetic treatment outcome has become an additional fundamental aim for the contemporary restorative practitioner. There is little doubt that the effective prevention, elimination and stabilisation of oral disease are essential prerequisites for successful oral rehabilitation.

Dental educators have responded to these needs by making available an array of resources, typically by means of traditional textual learning and hands-on courses. However, given the highly rapid pace of change and diverse developments in restorative dentistry, coupled with the current digital revolution (both in terms of information technology and social media), there is a need to deliver educational materials in a time-efficient, effective, user-friendly and economic manner – often at the 'touch of a button'!

In this context, many online video presentations are widely available, for example on YouTube, which allow the dental practitioner to visualise procedures rather than simply imagining the stages between steps shown on photos supplemented by text. However, it is important that such resources meet quality assurance requirements and concomitantly boast authenticity.

I have come to realise the advantage of such assured dynamic-graphic content through my 20 years involved in educating undergraduate and postgraduate dental students as well as in my own clinical practice. In this unique publication I have been joined by an international team of highly experienced clinical educators who have, with their vast experience, put together material that aims to cover the principles and procedures for an array of clinical techniques, which we as experienced clinicians and educators strongly believe are integral to providing successful restorative dental treatment. In doing so, we have included a comprehensive range of aesthetic dental procedures commonly executed in everyday practice.

This learning resource comprises a combination of several hours of recorded video accompanied by an illustrated handbook summarising the key points, making available a source of information that we feel will help you to learn in a quick, meaningful and 'bite-sized' manner, and which we hope you will also find helpful and enjoyable.

While concise, this handbook is evidence based and includes references and suggestions for further reading. Additionally, it contains some relevant still photographs of crucial points in the procedures. The clinical images used throughout this resource have been taken from the contributing authors' own dental practices and are from patients who have been treated by them.

Throughout this text, my co-authors and I have also tried to provide you with a number of useful, pragmatic clinical tips, which we feel may also help to tackle some of the minor (yet important) challenges that we as everyday practitioners encounter, but are seldom addressed.

The overall intention of this learning resource is to serve as a good accompaniment to traditional undergraduate and postgraduate learning materials, as well as to provide the general dental practitioner with a readily accessible form of relevant and appropriate information, combining the scientific and technical concepts in modern restorative dentistry.

This book is dedicated to those from whom we have learnt and to the many who continue on this journey.

**Subir Banerji**

# Acknowledgements

Undertaking a project such as this is not possible without acknowledging the help and support of the many who have contributed towards its production, both directly and indirectly.

We would like to thank our families for their support and patience during this time when many hours were spent writing and recording the content for this unique enterprise. Our contributors have given generously and selflessly.

We would also like to extend our warm thanks to our patients who have given their permission and consent, enabling the use of images and footage that allow us to illustrate the various techniques with a practical and pragmatic approach.

We would also like to acknowledge the support extended by the Wiley production team and the publishers to make this idea into a reality.

**Subir Banerji, Shamir B. Mehta and Christopher C.K. Ho**

## About the Companion Website

*Practical Procedures in Aesthetic Dentistry* is accompanied by a companion website:

www.wiley.com/go/banerji/aestheticdentistry

The website includes the following videos, corresponding to their listed chapter number:

2.2 Clinical Photography
2.3 Evaluation of the Aesthetic Zone
2.4 Clinical Smile Evaluation
2.5 Digital Smile Evaluation
2.6 Principles of Shade Selection
2.7 Treatment Planning for Aesthetic Dentistry
3.2 The Facebow Recording
3.3 Intra-occlusal Records
3.4 Semi-adjustable Articulators
3.6 Occlusal Stabilisation Splints
4.2 Crown Lengthening without Osseous Reduction
4.3 Crown Lengthening with Osseous Reduction
4.4 Management of Gingival Recession and Graft Harvesting
5.2 Teeth Isolation
5.4 Anterior Restorations
5.5 Posterior Restorations
5.6 The Finishing and Polishing of Resin Composite Restorations
5.7 Direct Resin Veneers
5.8 Repair and Refurbishment of Resin Composite Restorations
6.1 Tooth Preparation for Full Coverage Restorations
6.9 The Role of CAD/CAM in Modern Dentistry

Part I

Ethics

## 1.1

# Ethics in Aesthetic Dentistry

*Russ Ladwa*

## Principles

Ethics could be considered to be a moral code, giving a set of principles to guide behaviour. All of us who belong to the healing or caring professions are expected to look after our patients in their best interests, at all times. This is the obligation that society places on us, in return for the trust it places in our hands.

The doctor/patient relationship is underpinned by some fundamental principles, the first of these being 'beneficence' – that is, doing good and acting in the patient's best interests – and 'non-maleficence' – that is, doing no harm. This principle dates back to the Hippocratic oath, which also includes the exhortation *Primum est non nocere*, 'First and most importantly, do no harm'. This is further supported by a secondary principle of reserving more extreme measures to treat the more extreme conditions.

The two words 'aesthetic' and 'cosmetic' appear to be very commonly used in surgery and dentistry and are often interchangeable. 'Cosmetic' comes from the Greek word *cosmeticos* and generally implies temporary, superficial or reversible. 'Aesthetic' comes from the Greek word *aestheticos* and is concerned with the perception, the philosophy or the structure of beauty. With its deeper meaning, the term 'aesthetic' may appear to be favoured by the medical profession.

We live in an age where various cultural and social expectations associate beauty and appearance with attractiveness, youth, success and status.[1] Added to this, in the presence of a rapidly increasing amount of readily available information, the people who are seeking cosmetic procedures have rising demands and expectations. They may also see themselves more as consumers than as patients. Because aesthetic dentistry may be perceived as an issue to do with their 'wellness', they see it as their 'right' to have it done.

## Procedures

As dentists we have a problem and an ethical dilemma when faced with patients requesting cosmetic treatments that are purely elective and optional, merely in order to enhance the smile or appearance. This is especially the case when it is in the absence of any disease or functional disability or deficiency. The fact is that many procedures may involve considerable and irreversible harm to the existing biological tissues. It has been shown[2] that up to 30% of sound hard tissue may be removed for a porcelain veneer

*Practical Procedures in Aesthetic Dentistry*, First Edition. Edited by Subir Banerji, Shamir B. Mehta and Christopher C.K. Ho. © 2017 John Wiley & Sons, Ltd. Published 2017 by John Wiley & Sons, Ltd.
Companion website: www.wiley.com/go/banerji/aestheticdentistry

preparation, and between 62% and 73% of sound tooth structure may be removed during preparation for full ceramic crowns in anterior teeth.

There are several questions to ask of ourselves. First, do have we the required competence to perform the procedure? Competence may be considered as the sum total of knowledge (which must be up to date in terms of materials, techniques and methods as well as being evidence based) and skills (which consist of appropriate training and adequate experience).

Secondly, in terms of treatment planning, are there any other, less invasive options that would achieve almost the same or a similar objective and could be considered instead? Is the plan based on what is safe and appropriate for this particular patient? What will work and last the longest? What will cause minimal problems in the future? How can these problems be dealt with if and when they arise? Is the whole procedure to be done with minimally invasive measures and methods?[3]

When a patient is demanding a certain type of treatment, consent is a complex issue. Has the patient the mental capacity and the maturity to absorb, comprehend, analyse and assess all the information we offer? Did the patient give their consent freely, without any subconscious or subtle coercion on our part? As professional people we then have to ask some pertinent questions of ourselves. Did I give all the relevant options and facts with regard to the risks/benefits and failure/success and potential harm, in step with current acceptable professional standards? Where do I stand if a patient who is a bruxist, for whom I know gold would be the most conservative and long-lasting suitable material with which to restore the posterior teeth, refuses it?

The reality is that dentistry is a business too for many of us. Therefore there are further questions to ask. Did I or any of my team do anything by any form of communication (including any advertising in all its forms) to embellish or promote my qualifications or ability to encourage uptake of the treatment plan offered? Am I comfortable that I have no financial conflict of interest in the advice I have given? Would I be able to justify it to my peers? Would I be able to defend it to my profession's regulatory body? Would I be willing to carry out the proposed treatment on any member of my own immediate family?

In parallel with our patients' increased dental knowledge, intelligence and expectations, we have moved in medicine from the age of paternalism to one of collaboration. So it behoves us to work in a spirit of cooperation with our patients to help guide them and enable them to reach a proper and suitable decision, while at the same time respecting their autonomy.

However, if after having presented all the information honestly and fully, the patient still insists on having inappropriate or harmful work carried out, which we as the dentist disagree with and are uncomfortable undertaking, then not only are we professionally entitled to refuse, we should also feel at liberty to do so. It should be remembered that just as their culture and social environment influence patients, dentists also have our personal judgement coloured by our upbringing and family background. This is of the utmost relevance when facing a professional dilemma, because attitudes and behaviour go beyond education and competence. Therefore, our level in possibly engaging with aesthetic work with any downsides must be judged on each individual case and particularly in the patient's best interests. This ultimately becomes a matter for our individual conscience, guided by our internal moral compass. This is vital, as we need to retain the proper respect and trust of those we look after and care for, to belong and remain part of a worthy and noble profession.

## Tips

- Make sure you have covered all the treatment options, even those you may not consider within your area of expertise.
- Be prepared to refer the patient on if the option chosen is beyond your area of expertise or experience.
- Make sure to list the advantages and disadvantages of all the treatment options.
- It is good practice to have a consultation with your patient, follow it up with a written treatment plan and then allow the patient to have the opportunity to discuss that plan.
- It is good practice for the patient to be informed of all the likely costs not only of providing the treatment but also of any maintenance required over a period of time.

## References

1 Mousavi SR. The ethics of aesthetic surgery. *J Cutan Aesthet Surg.* 2010 Jan-Apr;3(1):38–40.
2 Edelhoff D, Sorensen JD. Tooth structure removal associated with various preparation designs for anterior teeth. *J Prosth Dent.* 2002 87:502–9.
3 Kelleher M, Djemal S, Lewis N. Ethical marketing in 'aesthetic' ('esthetic') or 'cosmetic dentistry' part 1. *Dental Update.* 2012;June:313–26.

# Part II

# Patient Assessment

## 2.1

# Patient History and Examination

*Subir Banerji and Shamir B. Mehta*

## Principles

The foundation for successful treatment planning is largely reliant on the ability of the clinician to attain an accurate and contemporaneous patient history and to carry out a meticulous clinical examination. All findings should be appropriately recorded. Treatment planning should aim to fulfil the patient's realistic expectations, provide an outcome that boasts functional and aesthetic success (spanning beyond the short term) and, where possible, utilise techniques that involve minimal intervention.

The initial assessment should take place in a relaxed setting, perhaps distinct from the operatory, and permit the patient to voice their views. Emphasis should be placed on actively *listening* to the patient's concerns and attitudes.

## Procedures

Begin by verifying the **essential patient data**, such as the patient's name, gender, date of birth, address and contact details. This may be attained by requesting completion of a pre-treatment evaluation document. The details can be checked by other members of your dental staff team, together with information concerning any relevant special needs.

Establish your patient's reasons for attendance, hence the nature of their **complaint and associated history**. There are three categories of 'dental aesthetic imperfections' that drive patients to seek aesthetic intervention, which may be broadly classified as matters relating to tooth colour, shape and/or position.[1]

A detailed **medical history** is mandatory. A template medical history form may prove helpful. It is beyond the scope of this text to discuss the relevance of the medical history and its impact on the provision of dental care. However, in brief, the patient's medical history (and status) may preclude them from attending necessary lengthy or frequent treatment sessions, require modification of the treatment protocol or may sometimes contraindicate certain types of treatment, as when there is an allergy to a material or product. Indeed, the underlying medical condition may also prove to be contributory to the aesthetic impairment, such as taking prescription medication that may induce

*Practical Procedures in Aesthetic Dentistry*, First Edition. Edited by Subir Banerji, Shamir B. Mehta and Christopher C.K. Ho. © 2017 John Wiley & Sons, Ltd. Published 2017 by John Wiley & Sons, Ltd.
Companion website: www.wiley.com/go/banerji/aestheticdentistry

gingival hyperplasia; or an eating disorder, hiatus hernia or gastric reflux, which may result in erosive tooth wear.

The condition of **body dysmorphic disorder (BDD)** is one to be particularly aware of. This may be considered a psychiatric illness characterised by a preoccupation with an imagined defect in appearance and may cause clinically significant distress or impairment in social, occupation or other important areas of functioning, with the preoccupation not being related to any other form of mental illnesses.[2,3] It would appear to be more common among patients seeking cosmetic and aesthetic treatments.

The patient's **dental history**, their attitude to dentistry and their oral health should be noted. Oral hygiene habits, past attendance habits and previous experience of dental care should also be detailed. Dental-phobic patients and those who lack the motivation to maintain a high standard of oral hygiene may be more suited to relatively simple, low-maintenance, minimally invasive forms of treatment. Patients with unrealistic expectations may require further counselling, especially prior to embarking on complex, irreversible forms of dental treatment.

The patient's **social habits** such as smoking and their level of alcohol consumption should be ascertained. Smoking and excessive alcohol consumption not only contribute to the initiation and progression of various forms of oral disease, they also may contraindicate certain forms of treatment, such as tooth whitening and implant therapy. A **diet history** should also be obtained, taking particular note of the frequency and quantity of refined carbohydrate intake, together with the consumption of acidic foods and drinks. Copious and frequent consumption of foods and beverages that may cause staining, including tea, coffee, red wine and turmeric, is a further factor to be considered when contemplating colour-enhancing treatments such as tooth whitening. The patient's occupation should also be noted, as it may affect their ability to attend on a frequent basis, or indeed have an aetiological role in the causation of their aesthetic concerns.

Now proceed to the **initial examination phase**. To be assured of completeness, you may wish to use an assessment template. Start with examination of the **extra-oral features**. This should include an assessment of the following:

- Temporomandibular joints and associated musculature
- Cervical lymph nodes and salivary glands
- Facial (and dento-facial) features such as facial proportions, symmetry, facial shape, profile and width, lip morphology and mobility
- Facial skin.

For details of how to carry out an evaluation of the temporomandibular joint and musculature, refer to Chapter 3.1.

A thorough **intra-oral examination** should be conducted in a systematic manner. It is common first to examine the **soft tissues** of the lips, cheeks, tongue, vestibule, soft palate, hard palate and floor of the mouth for the presence of any anomalies. The use of dental loupes with appropriate illumination is highly recommended.

Record the overall standard of **oral hygiene**; the use of plaque-disclosing tablets and the subsequent derivation of plaque scores may prove useful. The presence of any local factors that may encourage plaque and calculus accumulation and stagnation should also be identified, including overhangs and other defects in restorations. The presence and extent of extrinsic tooth stains should be noted also.

The **gingival tissues** should be examined for the presence of any inflammatory changes, including erythema, swelling, loss of stippling, blunting of the gingival papillae, bleeding on probing and the presence of any exudates. A **Basic Periodontal Examination (BPE)**[4] should be conducted on a routine basis. A full-depth, six-point periodontal chart may sometimes be indicated. It may also be important to document the levels of attachment to determine the amount of periodontal destruction and recession that has occurred. Other periodontal features to note include the presence of any tooth mobility, furcation involvement and any bleeding on probing.

Accurate charting of the dental hard tissues should record the presence and absence of teeth, dental caries, sound and defective restorations, tooth fractures, cracks, wear of abrasive, erosive, abfractive and attritional varieties and any tooth malformations. The extent and location of any caries should be noted, as should the type and extent of all dental restorations present. Dental restorations should be further assessed for their marginal integrity and adaptation, structural integrity, form, function and aesthetic appearance. The presence of any secondary caries, open contacts and other food traps and wear facets, present on either the remaining dental tissues or the functional surfaces, should be documented. The use of a sharp probe is helpful. Dry the hard tissues using air from the three-in-one syringe. It is helpful if the teeth are stain and plaque free.

It is important to carry out a detailed **occlusal assessment** to establish the ways in which the patient's occlusal scheme differs from what may considered to be the ideal and to determine the constraints the occlusal scheme may place on fulfilling the patient's aesthetic expectations. Details on the means of performing a detailed occlusal assessment may be found in Chapter 3.1.

The occlusal assessment should be followed by a detailed **evaluation of the aesthetic zone**. Further details may be found in Chapter 2.3.

For patients presenting with **tooth wear**, the pattern of wear should be accurately recorded. A number of indices have been described that may be used for the purposes of monitoring or indeed treatment provision. For more details refer to Part 9.

Finally, for patients who are edentulous or partially dentate, a record should be made of their **potential denture-bearing areas**, such as the size, shape, texture and mobility of the ridges and overlying mucosa. This may include the use of a classification system to categorise the space. For patients who have been provided with removable appliances previously, a detailed history and inspection of their appliances should be undertaken.

The role of **special tests** must not be overlooked. However, they should serve as adjuncts to the clinical examination. Commonly used special tests include the following:

- Dental radiographs/imaging techniques
- Vitality testing
- Diagnostic (and mounted, articulated or surveyed) study casts
- Diet analysis
- Dental photographs.

Following the methodical and detailed examination and collaborative evidence from any special tests and investigations, a **diagnosis** should be established to enable an appropriate treatment plan to be developed.

## Tips

- First impressions count. Remember that your patient will be forming an impression of you during this visit.
- Sometimes it is useful to have the initial appointment with a new patient over two visits. This enables the investigations, observations and data collected at the first appointment to be evaluated for discussion at the second.

## References

1 Chalifoux P. Practice made perfect; perception esthetics: factors that affect smile design. *Jour Esthet Dent* 1996;8:189–92.
2 American Psychiatric Assoc. *Diagnosis and statistical manual of diseases, DSM-IV*. Washington, DC: American Psychiatric Association Publishing; 1994. p. 466–9.
3 Phillips K, Dias S. Gender differences in body dysmorphic disorder. *Jour Nerv Ment Disease.* 1997;185:570–7.
4 Ainamo J. Assessment of periodontal treatment needs. Adaptation of the WHO Community Periodontal Index of Treatment Needs (CPITN) to European conditions. In: FrandsenA, editor. *Public health aspects of periodontal disease in Europe*. Berlin: Quintessence; 1983. p. 33–46.

## 2.2

# Clinical Photography

*Christopher C.K. Ho*

*Video: Clinical Photography*
*Presented by Christopher C.K. Ho*

## Principles

Photography is an essential diagnostic and communication tool for the aesthetic clinician. The old adage 'A picture paints a thousand words' is often quoted, and in aesthetic dentistry photographs help educate patients to understand the proposed treatment, are important clinical records and aid in the treatment planning process.

Historically we have witnesed the development from conventional to digital cameras. In the 1990s there was a rapid introduction of the intra-oral camera. It was the ability to show patients their dental problems 'tooth by tooth' that led to the rapid utilisation of this technology. However, the disadvantages were being able to show only a few teeth at a time, and the low resolution of subsequent picture reproduction.

The latest generation of digital photography with digital SLR and prosumer cameras is easy to use, provides good lighting and can take portrait and intra-oral shots from whole arch to two or three teeth with excellent resolution.

### Benefits of Photography

The benefits of photography include the following:

- **Improved patient communication**. Being able to display what is in a patient's mouth is a huge advantage compared to trying to describe their problem with words. If you let a patient see what is in their mouth, they can co-examine/diagnose their own situation.
- **Laboratory communication**. (Figure 2.2.1) Well-exposed clinical photographs can effectively communicate the optical characteristics of teeth and can show the shape, surface, morphology, value, shade, translucency and chroma. It was customary for ceramists to take a shade in person and convey it in words, but when building the crown trying to interpret what they wrote down was difficult and could be frustrating for both dentist and ceramist when colour matches were incorrect. Being able to access the images at any time makes the task of matching restorations much easier and can only improve the final result for both dentist and ceramist.

*Practical Procedures in Aesthetic Dentistry*, First Edition. Edited by Subir Banerji, Shamir B. Mehta and Christopher C.K. Ho. © 2017 John Wiley & Sons, Ltd. Published 2017 by John Wiley & Sons, Ltd.
Companion website: www.wiley.com/go/banerji/aestheticdentistry

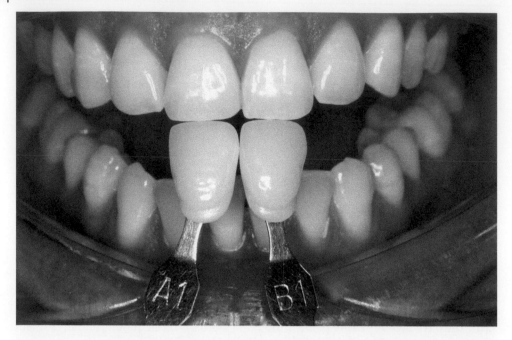

**Figure 2.2.1** Laboratory communication: use of shade guides conveyed in photograph to laboratory – note that the tabs are placed in the same vertical plane and angles as the teeth, with the incisal edge facing the incisal edges, as the ginigival portion of the tab is always shaded more like dentine.

- **Diagnostic tool and treatment planning aid**. Being able to recall images of a patient with the ability to magnify pictures enables the clinician sometimes to see what they may have missed in their clinical examination. The ability to look at images of patients, records and diagnostic models after they have left the practice also gives the clinician the ability to plan treatment for the patient as if they had the patient sitting in the chair.
- **Marketing library of before-and-after images**. Photos of patients who have undergone treatment can be both an educational and a powerful marketing tool.
- **Medico-legal considerations**. Unfortunately, with the increase in litigation that is evident in our community, it is advantageous to have photographic records of patients pre-treatment, during treatment and post-treatment.
- **Self-improvement**. Documenting your cases allows you to critique your own dentistry and helps you improve.

## Procedures

Given that a clinical digital camera for dental use is a must in any dental practice, what camera should you choose? The best option is a SLR single-lens reflex camera with an 85–105 mm macro lens and a dual-point or ring flash. There are many choices available and your decision should be made on the basis of functionality, weight and cost. Some of the considerations in relation to individual components are discussed in what follows.

Components of the Camera

### Lens

Many prosumer 35 mm zoom lenses have 'macro' settings, which allow you to focus close up, but not nearly as close as you need for clinical dental photography. In order to focus very closely, you need a **true macro lens**. This allows you to focus down to a 1:1 magnification, which works out to an area approximately 3 cm wide.

Intra-oral photography needs a fair amount of working distance and distortion-free headshots. A macro lens in the range of 85–105 mm is ideal, such as the Nikon AF-S DX Micro-NIKKOR 85 mm f/3.5G ED VR 85 mm lens, or the Canon EF 100 mm f2.8 USM macro lens. This focal range is also perfect for taking photos up to head size.

### Flash

There are different types of flash available: point, ring and dual point. The point flash (often within the camera) is a directional flash and offers more natural lighting, with increased shadows and more depth and contrast. These shadows help your eye see three-dimensional depth and surface texture.

The ring flash (Figure 2.2.2) is a circular flash that encircles the lens barrel and fires in all directions. This gives an even distribution of light with fewer shadows, but less contrast and depth. The images from ring flashes have more of a flat, even look to them. The ring flash is extremely useful for photographing areas where access is difficult and where uniform illumination is required, such as for occlusal and posterior photos.

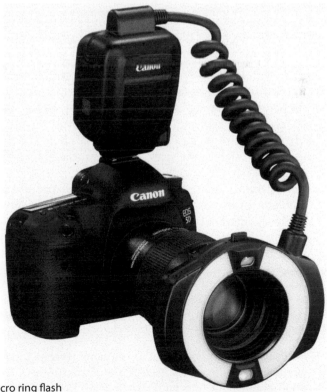

Figure 2.2.2  Canon MR-14EX macro ring flash

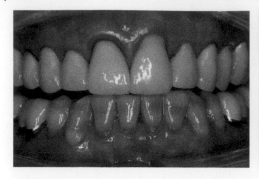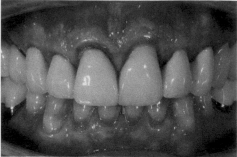

Figure 2.2.3 Photo taken with a ring flash (left) compared to one with a dual-point flash (right) – note the difference in the second image, with more depth, texture and a three-dimensional effect

The dual-point flash has the ability to change the angle of the flash, reduces reflection and can give you better depth and capture more texture and form. It is more difficult to get as predictable a posterior shot. It is also not as easy to stay consistent, because of the many ways to manipulate the twin flash. You need to set up a system for yourself to take particular shots in certain positions while the ring flash stays put in the same position all the time.

Figure 2.2.3 illustrates the difference between photos taken with ring and dual-point flashes.

### Camera Body

With a digital-based camera the image is electronically captured and storage of images is via recording media like compact flash or smart media cards.

### Accessories

- **Retractors.** Plastic is favoured over metal, since there is minimal reflection off plastic retractors. There are cheek retractors that retract the cheeks, as well as occlusal retractors that retract the lips and labial sulcus for occlusal shots.
- **Mirrors.** These are necessary for occlusal shots and certain lateral shots. They come in different shapes and sizes. The best surfaces for mirrors are rhodium coated and made of glass.
- **Backgrounds.** These can be used to frame extra-oral shots and different colours can highlight a patient's face and skin tone. This can be as simple as a painted wall colour to give a different background or special curtains that can be specifically purchased for this purpose. Intra-oral black backgrounds can allow better contrast and enable the translucency of teeth and restorations to be displayed (Figure 2.2.4).

### What Photographs Do You Need?

Images taken in dentistry can be full-face images, retracted and non-retracted smiles and occlusal shots.

- **Full face.** This image is shot at the same level as the patient and should cover their whole head. This vertical angle is important for the majority of images taken in dental photography. The interpupillary line and long axis of the teeth are used to align the camera.

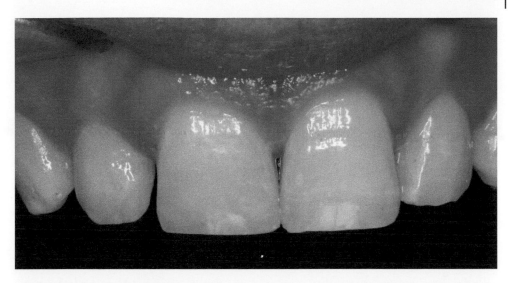

Figure 2.2.4 Contrasters or black cardboard can be used to provide a black background, allowing excellent display of characterisations

- **Full smile.** A non-retracted natural smile should be taken. The incisal plane of the upper teeth should be in the middle of the image.
- **Full smile – right and left lateral view.** This view shows the lips as well as the teeth visible for this angle. The upper lateral incisor is centred on the slide. The contralateral central incisor should be visible and possibly the lateral incisor and canine too.
- **Upper and lower teeth frontal retracted view.** The upper and lower teeth are slightly parted so that the incisal edges are visible. The midline of the face should be in the centre of the picture and the occlusal plane in the centre horizontally.
- **Upper and lower right and left lateral retracted view.** The image is centred on the lateral incisor so that it is in the centre of the picture. The retractor is pulled to the side of which the picture is being taken, while the contralateral retractor is loosely held.
- **Upper and lower occlusal retracted view (use mirror).** This is a reflected view from a high-quality mirror, with as many teeth as possible included. Keep the mirror clear of fogging. The mouth should be opened as wide as possible to allow the best mirror position. In the lower jaw it is exactly the same as with the upper teeth, but the patient needs to be asked to keep their tongue back so that it does not obscure the teeth.

## Tips

- The author prefers manual retractors that are controlled by the patient. It is preferable for the patient to hold these, as they will apply retraction that is appropriate without the retractors being stretched too far, as can be done by a staff member.
- One of the problems with the use of mirrors intra-orally is their tendency to fog up. To prevent this from happening, either the mirror can be warmed up or an assistant can blow air from a three-in-one syringe over the mirror to prevent condensation appearing.
- All images should exhibit little or no saliva and should be free of other distracting effects, for instance fingers. It is best to take photos before any treatment is begun, such as impressions, scaling or occlusal articulation, so that there are no distractions within the image.

## 2.3

# Evaluation of the Aesthetic Zone

*Subir Banerji and Shamir B. Mehta*

*Video: Evaluation of the Aesthetic Zone*
*Presented by Subir Banerji and Shamir B. Mehta*

## Principles

The terms 'aesthetic zone' and 'smile zone' are commonly used to denote the appearance of the teeth and smile. This zone has been shown to influence significantly factors such as social acceptability, self-confidence and professional prospects. It is paramount to undertake a meticulous assessment of the aesthetic zone during patient examination, so that you may best determine which features may require addressing while developing the treatment plan.

It is important in the first instance to gain an insight into the personal perceptions of your patient concerning their dental and facial aesthetics and their expectations; a template questionnaire may prove helpful here.[1]

There are certain proportions of both a facial and dento-labial variety that are accepted as being visually pleasing.[2] These are can be referred to as **universal concepts in dental aesthetics**. It is important to record the presence of any harmony or disharmony that exists between the varying components of the smile zone in relation to these accepted parameters.

The **Golden Proportion** is a mathematical concept applied in architectural design and engineering to study design proportionality in the beauty of art and nature. It suggests an ideal mathematical proportion of 1:1.618. In terms of the anterior maxillary dentition, this would imply that the maxillary central incisor should be 1.618 times wider than the maxillary lateral incisor, which in turn would be 1.618 times wider than the maxillary canine when viewed from a frontal direction. Thus, the width of the maxillary canine according to this concept should be 62% of the width of the lateral incisor. However, the Golden Proportion has been described to exist in fewer than 20% of all natural dentitions examined.

A plethora of studies have also investigated the average dimensions of maxillary central incisor teeth, which undoubtedly are the most dominant teeth in the aesthetic zone. The average lengths and widths of the latter have been reported to be 10–11 mm and

*Practical Procedures in Aesthetic Dentistry*, First Edition. Edited by Subir Banerji, Shamir B. Mehta and Christopher C.K. Ho. © 2017 John Wiley & Sons, Ltd. Published 2017 by John Wiley & Sons, Ltd.
Companion website: www.wiley.com/go/banerji/aestheticdentistry

8–9 mm, respectively.[3] The latter would infer that an average maxillary central incisor would have a length to width ratio of 1.2:1. It is also frequently stated that the central incisor length should be approximately one-sixteenth of the facial height.

## Procedures

Clinical evaluation of the aesthetic zone can be subdivided into an assessment of the following:

- Facial features
- Lips and facial skin
- Dento-labial and dento-facial relationships
- Teeth and gingivae.

With your patient comfortably seated upright in the dental chair, adopting a natural head pose, and you seated at the same height, their face when observed from a **frontal** direction can be **apportioned** into three separate zones. The 'upper third' spans the area between the hairline/forehead and the ophriac line (brow line); the 'middle third' extends from the ophriac line to the interalar line (base of the nose); and the 'lower third' includes the area between the interalar line and the tip of the chin. You may choose to use some wooden spatulas to assist you with this task, or consider simple software to delineate these zones on a digital photograph. For a 'well-proportioned' face these zones should roughly divide into equal dimensional segments. This may be a useful guide to apply when treatment planning for patients who have lost occlusal vertical height.

Maintaining the frontal view, next assess your patient for **facial symmetry**, first in the vertical plane across the facial midline (an imaginary line connecting the nasion, a point between the eyebrows and the base of the philtrum), and then horizontally across the interpupillary line. Aesthetic harmony is said to be present where the vertical and horizontal reference planes are perpendicular to each other, and the dental midline is coincident with the facial midline. The interpupillary line will also provide you with a key reference axis in determining the ultimate position of the incisal, gingival and occlusal planes.

Now, adopting a lateral view, observe your patient's **lateral facial profile**, ideally with their Frankfort plane parallel to the floor. You will typically notice one of three forms of facial profile: normal, convex or concave.

Reverting now to the frontal view, determine your patient's **facial shape and width**. Four types of basic facial shape are commonly described: ovoid, square, tapering and square-tapering (Leon Williams Classification). Associations have been made between facial shape and personality. Next, carry out a brief assessment of your patient's **facial skin**.

Now, progressing to the labial assessment, determine your patient's level of **lip thickness and lip symmetry**. Full lips are often associated with the dominance of the upper central incisors in the aesthetic zone. **Lip mobility** refers to the amount of lip movement that occurs when a patient smiles. The amount of anterior tooth displayed should be determined, with the lips in both resting and dynamic positions. The resting position of the lips has been classically used to determine the ultimate position of the incisal edges of the anterior maxillary teeth when undertaking prosthodontic rehabilitation.

Ask your patient to make the sound 'E'. The term **lip line** or **smile line** refers to the relationship that exists between the inferior border of the upper lip and the teeth and gingival soft tissues on smiling. You are likely to observe one of three types of lip line:

- **Low smile line** – where motility of the upper lip exposes the anterior teeth by no more than 75%, with no display of gingival tissue.
- **Medium smile line** – where lip movement results in the display of between 75% and 100% of the anterior teeth as well as the interdental papillae.
- **High smile line** – which exposes the teeth in full as well as the gingival tissues beyond the gingival margins, often referred to a 'gummy smile'.

Now analyse the **width of your patient's smile**. It is has been reported that a smile displaying 10 maxillary teeth (up to and including the second premolar teeth) is the most observed common smile width pattern. Where a large negative space exists between the buccal surfaces of the posterior maxillary teeth and the labial commisures when smiling (known as the buccal corridor), aesthetics may appear to be suboptimal.

You should also evaluate your patient's **smile arc**. This refers to the relationship between the curvature of the lower lip and the curvature of the incisal edges of the maxillary incisor teeth in a posed smile. Ideally, the curvature of the lower lip should be parallel to that of the incisor edges and the superior border of the lower lip should be spatially positioned slightly inferior to the incisal edges. You may choose to undertake phonetic tests such as enunciation of 'F' and 'V' sounds to help you verify the correct spatial relationship between the incisal edges of the anterior maxillary teeth and the lower lip.

Finally, determine the relationship between your patient's dental midline and facial midline. Here, the maxillary centre line is best assessed against the midpoint of the philtrum. A discrepancy of up to 2 mm between the maxillary midline and facial midline is generally considered to be aesthetically acceptable. Your patient's mandibular midline should ideally be coincident with the maxillary midline. However, that has been observed to occur physiologically in only a quarter of the population.

Now divert your attention to the assessment of your patient's teeth. **Teeth** should be evaluated for variations in colour:

- Hue – basic colour
- Chroma – saturation of the basic colour
- Value – brightness.

Also determine the **form** of your patient's maxillary central incisors (ovoid, square or triangular). Do they reflect the personality, sex, age and strength index of your patient? Maxillary lateral incisors also often display considerable variations in morphology. Peg-shaped lateral incisors are commonly encountered, and may be present unilaterally or bilaterally. The mandibular anterior dentition should also be assessed, with particular attention given to the profile of the incisal edges.

Now, from a frontal view, assess the **symmetry and axial inclination** of your patient's teeth. It has been suggested that a key determinant in attaining a highly aesthetic smile is to some extent dictated by the attainment of symmetry between the central incisor teeth. When viewed from the front, the axial inclinations of the anterior maxillary teeth have a tendency for a mesial tilt or inclination towards the vertical midline.

**Contact areas**, **connectors** and **embrasures** should be closely assessed. An embrasure is the triangular incisal space that exists inferior to the contact point. Embrasure spaces should ideally increase in size when progressing distally away from the midline. Similarly, contact points should be positioned in a more apical location when moving distally from the midline in a symmetrical manner. The connector may be defined as the area between two adjacent teeth that seem to touch in a frontal view. Connectors should ideally be symmetrical across the dental midline.

Finally, assess your patient's **gingival aesthetics**. For optimal aesthetics to exist, the gingival levels of the anterior maxillary segment should be symmetrical about the midline, with the horizontal gingival levels of the central incisor and canine teeth being placed slightly more apical (by approximately 1 mm) than that of the lateral incisors. The presence of 'black triangles' between the teeth is usually considered to be highly unattractive.

## Tips

- Make the undertaking of aesthetic evaluations part of your routine examination.
- Take time to discuss the outcomes with your patient.
- Beware of racial and cultural variations in aesthetics.

## References

1 Jornung J, Fardal O. Perceptions of a patient's smile: a comparison of patients' and dentists' opinions. *Jour Am Dent Assoc*. 2007;138:1544–53.
2 Ahmad I. Anterior dental aesthetics: facial perspective. *Br Dent J*. 2005;199:15–21.
3 Summit J, Robbins J, Hilton T, Schwartz R. *Fundamentals of operative dentistry: a contemporary approach*. 3rd ed. Chicago, IL: Quintessence; 2006. p. 68–80.

## 2.4

# Clinical Smile Evaluation

*Subir Banerji and Shamir B. Mehta*

*Video: Clinical Smile Evaluation*
*Presented by Subir Banerji and Shamir B. Mehta*

## Principles

In Chapter 2.3, the idea of a universal concept in dental aesthetics and beauty was briefly alluded to. While it may be comparatively straightforward to implement aesthetic changes in relation to universally determined concepts, it may not be as simple where more subjective variables are concerned.

It is important to gain an insight into your patient's *exact* needs. This may be attained initially by interviewing the patient. A detailed smile evaluation questionnaire may also prove helpful.

In order to develop predictability, there is a need for a technique that permits the opportunity for all dentists to enable reversible visualisation of any planned aesthetic changes, gain informed consent and avoid unrealistic expectations. One such technique is the 'intra-oral mock-up' or 'dry and try'.

## Procedures

Commence with the selection of an appropriate shade of resin composite. The teeth should ideally be clean and moist, and you should take note of the background illumination.

Isolate the anterior maxillary teeth. Cotton wool rolls, a split dam technique or an alternative soft tissue retraction procedure may prove helpful. The teeth are air dried, but no effort should be made to prepare them for adhesive bonding.

Where an increase in the length of the central incisor teeth is desired, first measure the width of the tooth using a Michigan O probe with Williams markings. Apply resin composite to one of the maxillary central incisor teeth; the amount of material added should generally aim to attain a rough length to width ratio of 1.2:1. Accordingly, for an average-width maxillary central incisor with a width of 8–9 mm, a length of 10–11 mm would be deemed suitable. Where the pre-existing width may present itself as an unsuitable marker, you may also choose to measure the length of the resting vertical dimension of your patient's face. The length of a central incisor should be approximately one-sixteenth of this length. The resting position of the upper lip should also be applied

*Practical Procedures in Aesthetic Dentistry*, First Edition. Edited by Subir Banerji, Shamir B. Mehta and Christopher C.K. Ho. © 2017 John Wiley & Sons, Ltd. Published 2017 by John Wiley & Sons, Ltd.
Companion website: www.wiley.com/go/banerji/aestheticdentistry

as a useful guide to determining a suitable length. Depending on your patient's age, there should be between 0.0 mm and 3.5 mm of incisal edge display with the upper lip assuming its resting position. Where a decrease in the length of the selected tooth is desired, use a surgical marker pen to mark the desired length to attain the appropriate proportions. Figure 2.4.1 is an example of a patient presenting with a worn anterior dentition, where an intra-oral mock-up has been carried out as described.

Now ask your patient to say the letter 'F' or 'V' and observe the relationship between the incisal edge and upper border of their lower lip. Ideally, the incisal edge should be contoured to follow the profile of the upper border of the lower lip, with a constant spatial distance of approximately 3 mm. Having re-established the relationship of the incisal edge to the 'smile arc' during a posed smile, repeat these steps on the contralateral tooth. It is generally thought that a male smile presents with a straighter line, while a female smile is more curved.

Using a set of wooden spatulas, determine the relationship between the incisal edges of the maxillary anterior teeth and the interpupillary line. Ideally, parallelism should exist; hence material may be added or subtracted to develop this form of spatial relationship. Where the interpupillary line is canted (a disparity exists in the horizontal plane between the eyes), use an alternative reference plane, such as the horizon.

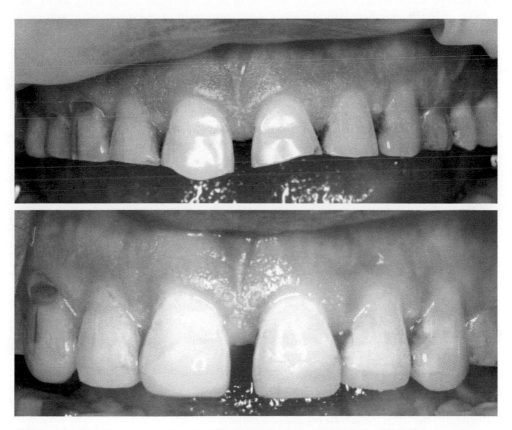

Figure 2.4.1 Worn anterior maxillary dentition – an intraoral mock-up has been carried out using direct resin composite from which a diagnostic wax-up is produced

Now view the profile of the maxillary incisor teeth in a lateral direction. Material should be added or removed to develop a lateral profile that presents itself with two or three planes on the labial (facial) surface. Look at the lip support attained; a naso-labial angle of 85–105° should be developed where a 'normal profile' is required.

Consider contouring the mock-ups at this stage to crudely reflect the patient's age, sex, personality and strength index, culminating in an ovoid, square, tapering or square-tapering profile (Leon Williams Classification). Invariably, the latter will involve adjustment of the mesial and distal incisal edges.

For cases where there may have been considerable loss of incisal edge tissue, thought should be given to the position of the contact area, which should be ideally positioned in the incisal third of the maxillary central incisor tooth, 6 mm coronal to the crestal bone, so as to develop the ultimate papillary infill and the elimination of unwanted black spaces.[1]

For cases where there is a need to alter the width of the maxillary central incisor teeth (such as in diastema closure), resin composite may be added to the interproximal surface(s). The width to length ratio may be applied as discussed earlier.

Now observe the relationship between the maxillary dental midline and the facial midline. Ideally, the discrepancy should be no greater than 2 mm.[2]

Once the maxillary central incisor teeth have been formed to the desired morphology (or indeed where such teeth may be deemed to be aesthetically acceptable), attention is diverted to the maxillary lateral incisor teeth. Add resin to the incisal edge (assuming an alteration in the length is indicated), such that the incisal edge is placed a couple of millimetres apical to that of the central incisor; develop the profile of the incisal edge in accordance with the patient's smile arc.

In going from the midline, the axial inclination of the maxillary anterior teeth should assume a 'mesial tilt'; this will usually involve the mesio-incisal corner being slightly more coronal than the disto-incisal corner. The mesial contact point should be placed slightly more apical than that formed between the central incisors.

For cases where an alteration in the width of the lateral incisor is desired, the concept of the Golden Proportion may be applied. In such instances, assuming that the width of the maxillary central incisor is of the desired dimensions, the width of the maxillary lateral incisor should be 62% of this dimension or, conversely, the ratio of the width of the central incisor should be 1.618:1 of the lateral incisor when viewed from a frontal direction. The use of a Golden Proportion gauge (Golden Mean gauge, as seen in Chapter 9.4) may be helpful in this exercise. The profile of the contralateral maxillary lateral incisor should now be developed to roughly mimic that of the above. The embrasure space formed between the central and lateral incisors, and indeed that of the canine teeth, should progressively increase in size in progressing distally from the midline.

Now add resin to the maxillary canine teeth, applying the concepts already discussed, with the aim of maintaining symmetry across the midline. The average length of a maxillary canine should be 11–13 mm. The connector areas (area between two adjacent teeth that appear to touch when viewed frontally) should follow the 50–40–30 rule, such that the connector area between the central incisors is 50% of the length of their clinical crowns, and those between the central and lateral incisors are 40% and 30% of the length between the lateral incisor and canine, respectively.[3]

Focus your attention on the gingival aesthetics. Where there is a need for alterations, add resin to areas to simulate the effect of crown lengthening, such that the horizontal levels of the central incisor teeth and canines are in the same plane, with symmetry across the midline and approximately 1 mm apical to the lateral incisor.

Now observe the width of your patient's smile. The presence of black spaces between the cheeks and teeth (negative buccal corridor) may look particularly unaesthetic. Thus, if needed, add resin to the buccal cusp tips of the premolar teeth to assess the effect of reducing this dimension.

Last, observe the mandibular teeth in relation to the maxillary. You may consider adding resin to the mesial surfaces of the lower central incisors, with the aim of attaining a congruent vertical reference with the maxillary centre line, although coincidence of these planes has been reported to exist in only 25% of the population.[4]

It is worthwhile now showing these crude changes to your patient. It is advisable to take high-quality photographs of the mock-up, and perhaps consider taking a video recording to assess the effects of dynamic aspects such as the patient's speech.

Take an over-impression of the mock-up using alginate or silicone putty. Then remove the resin composite material. Now, take an impression of the existing dentition and surrounding soft tissues. These records should be dispatched to the laboratory with a detailed occlusal prescription, aesthetic prescription and the photographic records, together with any feedback for your patient so that an aesthetic and functional diagnostic wax-up may be formed.

Carefully appraise the wax-up when it arrives from the laboratory (Figure 2.4.2). If you are satisfied, take an impression of the wax-up and use this to fabricate an intra-oral mock-up. Figure 2.4.3 shows an intra-oral mock-up derived using the wax-up in Figure 2.4.2. Critically appraise the 'trial smile' prior to demonstrating it to your patient, as also shown in Figure 2.4.3.

You may also choose to have your technician provide your patient with a 'clip-on smile' that mimics the prescription, so that they have a further opportunity to appraise and discuss these changes with family and friends.

You will now have given the patient the chance to crudely 'test-drive' their planned smile. You will also have had a chance to make a note of their level of expectation!

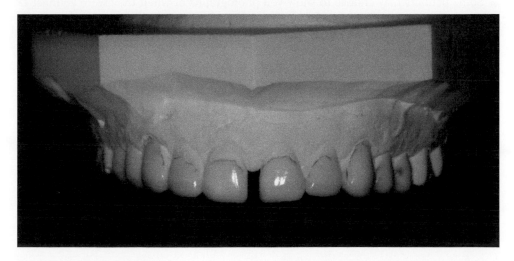

Figure 2.4.2 Diagnostic wax-up

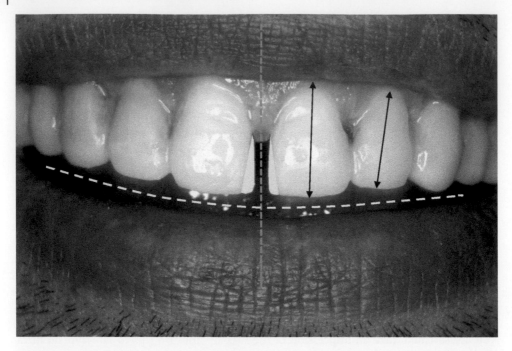

Figure 2.4.3 The wax-up has been indexed and 'copied' using a bis-acryl-based temporary crown and bridge material – the markings demonstrate the critical appraisal of the wax-up to verify the smile arc, axial inclination, symmetry, morphology and proportions

## Tips

- During the appraisal of the intra-oral mock-up, encourage your patient to bring in their partner or friend in order to ask their opinion as well.
- Some patients may choose to show you photographs of when they were younger or even pictures of celebrities – be mindful to keep their expectations realistic!

## References

1 Tarnow DP, Magner AW, Fletcher P. The effect of the distance from the contact point to the crest of bone on the presence or absence of the interproximal dental papilla. *J Periodontol.* 1992 Dec;63(12):995–6.
2 Johnston C, Burden D, Stevenson M. The influence of facial midline discrepancies on dental attractiveness ratings. *Eur Jour Ortho.* 1999;21:517–22.
3 Dias N, Tsingene F. SAEF-smile aesthetic evaluation form: a useful tool to improve communication between clinicians and patients during multidisciplinary treatment. *Eur Jour Esthet Dent.* 2011;6:160–75.
4 Miller E, Bodden W, Jamison H. Dentofacial perspective. *Br Dent Jour.* 2005;199:81–8.

## 2.5

# Digital Smile Evaluation

*Andrea Shepperson*

*Video: Digital Smile Evaluation*
*Presented by Andrea Shepperson*

## Principles

Concepts of smile design and dento-facial aesthetics have been an integral feature of dentistry since early denture design. Essential design criteria have been developed, beginning with an evaluation of facial aesthetics and moving to dento-facial relationships. Design begins with full-face evaluations, determining where teeth should sit in the face to provide balance and harmony. Once fundamental tooth position is determined, micro-aesthetic elements are applied that consider tooth form and arrangement, tooth proportion, axial alignment, gingival scallop and colour. These universally recognised principles are well documented in both early denture and prosthodontic texts, and more recently in books and online references outlining systematic evaluation in case planning.[1-5]

Advances in digital photography and software functionality allow convenient and accurate conceptual evaluation of dento-facial aesthetics on a computer.

Ratios, proportions, guidelines and smile simulation are simple to convey with accuracy and become a useful and efficient tool for communication between dentist, laboratory technician and patient.[6,7]

## Procedures

### Digital Smile Evaluation

#### Photography
Digital smile evaluation requires a standard series of digital photographs using a high-resolution digital camera with macro lenses. A selection of appropriate retractors and mirrors captures quality images for evaluation. The use of a black contrasting device in intra-oral views provides a dark background on which to evaluate micro-aesthetic elements and visualise lines and design guides.

*Practical Procedures in Aesthetic Dentistry*, First Edition. Edited by Subir Banerji, Shamir B. Mehta and Christopher C.K. Ho. © 2017 John Wiley & Sons, Ltd. Published 2017 by John Wiley & Sons, Ltd.
Companion website: www.wiley.com/go/banerji/aestheticdentistry

### Cloud-Based File Sharing

Clinicians, specialists and technicians share design information via the cloud, synchronising design updates and shared data. The result is a continuous workflow by all parties involved in the final case. Geographical location is no longer a barrier to effective communication.

### Facial References

Traditional communication of facial references occurs with the use of a facebow or simple stick-bite tool to transfer vertical and horizontal reference planes to dental casts. Articulation of casts, based on these references, allows a technician to design tooth alignment relative to the face and to develop incisal or occlusal planes in reference to articulator mounting platforms, which mimic facial planes.

Digital smile evaluation uses a digital facebow – horizontal and vertical guidelines drawn on a screen with the ability to re-orientate or rotate a photograph to determine the ideal vertical and facial planes (Figure 2.5.1).[7]

Smile design begins with full-face photographs of the patient. Standard full-face photos should include the following:

- Lips in repose with lips slightly parted
- A natural smile
- A full 'eeee' smile with maximum gingival display
- An optional additional full-face view with intra-oral retractors and teeth apart, to highlight undulations in the occlusal plane.

These photographs allow a number of simple facial parameters to be assessed:

- Orientation of the dental and facial midlines
- Facial proportions or thirds.

Lines can be drawn onto full-face images to provide a guide for more harmonious relationships, and these become a blueprint for the technician to align casts using a virtual

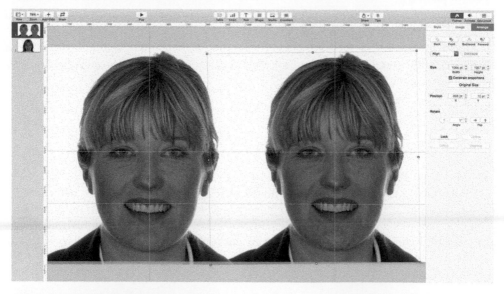

Figure 2.5.1 The digital facebow analysis allows fine adjustment to head position to create accurate horizontal and vertical facial references

or digital facebow. In its simplest form this is only a two-dimensional reference. However, advances in intra-oral scanning and interfaces between computer-aided design (CAD) technology and digital photography and smile evaluation have allowed three-dimensional referencing of virtual casts in relation to the face.

### Dento-facial References

Full-face photographs also allow determination of dento-facial references. These include:

- Tooth display in repose
- Smile line and contour – the alignment of the incisal edges and cusp tips in relation to the lower lip
- Gingival display – lip position in relation to gingiva in a full smile
- Horizontal references created by incisal edges of maxillary anterior teeth (the incisal plane)
- Alterations in the occlusal plane that highlight wear patterns and over-erupted teeth.

Tracings, measurements, lines and curves provide clear visual references and detail that may be overlooked in analogue planning. Repositioning lines and curves is simple in the digital evaluation. Waxing or surgical guidelines are clearly evaluated and communicated.

### Tooth Proportion

Tooth proportion is an important assessment for reconstruction of worn teeth and alteration of gingival height. Teeth have pleasing height to width ratios and these have traditionally been measured with callipers and calculations done mathematically from dental casts. The use of rectangles in fixed ratios in digital planning is a fast and effective tool for assessing desired tooth proportion. The transfer of information to the technician is very precise and allows accurate determination of the wax-up and final restorative parameters (Figures 2.5.2, 2.5.3, 2.5.4 and 2.5.5).

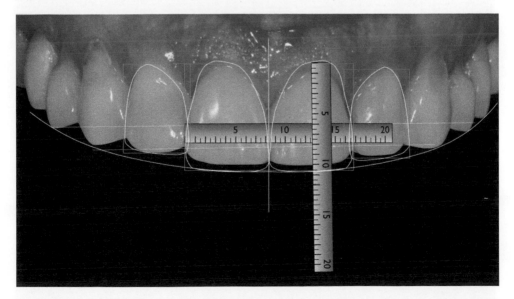

Figure 2.5.2 Optimal height to width ratios and calibrated digital rulers provide valuable information for the technician in establishing the diagnostic wax-up and final case

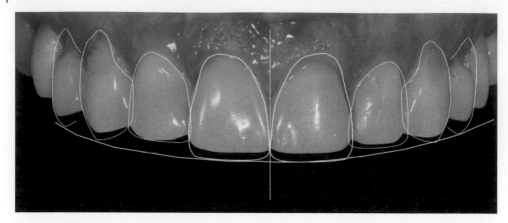

Figure 2.5.3 Tooth form and arrangement are finalised to design guidelines

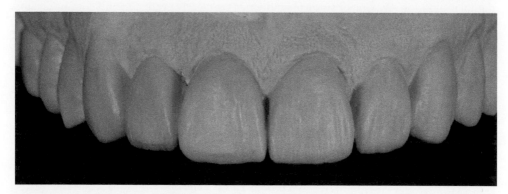

Figure 2.5.4 The laboratory technician is able to develop accurate changes based on the digital prescription

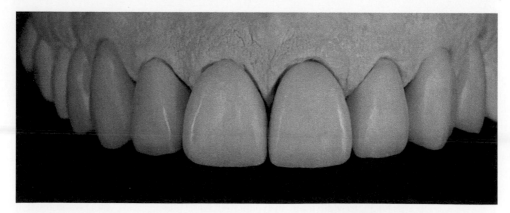

Figure 2.5.5 The final veneers mimic previously established and verified digital design guidelines

**Tooth Alignment**

The arrangement of teeth, axial inclination, overlap and rotation and orthodontic correction can be simulated in digital smile planning. Information can be shared among interdisciplinary team members to convey treatment goals.

**Tooth Form**

Digital planning tools offer a library of tooth forms to match and harmonise with the patient's face and morpho-psychology. These can be interposed and changed to evaluate the impact on the face as a whole, and act as another communication tool for both patient and technician.

**Tooth Colour**

Simulations and tooth libraries allow alteration of tooth colour and value through simple digital sliders that adjust colour temperature, brightness and contrast and saturation. Patients can preview and comment on desired shades.

**Video in Digital Smile Evaluation**

Most modern DSLR cameras include high-definition (HD) video functionality and this is also readily available on smart devices and compact video cameras. Digital smile evaluation increasingly includes digital video. This allows a functional evaluation of the face and smile that may reveal details not noted in still images. Lip mobility, chewing and speaking patterns and posturing habits can be recorded and provide insights that can otherwise be overlooked. They also provide a valuable medico-legal record of what was discussed and agreed between dentist and patient.

**Calibration**

Any digital data needs to be calibrated from the 'live' case. For example, the combined width of the maxillary central incisors, determined with callipers, provides a precise and reproducible hard-tissue measurement that can be translated to a digital ruler. Digital ruler ratios are set at calibration and fixed for any additional virtual measurements on photographs.

**Digital Diagnostic Wax-Up**

Digital smile evaluation is a design and communication tool that allows a technician to create a three-dimensional (3D) diagnostic wax-up or mock-up on articulated casts based on the two-dimensional (2D) elements prescribed by the digital design. It also permits a virtual wax-up by placement of tooth-coloured forms on a photograph to simulate an intra-oral mock-up. Some dental companies provide a smile simulation service that creates a before-and-after representation of the digital wax-up. This has always been a guide only and lacks the precision of a 3D physical wax-up on study casts.

CAD software creates a virtual wax-up by placing teeth on a scanned cast and modifying shapes. Some software manufacturers have integrated photographic digital design with 3D scanning (DSD Connect, DSD Technology, Razvad, Romania). The digital design proposal can be milled as a model from which silicone keys are made to produce a mock-up in the mouth. Alternatively, provisional restorations can be milled and inserted into the mouth, providing a working mock-up to assess aesthetics and function.

The final determinant of a harmonious design is by reproduction of the new smile intra-orally. The mock-up or trial smile permits 'live' design evaluation in a functioning patient. It is an important step for patient and planning approval before any irreversible dentistry commences.

### Functional Relationships

The final smile design elements may be constrained by functional relationships such as eating, talking and functional habits.[8-10] A definite test of any smile design process, either digital or analogue, is to trial the design intra-orally.

A series of functional and phonetic tests will indicate modifications to tooth length, orientation, arrangement and inclines.

Phonetic tests include the following:

- **'F' (fricative) sounds.** The patient is asked to count from 40 to 50. The incisal edges of the maxillary central incisors should just engage the wet/dry line of the lower lip. If the patient has noisy and imprecise 'F' sounds, then the teeth may be too long and they require shortening until the patient can speak comfortably.
- **'S' (sibiliant) sounds.** The patient is asked to count from 60 to 70. The mandible moves anteriorly to allow the tongue to form a seal behind the maxillary teeth when phonating 'S' sounds. If the palatal surfaces of the wax-up do not allow sufficient room and are too bulky, the patient will feel interferences as the lower teeth collide with the palatal surfaces of the upper front teeth.

### Chewing

Anterior tooth relationships need to provide light contact in the maximum inter-cuspation position.[9,10] They also need to allow room to move within the envelope of function when the patient eats or swallows. If palatal inclines have excess volume or there is an increase in overbite, then the patient may experience functional interferences.

Dental design software now includes elements of virtual articulation, allowing some reproduction of mandibular movements and a correlation of the intra-oral environment.

Currently there are limitations to this technology so that it does not accurately reproduce an intra-oral environment. It is necessary to make a copy or clone of the functionally refined intra-oral mock-up or provisional restorations. An impression or scan is made of the trial restorations after phonetic and functional adjustments[11-13] have been made in the mouth. This model forms a customised template for the design of the final restorations and occlusal scheme, to avoid the introduction of interferences in the envelope of function.

## Tips

- Learn accurate photographic techniques for data capture.
- Purchase a quality camera and accessories. Most dentists invest in a quality DSLR with macro lenses and purchase dental-specific mirrors, retractors and contrasters.

- Become familiar with the rules and ratios of universally accepted guidelines for facial and dental harmony.
- Attend courses on digital smile planning.
- Use digital smile planning to enhance communication with the patient, laboratory and colleagues, including specialists.

## References

1 Rufenacht C. *Fundamentals of esthetics*. Chicago, IL: Quintessence; 1990.
2 Fradeani M. *Esthetic analysis: a systematic approach to prosthetic treatment*. Chicago, IL: Quintessence; 2004.
3 Magne P, Belser U. *Bonded porcelain restorations in the anterior dentition: a biomimetic approach*. Chicago, IL: Quintessence; 2002.
4 Bhuvaneswaran M. Principles of smile design. *J Conserv Dent*. 2010;13(4):225–32.
5 Morley J, Eubank J. Macroesthetic elements of smile design. *J Am Dent Assoc*. 2001 Jan;132(1):39–45.
6 Lin WS, Zandinejad A, Metz MJ, Harris BT, Morton D. Predictable restorative work-flow for computer-aided-design/computer-aided-manufacture fabricated ceramic veneers utilizing a virtual smile design principle. *Oper Dent*. 2015 Jul–Aug;40(4):357–63.
7 Coachman C, Van Dooren E, Gürel G, Landsberg CJ, Calamita MA, Bichacho N. Smile design: from digital treatment planning to clinical reality. In: Cohen M. *Interdisciplinary treatment planning, vol. II: comprehensive case studies*. Chicago, IL: Quintessence; 2011. p. 119–74.
8 Gibbs CH, Lundeen HC, Mahan PE, Fujimoto J. Chewing movements in relation to border movements at the first molar. *J Prosthet Dent*. 1981;46:308–22.
9 Lundeen HC, Gibbs CH. *The function of teeth: the physiology of mandibular function related to occlusal form and esthetics*. Gainesville, FL: L & G; 2005.
10 Bakeman EM, Kois J. The myth of anterior guidance. *J Am Acad Cosmetic Dent*. 2012 Fall;28(3):56.
11 Gürel G. Applying foundational principles to digital technologies: ensuring success in aesthetic dentistry. *Dent Today*. 2014 May;33(5):144–8.
12 Gürel G. Discovering the artist inside: a three-step approach to predictable aesthetic smile designs, part 1. *Dent Today*. 2013;32:74–8.
13 Gürel G. Discovering the artist inside: a three-step approach to predictable aesthetic smile designs, part 2. *Dent Today*. 2013;32:126–31.

## 2.6

# Principles of Shade Selection

*Christopher C.K. Ho*

*Video: Principles of Shade Selection*
*Presented by Christopher C.K. Ho*

## Principles

Shade selection is an important procedure providing patients with an aesthetic restoration that harmoniously blends to the remaining dentition. Knowledge of the scientific basis of colour, from understanding light to interpreting the artistic aspects of shade selection, ensures a successful result.

Shade selection involves the perception of colour, which depends on three entities:

1) Light source (illuminant)
2) Object
3) Detector (ocular or instrumental).

### Illuminant

The colour of an object can be influenced by the illuminant, for instance tungsten light may cast a yellow colour compared to daylight. The property of influencing the colour of objects is called 'colour rendition'. There are three main illuminants within any dental practice: natural, incandescent and fluorescent. Incandescent lighting is predominantly red/yellow and lacking in blue, while fluorescent lighting is high in blue tones and low in red. Initial shade selection should initially be made with daylight or colour-corrected lighting, and then the shade should be matched under different lights to avoid metamerism (the phenomenon that occurs when shades appear to match under one lighting condition and not another).

### Object

Colour possesses three dimensions: value, hue and chroma. A high-value object often reflects most of the light falling onto its surface and appears bright. The converse is true with a dark object, which absorbs most of the light and appears dull or of low value. Hue is the wavelength of light, and is dependent on the spectral reflectance from an object. Chroma is the concentration of colour or colour intensity.

*Practical Procedures in Aesthetic Dentistry*, First Edition. Edited by Subir Banerji, Shamir B. Mehta and Christopher C.K. Ho. © 2017 John Wiley & Sons, Ltd. Published 2017 by John Wiley & Sons, Ltd.
Companion website: www.wiley.com/go/banerji/aestheticdentistry

### Detector

The third part of the stimulus for colour is the spectral response of the detector, or the eye.

The difficulty of shade selection is that clinicians must be able to interpret a multilayered structure of varying thicknesses, opacities and optical surface characteristics. This can affect the way in which the eye perceives colour.

The basic hue of the tooth is determined by the colour of the underlying dentine, while value is a quality of the enamel overlay. Muia explains: 'The dentine imparts all the colour. Enamel is like a fiberoptic structure conducting light through its rods.'[1] Chroma is the saturation of colour in the dentine, but is influenced by the value and thickness of the enamel. Teeth are often termed 'polychromatic' and have variations in hue, value and chroma that give three-dimensional depth and characteristics. A young dentition is characterised by opaque, high-value enamel, which blocks the underlying dentine. As teeth age, the enamel becomes more translucent and dull (low value), revealing the underlying dentine. This layering can make reading of tooth colour difficult, since the value of the enamel and surface lustre often complicate colour evaluation of the underlying dentine.

### Types of Shade Guides

The most popular shade guides are the following:

- Vita Classic
- Vita Toothguide 3D-Master
- Vita Linearguide 3D-Master (Figure 2.6.1)
- Chromascop
- Custom guides.

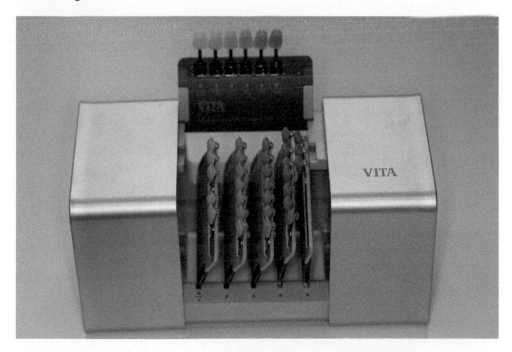

Figure 2.6.1 Vita Linearguide 3D-Master (VITA Zahnfabrik, Bad Säckingen, Germany)

A number of related factors in selecting shades must also be understood to achieve a successful result. These factors include translucency, contour, surface texture and lustre. Selecting the basic shade or colour is only the first step.

### Translucency

There are various patterns of translucency, which may also affect value, as increasing translucency decreases value. The amount, location and quality of translucency vary with the individual and their age. Young teeth often have greater incisal translucency, with the enamel appearing transparent. With age, from daily functions like eating and brushing, the enamel becomes thinner and allows the underlying dentine to appear. This is seen in the teeth becoming lower in value and higher in chroma.

### Surface Texture

Surface texture influences aesthetics by modifying the amount and direction of light reflected off the facial surface. Texture should be designed to simulate the reflectance pattern of the adjacent natural teeth. Young teeth may have a lot of characterization with stippling, ridges, striations and lobes. These features may be worn away with age, leaving smoother, highly polished surfaces.

## Procedures

- Shade selection should be completed before preparation, as teeth can become dehydrated and result in higher values.
- Shades should be done when the dental team is not fatigued, so not at the end of the day.
- Ensure that surgery surroundings are of neutral colour so that there is no colour cast onto the teeth.
- Ask the patient to remove any lipstick and not to wear lurid clothing or any items that may distract attention from the teeth.
- Make sure that teeth are clean and unstained before attempting shade selection.
- The patient should be in an upright position at a level similar to the operator and the shade guide should be at arm's length. This ensures that the most colour-sensitive part of the retina will be used.
- Observations should be made quickly (within 5 seconds) to avoid fatigue. The eye cannot discriminate for longer than this and the cones become sensitised to complement the observed colour.
- Blue fatigue can accentuate yellow sensitivity, so dentists can look at a blue object, bib and so on, while resting the eyes.
- Use colour-corrected light illumination, which should be of a diffuse nature.
- Choose the basic shade at the middle of the tooth. Viewing tabs through half-closed eyes can decrease the ability to discriminate colour, but increases the ability to match value. Look at the other parts of the teeth, dividing the teeth into nine sections from apical to incisal, and mesial to distal.
- Examine the teeth for translucency and any characterisations, such as craze line or hyopcalcification.

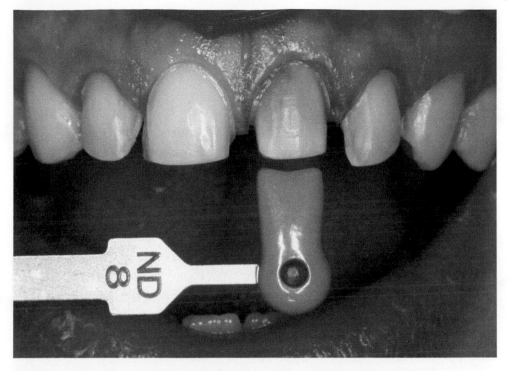

Figure 2.6.2 Stump shade taken to determine colour of the underlying tooth preparation

- Create a shade/chromatic map, divided into different sections to ensure correct placement of different effects, characterisations and shades.
- Photograph teeth and tabs using different lighting conditions to minimise metamerism, for example flash (5500K) and natural daylight (6500K).
- Send the digitised images and shade map to the ceramist.

Stump Shade Selection

With the increasing use of translucent all-ceramic restorations, it is important to communicate the prepared tooth or 'stump' shade to the ceramist so that they can build the restoration with the right opacity/translucency (Figure 2.6.2). It may be necessary to use a more opaque ceramic to block discoloration. For instance, many of the new materials such as lithium disilicate are supplied with varying opacity/translucency, or zirconia-based restoration may be a better choice than a glass-based ceramic.

## Tips

- It may be best to remove the necks of shade tabs where possible, as their colourants may introduce errors.
- The development of new shade-matching systems may herald a major advance in clinical practice.

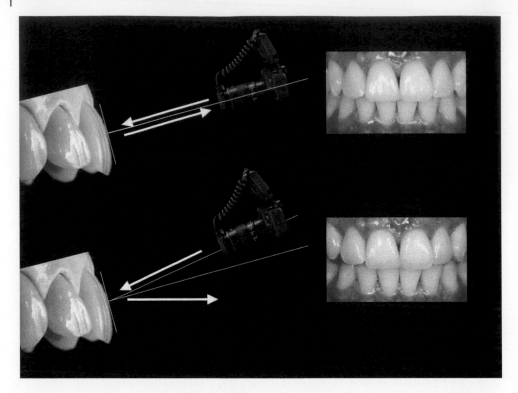

**Figure 2.6.3** Photographing the teeth from above the plane perpendicular to the labial surface allows less specular reflection, revealing the characteristics of the teeth

- Often when taking photographs for shade matching the flash is reflected from the labial surface of the teeth, hence the specular reflection masks the characteristics of the teeth. It can be helpful to take the photograph from slightly above the patient, angling the camera down so that the flash is reflected differently (Figure 2.6.3).

## Reference

1 Muia P. Paul Muia explains his four dimensional tooth color system. *Quintessence Dent Technol.* 1983 Jan;7(1):57–62.

## Further Reading

Ahmad I. *Dental photography: a practical clinical manual.* Chicago, IL: Quintessence; 2004.

Ahmad I. *Protocols for predictable aesthetic dental restorations.* Oxford: Blackwell Munksgaard; 2006.

Hammad I. Intrarater repeatability of shade selections with two shade guides. *J Prosthet Dent.* 2003;89(1):50–53.

Rosenstiel SF, Land MF, Fujimoto J. *Contemporary fixed prosthodontics.* Chicago, IL: Mosby; 1995.

Shillingburg HT, Hobo S, Whitesett LD, Jacibi R, Bracketts SE. *Fundamentals of fixed prosthodontics.* 3rd ed. Chicago, IL: Quintessence; 1997.

Vanini L, Mangani FM. Determination and communication of colour using the five colour dimensions of teeth. *Pract Proced Aesthet Dent.* 2001;13(1):19–26.

## 2.7

# Treatment Planning for Aesthetic Dentistry

*Subir Banerji and Shamir B. Mehta*

*Video: Treatment Planning for Aesthetic Dentistry*
*Presented by Subir Banerji and Shamir B. Mehta*

## Principles

The principles for treatment planning where aesthetic dental procedures are being considered follow the same basic tenets as for any other form of restorative care provision. Effective planning should aim to help restore oral health and function, with a concomitantly acceptable aesthetic outcome.

Predictability is a key determinant for long-term success in restorative dentistry. That success is based on the implementation of a sound, sequenced and logical plan derived from the information gathered from the patient's history and examination, taking into account the wishes of the patient and the skills of the dental operator. The need for the clinician periodically to assess the efficacy of each stage of the treatment plan (prior to progressing to the next stage), as well as the importance of maintenance and monitoring, are readily overlooked during treatment planning, highlighting the flexible nature of the process (especially with more complex casework).

The importance of effective dentist–patient communication, good record keeping and obtaining informed consent to treatment cannot be overstated.

## Procedures

Start by compiling a 'problem list' from the information you have gathered. This diagnostic information should be ordered as described in this chapter. Your primary consideration should be the management of any presenting emergency, hence this is termed the **acute stage**. An effective, empathetic approach can prove to be an excellent practice builder. Treatment may range from the simple application of a proprietary varnish to seal patent dentinal tubules, the placement of a splint to treat an incomplete fracture, prescription of chemical-therapeutic agents, the placement of a composite bandage to treat a fractured tooth, extirpation of an inflamed dental pulp or drainage of a swelling to the extraction of a symptomatic tooth.

*Practical Procedures in Aesthetic Dentistry*, First Edition. Edited by Subir Banerji, Shamir B. Mehta and Christopher C.K. Ho. © 2017 John Wiley & Sons, Ltd. Published 2017 by John Wiley & Sons, Ltd.
Companion website: www.wiley.com/go/banerji/aestheticdentistry

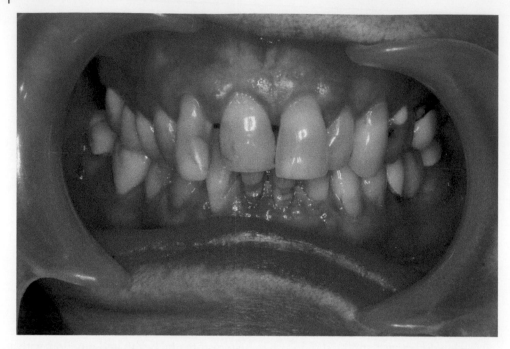

Figure 2.7.1 This patient has a failing upper right lateral incisor and the presenting complaint is the extreme mobility of this tooth

Many clinicians would contest the notion of the existence of an 'aesthetic dental emergency', although a missing anterior crown or an anterior dental restoration may prove to be socially debilitating! Successful treatment planning does involve a level of pragmatic flexibility. It may be desirable to deal with this emergency in a reversible manner, an example of which is shown in Figures 2.7.1 and 2.7.2.

Active restorative intervention can only be successful beyond the short term where the patient and clinician have collectively been effective in preventing the aetiological factor from causing further deterioration of the patient's oral health. The importance attached to the **preventative phase** can often be overlooked. Preventative care prescription is naturally tailored to the underlying pathology and may range from diet advice, habit and lifestyle modification, oral hygiene instruction, fluoride application, the protection of surfaces with sealant-type restorations and the provision of an occlusal splint to referral to a medical practitioner where an underlying medical condition may be aetiological.

It is vital to assess the efficacy of the preventative phase. This may involve an evaluation of habit changes, plaque and bleeding on probing scores, periodontal pocket assessments, the outcome of further investigations and compliance with any prescribed treatment(s). The period of evaluation may be variable, ranging from a few weeks to several months, depending on the nature and extent of the pathology (or aetiological factor) and the compliance of your patient.

The next phase involves **stabilisation** of the effects of the pathology. This may entail the management of any of the following:

- Carious lesions
- Active periodontal disease

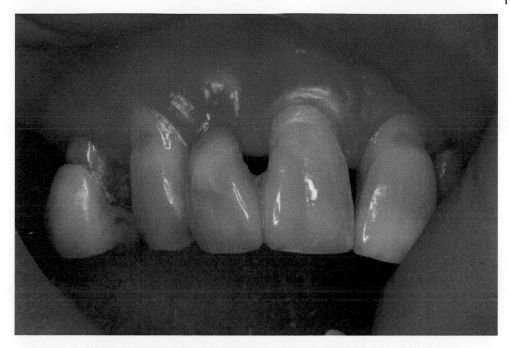

Figure 2.7.2  The tooth was extracted, root sectioned, adjusted palatally to accommodate the occlusion and immediately splinted to the adjacent tooth with composite resin to address the 'aesthetic dental emergency'. The image here shows the area after a period of healing of the soft tissues has taken place. A more definitive alternative can now be considered after the comprehensive treatment plan has been developed

- Occlusal pathology
- Soft and non-dental tissue lesions
- Non-carious hard-tissue pathology.

Teeth diagnosed as having a 'hopeless prognosis' should be extracted. Assessment of prognostic outcome may be based on an evaluation of the following:

- Quantity and quality of the remaining tooth structure
- Periodontal support
- Endodontic status
- History of the affected tooth
- Your experience and skills with treating the presenting condition (although this may be rather misleading), as referral may be need to be sought.

Where your patient has extensive carious lesions, you may choose to apply a 'quadrant by quadrant' approach, which will reduce the frequency of local anaesthetic administration and may prove to be time and cost effective. You may also consider the prescription of direct restorations, which may sometimes be provisional. For the latter purpose the prescription of glass-ionomer cements may prove helpful because of their documented merits. Secondary carious lesions and leaking or failed restorations should also be addressed. Non-carious lesions may equally require intervention.

Periodontal treatment at this stage is usually non-surgical, including prophylaxis, supra- and subgingival scaling, and the correction of plaque-retentive factors such as poorly contoured and/or overhanging restorations, as well as areas of cavitation.

Endodontic treatment should be completed, and suitable core materials placed to provide an effective coronal seal and coronal support for a definitive complex restoration. Any simple occlusal therapy (preferably of the non-invasive variety), such as the prescription of an occlusal splint or the addition of dental materials to correct any occlusal anomaly, should also be undertaken during this phase.

After a suitable time interval, re-evaluate your patient's compliance with the preventative and stabilisation stages. It is at this juncture that you may give consideration to the aesthetic desires of your patient – their 'wish list'. Are their expectations realistic? If not, then further counselling may be required, perhaps referring the patient to another dental or indeed medical colleague. If, however, you feel that their expectations are predictably achievable, then carry out a detailed evaluation of the aesthetic zone and a comprehensive occlusal examination, as described in Chapters 2.3 and 3.1, respectively. From those exercises, proceed to forming a 'problem list' and place this in light of the 'treatment goals', after taking into account any constraints from the patient's medical or dental health.

It is very tempting to impose your 'favourite' methods for treating any aesthetic matter according to your skill set. However, it is far more prudent to take a more holistic approach, based on a fair and robust exploration of the possible options. This may require further diagnostic measures, such as smile evaluation techniques as described in Chapter 2.4.

Now you can discuss possible options and ultimately decide on a definitive plan. This requires a comprehensive appraisal of the merits and drawbacks of *each* option; contingency planning should be placed in an appropriate context.

Make sure that you give your patient the time and space to contemplate the options discussed and, if necessary, allow them to seek a second opinion. Each option should be presented in a comprehensive written format and a signed copy of this plan retained in the dental records. Clarity should be provided about the time and financial commitments involved.

Having verified the plan, attained written consent and ascertained successful stabilisation, the next stage involves the provision of **definitive restorations**. This may include the replacement of provisional restorations with definitive direct restorations, as well as the replacement of aesthetically compromised restorations, such as an unattractive anterior direct resin restoration.

Assess the need for surgical periodontal procedures, including grafting, guided tissue regeneration, pocket elimination, root amputation and so on. Teeth with poor prognostic outcome, or the need to create space for orthodontic tooth move-ment, may necessitate dental extractions. You may also contemplate other surgi-cal procedures such as the extraction of retained root apecies, the management of unerupted teeth or pre-prosthetic surgery prior to the preparation to receive fixed or removable prosthodontics. Direct resin restorations may also be placed to treat cases of tooth wear. These are often referred to as 'immediate composite restora-tions' to protect work surfaces, and to evaluate aesthetic and occlusal tolerance to proposed changes. Procedures such as vital and non-vital tooth bleaching are appro-priate at this stage, and are often undertaken prior to the placement of definitive restorations.

Now determine the success of the previous phase. This may indicate the need for indirect **definitive complex restorations** such as crowns (full and partial variety), onlays or veneer restorations to restore teeth, where the direct approach may prove not to meet the functional and aesthetic needs of the patient and their tooth/teeth. Treatments may range from relatively simple conformative techniques to re-organised rehabilitation. Edentulous spaces may also be restored using removable prostheses, fixed bridgework or dental implants (sometimes in combination). Orthodontic treatment may be required to assist with restorative procedures, such as the uprighting of a tilted tooth, space opening or space closure, or be prescribed to meet the aesthetic needs of the patient, where crowding or spaces are present.

Finally, place your patient on a periodic programme of **monitoring and maintenance**.

## Tips

- Allocate appropriate time for these key stages, and make sure that they are suitably remunerated.
- It is crucial to obtain informed consent from your patient prior to embarking on the provision of any treatment and to provide written treatment plans where necessary.

## Further Reading

FGDP(UK). *Clinical examination and record-keeping: good practice guidelines.* London: Royal College of Surgeons of England; 2009.

Newsome P, Smales R, Yip K. Oral Diagnosis and treatment planning, part 1. Introduction. *Br Dent J.* 2012;213:15–19.

**Part III**

**Clinical Occlusion**

## 3.1

# Clinical Occlusion: Assessment

*Subir Banerji and Shamir B. Mehta*

## Principles

In order to attain longer-term success with restorative care, it is paramount to develop a fundamental appreciation of clinical occlusion. However, clinical occlusion is a subject in dentistry over which many operators unfortunately develop deep anxiety! Sometimes the applied nomenclature and the manner in which various concepts are portrayed can be confusing, in particular the means by which they may relate to practical procedures and their functional relevance. The aim of this part of the book is therefore to keep matters simple, succinct and relevant to everyday clinical practice.

Failure to provide a mechanically sound masticatory system that is conducive to optimal function with desirable levels of load distribution and minimal concomitant trauma to the investing structures will culminate in premature restorative failure. There is also a risk of causing iatrogenic damage to the residual tissues, as well as possible instability concerning the spatial position of a tooth or teeth within the dental arches.

The clinician must therefore be aware of the concept of the **ideal occlusal scheme**. An assessment of the patient's existing occlusal scheme should be carried out with reference to this standard. The assessment should take into account both **static** and **dynamic** components of the patient's occlusal scheme.

As part of good clinical practice, a preliminary occlusal assessment should be carried out when undertaking a routine patient examination. However, there are certain circumstances where a more detailed evaluation may be indicated. These would include the following:

- The presence of pathological tooth wear
- A history of recurrently fracturing teeth or restorations
- Where restorations involving the occlusal table are being planned (of both the direct and indirect varieties)
- Presence of temporomandibular joint disorders
- Instability within the dental arch, such as increased tooth mobility or movement.

This chapter will address the clinical stages involved as part of the occlusal assessment.

*Practical Procedures in Aesthetic Dentistry*, First Edition. Edited by Subir Banerji, Shamir B. Mehta and Christopher C.K. Ho. © 2017 John Wiley & Sons, Ltd. Published 2017 by John Wiley & Sons, Ltd.
Companion website: www.wiley.com/go/banerji/aestheticdentistry

## Procedures

A thorough examination of the temporomandibular joints is recommended. Ask your patient to point to any areas of their head or face that may be symptomatic on maximal opening – if they point to a muscular area, it may be suggestive of muscular dysfunction.

A note of the presence of any mandibular deviation on opening and closing movements is useful. The maximum degree of mandibular opening should be determined by measuring the interincisal distance; any distance less than 35 mm is considered to be restricted. The maximum degree of lateral movement should also be determined; the normal is accepted to be about 12 mm.

Bilaterally palpate the masticatory muscles by pressing them between your thumb placed extra-orally and index finger intra-orally, and observe the presence of hypertrophy, tenderness or discomfort, particularly in areas of muscle insertion. The anterior and posterior temporalis muscles and the superficial and deep masseter muscles are perhaps the most relevant in this context. However, you may also wish to assess the anterior digastric, sternomastoid, trapezius and medial and lateral pterygoid muscles.

Make a note of the appearance of your patient's face: a square profile, usually due to hypertrophy of the masseter muscles, may be suggestive of a tendency towards a parafunctional tooth-clenching habit. It is commonplace also to describe the skeletal profile.

A detailed intra-oral occlusal evaluation should take into account both static and dynamic features. The former are traditionally noted during the classical orthodontic assessment. The **static occlusal examination** should take note of the presence of any of the following features:

- Tooth rotations, tilting, drifting, supra-eruption
- Crowding
- Spacing
- Overjet
- Overbite (including open bites and cross-bites)
- Occlusal vertical dimension (freeway space).

The assessment of these features will help to establish the presence of any malocclusions and further categorise the interarch occlusal relationships (such as the incisor, canine and molar segment classifications).

Assess your patient's teeth for any signs of faceting, fractures, dental caries or mobility. It is worthwhile also to make a note of the plaque and calculus levels, signs of gingivitis, loss of attachment and the overall periodontal health. Signs of occlusal instability may be associated with the presence of recurrently fracturing teeth (or restorations), changes in tooth shape or position (drifting, tilting, rotation or spacing), wear facets and tooth mobility (fremitus). Indentations on the lateral borders of the tongue and/or the buccal and labial mucosa may be indicative of a bruxist tendency.

It is worthwhile carrying out a **freeway space (FWS)** assessment, particularly where your patent may present with a worn dentition. A plethora of different methods have been described in the contemporary literature on how best to determine the FWS. The use of a Willis gauge measuring the difference between the **resting vertical dimension (RVD)** and **occlusal vertical dimension (OVD)** is very commonly applied. For this procedure, encourage your patient to sit upright in the dental chair and to relax. Ask them to moisten their lips gently and place the lips together. Ascertain their RVD. Now, ask them to close the lips together and make a note of their OVD.

Then proceed to the **dynamic occlusal examination**. With the dental chair in a reclined position, start by establishing the **intercuspal position** (ICP), also commonly referred to as the maximal intercuspal position (MIP) or centric occlusion (CO). This is the position when the maxillary and mandibular teeth are maximally meshed together. Intercuspal contacts can be recorded using articulating foil that is 8 μm in thickness. Contacts may be marked up using proprietary articulating paper. A photographic record can also prove helpful.

It is generally accepted that when undertaking a limited number of restorations that may involve modification of the anatomical form of the occlusal table, the occlusal end-point should conform to the existing intercuspal position, unless of course it may be deemed unstable (indicated by the presence of occlusal instability) or there are signs or symptoms of temporomandibular joint dysfunction or masticatory muscle fatigue.

The ease with which your patient's mandible can be manipulated into its **retruded arc of closure** should also be established. Where your patient may have established protective neuro-muscular reflexes, this may not be readily achievable. **Centric relation (CR)** refers to the maxilla–mandibular relationship at the point where the condyles are located in the most anterior–superior position in the glenoid fossae. The **retruded contact position (RCP)** in this context refers to the position of the mandible when first tooth contact occurs on a retruded arc of closure – or the **terminal hinge axis**. The latter is used to describe an imaginary horizontal line that passes through the rotational centres of each of the condylar processes. It is good practice to make a record of the RCP.

In the sagittal plane the mandible can only exhibit **rotational** and **translational movement**; it has been suggested that rotation is limited to about 12 mm of incisor separation before translational movements commence. When recording this position it is imperative that your patient is relaxed, as discussed further in Chapters 3.3 and 3.6.

It is important to document your patient's **anterior guidance**. Where the occlusal scheme is considered to be stable (**mutually protective**), when the patient displays a protrusive mandibular movement, the contact formed between the palatal surfaces of the anterior maxillary teeth and their antagonists coupled with the inclination of the condylar path should collectively aim to separate (or disclude) the posterior teeth from each other. This avoids any harmful occlusal contacts that may otherwise culminate in cuspal fractures, repeated restoration fracture, recurrent decementation of indirect restorations, pathological tooth wear or fremitus. However, in the position of maximum intercuspation, only light occlusal contacts should exist between the anterior segments, with occlusal loading primarily taking place between the posterior teeth.

The steepness of the anterior guidance provided by the anterior teeth should also be recorded, whether steep, moderate or shallow. The effect of altering the anterior guidance on the posterior dentition must be carefully evaluated where the clinician may be contemplating an alteration in the anterior guidance, such as the prescription of multiple anterior crowns. Ideally, the anterior guidance should be **shared** between the anterior teeth to optimise stress distribution.

Occlusal contacts when undertaking **mandibular lateral excursive movements** should also be determined. Lateral guidance may be provided by the canine teeth (**canine guidance**) or by the posterior teeth (**group function**). The morphology of the canine tooth makes it a very suitable candidate to provide guidance during lateral excursive movements. Indeed, it has been shown that canine guidance is the most common type of occlusal arrangement found in the natural dentition. The presence of a canine-guided occlusion helps to permit posterior tooth disclusion on lateral excursion, which may otherwise lead to similar disastrous consequences to those already discussed.

A number of alternative occlusal schemes have been described in the literature, such as a **balanced occlusion (bilaterally balanced occlusion)** or a **unilaterally balanced occlusion**.

Make a note of the presence of any **occlusal interferences** (undesirable contacts that occur between opposing teeth in any mandibular position), which may cause mandibular displacement on either the working side (the side towards which the mandible moves during a lateral excursive movement) or the non-working side (the side away from which the mandible moves in lateral excursion). When undertaking restorative rehabilitation involving a re-organised approach, in the ideal situation lateral guidance should be provided by the canine teeth, with the absence of any occlusal interferences.

The use of articulated study casts to analyse the patient's occlusion can be invaluable.

## Tips

- Try to develop the habit of undertaking a detailed occlusal assessment for every new patient, to establish a baseline.
- Try not to get confused by complex terminology.
- An occlusal scheme that offers canine-guided disclusion is a simple end goal (provided that the canine is deemed suitable to carry the load).

## Further Reading

Mehta SB, Banerji S, Millar BJ, Suarez-Feito, J-M. Current concepts on the management of tooth wear: part 1. Assessment, treatment planning and strategies for the prevention and the passive management of tooth wear. *Br Dent J.* 2012;212:17–27.

Rosenstiel S, Land M, Fujimoto J. *Contemporary fixed prosthodontics.* 4th ed. St Louis, MO: Mosby; 2006.

Shillingburg H, Sather D, Wilson E, et al. *Fundamentals of fixed prosthodontics.* 4th Ed. Chicago, IL: Quintessence; 2012.

Wilson NHF. *Principles and practice of esthetic dentistry: essentials of aesthetic dentistry,* Vol. 1. London: Elsevier; 2014.

## 3.2

# Facebows: The Facebow Recording

*Subir Banerji and Shamir B. Mehta*

*Video: The Facebow Recording*
*Presented by Subir Banerji and Shamir B. Mehta*

## Principles

This chapter focuses on the **facebow**, a rigid but adjustable device that relates the maxillary occlusal surface to an **anatomical reference point**. The facebow recording is often the first procedure undertaken when mounting study casts on a dental semi-adjustable articulator. Its primary purpose is to permit mounting of the maxillary cast on the articulator. In addition, the facebow also provides a guide to the width between the condyles, referred to as the **intercondylar width**, which has further practical significance, as discussed in Chapter 3.4. Facebows are also referred to as **hingebows** in the literature; the indications for the use of a facebow therefore indirectly relate to the need to use a dental articulator and are discussed in Chapter 3.4.

Typically, two **reference points** are chosen when attaining a facebow record: a **posterior** one, typically the **terminal hinge axis**, an imaginary line that runs between the heads of the mandibular condyles (which relates to the condylar elements of the articulator). A second, more **anterior reference point** is also usually selected, which may vary between different articulators. Both anterior and posterior reference points should be replicable during further subsequent appointments. Typical anterior reference points include the nasion or the inner canthus of the eye.

Facebows generally fall into the category of being either **arbitrary** or **kinematic**. Arbitrary facebows, as the name perhaps suggests, are less accurate in the manner in which they relate to the terminal hinge axis. However, they are suitable (and have been proven to be so) for most routine restorative dental procedures. They effectively approximate the position of the terminal hinge axis, typically to the position external to the auditory meatus (which is erroneous by definition). Facebows that utilise the external auditory meatus as the reference point are commonly referred to as **earbows**.

In contrast, the use of a kinematic facebow requires the terminal hinge axis to be more accurately determined, which may be more relevant where there is a need to copy the precise opening and closing movements of the mandible on the dental articulator, such as in a complex restorative reconstruction involving an alteration of the existing vertical and horizontal occlusal relations.

*Practical Procedures in Aesthetic Dentistry*, First Edition. Edited by Subir Banerji, Shamir B. Mehta and Christopher C.K. Ho. © 2017 John Wiley & Sons, Ltd. Published 2017 by John Wiley & Sons, Ltd.
Companion website: www.wiley.com/go/banerji/aestheticdentistry

The **facebow fork** or **bite fork** is an item of equipment that is used to record the maxillary occlusal surfaces using a variety of different media. These materials should offer dimensional stability, a suitable working time and ease of use. Typically applied recording materials include impression compound, greenstick, polyvinyl siloxane (PVS) bite-registration materials (such as Stonebite, Dreve Dentamid GmbH, Unna, Germany) or extra-hard wax, such as Moyco beauty wax (Integra Miltex, Rietheim-Weiltheim, Germany). The record attained using the bite fork is then inserted into the facebow, permitting attainment of the registration required.

The assembly is then transferred to the articulator (in part or whole) depending on the apparatus being used. The maxillary cast is positioned on the occlusal record, which has been related to the terminal hinge axis on the articulator, and the cast attached to a mounting plate on the articulator using a suitable mounting stone/plaster.

## Procedures

There are many articulators available in the marketplace. The procedure described here relates to the use of the Denar Mark II System (Whip Mix Corporation, Louisville, KY, USA), utilising the Denar Slidematic facebow. This is an example of an arbitrary facebow; the articulator is of the **arcon**, **semi-adjustable** variety (see Chapter 3.4).

If you have the Denar Slidematic facebow kit at your disposal, open the kit and you will find, among many other items, a **reference point locator** (sometimes referred to as a reference plane locator). This is used to identify the anterior reference point for facebow transfer, which will be **43 mm** from the incisal edge of either the central or lateral incisor towards the inner canthus (corner) of the patient's right eye.

With your patient sitting upright, simply place the flat aspect of the reference point locator on the incisal edge of either of the right incisor teeth (for an edentulous patient use the lower border of the upper lip at rest). Using the felt-tip pen provided, place a mark (dot) on the patient's face below the inner canthus of the right eye, where the pointed end of the reference locator touches your patient's face. You may choose to measure and record the distance between this reference point and the inner canthus of the right eye, in the event that the anterior reference point is lost through a dental extraction or restorative intervention of one of the reference incisor teeth.

Place your chosen material for recording the occlusal surface of the maxillary arch on the bite fork. Take care to make sure that the recording material is placed on the correct side of the bite fork, with the shaft projecting from your patient's right. The material should cover all aspects of the bite fork. If you are using a thermoplastic material such as wax or impression compound, check that the temperature of the material is low enough to avoid scalding your patient's lips and face.

Carefully insert the loaded bite fork into your patient's mouth and centre it over the maxillary cusp tips. Lightly compress the fork to attain an impression; some protocols advocate instructing your patient to bite down gently into the recording medium. The index ring on the fork should ideally line up with your patient's midline. The objective (according to the manufacturer) is to produce a 'slight impression' of the cusp tips, primarily avoiding fossae.

It is not essential to record every cusp; the level of detail required should be enough to permit the seating of an accurate maxillary cast in a stable manner. A record that is very shallow will not permit accurate and reproducible seating of the cast. In contrast, a record that is too deep will not permit accurate repositioning, as the cast is not a precise duplication of the teeth.

If you are using a wax-based material or impression compound, cool the material using a three-in-one air gun and subsequently remove the record from your patient's mouth and chill it under cold water. Clearly, this stage is not necessary with the use of PVS materials. Assess the record and re-seat it to assess for distortion and stability. Does it rock when you re-position the bite fork and support it with your index finger on either side? Where the record may reveal unwanted details such as pits and fissures, carefully trim these away prior to re-seating using a scalpel. If there are any perforations through the registration medium (with metal display), your cast will not seat accurately. Under such circumstances, start again.

It is good practice to have the maxillary cast at your disposal prior to the facebow recording. In this way, you can also check that the cast seats accurately in the bite fork.

Now, with the bite fork in situ, ask your patient for assistance with its support. You may choose to request that they place their thumbs on either underside of the bite fork, or alternatively you may ask your assistant to firmly hold the bite fork in position.

Fasten the reference pin to the underside of the facebow and loosen all of the toggles and clamps. Slide the clamp marked '2' over the protruding end of the bite fork towards your patient's face. This clamp should be positioned over the shaft on the right side of your patient. Place each of the calliper ends into your patient's external auditory opening (similar to a stethoscope). It is helpful if your dental assistant guides you with the side you are facing away from. If you have elected for your assistant to support the bite fork in the patients mouth then you can ask your patient to position the earpieces, particularly if placement proves to be tricky and uncomfortable, and especially where both ears are at slightly different levels.

Next, release the anterior reference pointer and position it so that it points towards the anterior reference point marked earlier. Slide the facebow from up to down, such that the tip of the reference pointer contacts the reference point; at this point the bow will be horizontal to the Frankfort plane. Tighten the screw on clamp '1', which is the vertical reference pin, and then the screw on clamp '2', the horizontal reference pin. If you have got it correct, the digits 1 and 2 should be facing in your direction.

Tighten the toggles and clamps until the recording apparatus is secure. You will notice the presence of a scale on the superior surface of the facebow. Make a note of the measurement on this scale as an indication of the intercondylar width. This can also be used to position the condylar pillars of the articulator.

Finally, loosen the calliper screw and remove the facebow from your patient's ears. Slide the bite fork (now attached to the earbow) out of your patient's mouth and disinfect the recording. With this system, the facebow and bite fork assembly can be separated and carefully transported, ready for transference to the dental articulator.

## Tips

- Practise the use of a facebow on your dental nurse, or a relative or friend.
- Make sure that your dental technician is confident and competent with the use of your chosen system.

## Further Reading

Rosenstiel S, Land M, Fujimoto J. *Contemporary fixed prosthodontics*. 4th ed. St Louis, MO: Mosby; 2006.

Shillingburg H, Sather D, Wilson E, et al. *Fundamentals of fixed prosthodontics*. 4th ed. Chicago, IL: Quintessence, 2012.

The Denar Mark II System, Technique Manual. Whip Mix Corporation, Louisville, KY, USA. www.whipmix.com

# 3.3

# Intra-occlusal Records

*Subir Banerji and Shamir B. Mehta*

*Video: Intra-occlusal Records*
*Presented by Subir Banerji and Shamir B. Mehta*

## Principles

In this chapter, the means by which the occlusal surfaces of the mandibular cast relate to those of the maxillary cast will be described, thereby permitting the mounting of a set of casts against each other on the articulator. In order to accomplish this, there is a need to attain an accurate **intra-occlusal record**. Inter-occlusal records may either provide a record of the **intercuspal position** (**ICP**, synonymously termed the position of maximum intercuspation or MI) or of the **centric relation (CR)**.

The CR record aims to record the relationship of the mandibular arch to that of the maxillary arch when the condyles are seated in their most anterior–superior positions in the glenoid fossae. In this position, opening and closing movements of the mandible take place in a rotational manner (as opposed to translation) for the first few millimetres and would correspond to rotational movements occurring at the dental articulator's condylar housing.

Unlike the intercuspal record, which records the position where the antagonistic occlusal surfaces are maximally meshed together, the CR record is attained *regardless of any given position of tooth contact*. The CR record is often referred to as being a fixed and reproducible record in the literature; fixed in this context is in reference to a fixed anatomical position (independent of the occlusal surfaces), which is reproducible between that of the patient's condyles and the condylar housing of the dental articulator, where rotational movements of the condyles will take place against the corresponding articular eminences.

**Lateral excursive** and/or **protrusive mandibular** records may also be taken in conjunction with the CR record in order to programme the condylar guides on the articulator, which would relate to the anatomical limits of the movements of the condyles in their glenoid fossae.

An intercuspal record is generally taken when mounting a set of **working casts** where the occlusal scheme is stable, often where relatively simple restorations are being considered; hence the need to conform to the existing occlusal scheme. The use of casts mounted in CR for this purpose may culminate in an undesirable occlusal interference.[1]

*Practical Procedures in Aesthetic Dentistry*, First Edition. Edited by Subir Banerji, Shamir B. Mehta and Christopher C.K. Ho. © 2017 John Wiley & Sons, Ltd. Published 2017 by John Wiley & Sons, Ltd.
Companion website: www.wiley.com/go/banerji/aestheticdentistry

The CR record, in contrast, is advocated when fabricating **study casts**, thereby permitting evaluation of the retruded contact point (RCP), also referred to as the centric relation contact position (CRCP), which is the first point of tooth contact while the mandible is in CR. Evaluation of the RCP may otherwise be very difficult in the presence of the patient's soft tissues and protective neuro-muscular reflexes.

Approximately 90% of patients have a slide between RCP and ICP; casts mounted in CR can readily elucidate this. In this case, any **premature tooth contacts**, also termed **deflective contacts** (which will guide the patient's mandible from CRCP to ICP), can be noted, and the need for any occlusal correction determined prior to embarking on complex prosthodontic treatment plans.

For patients with pathological tooth wear, where active restorative intervention is being considered, the discrepancy between RCP and ICP may result in a level of inter-occlusal clearance. This may be utilised to place restorative materials when re-organising the occlusion without a need for increasing the occlusal dimension or subtractive tooth preparation to accommodate future restorations.[2]

The use of CR as a position independent of tooth contact would also seem sensible when undertaking a complex occlusal rehabilitation, where re-organisation of the occlusal scheme is planned, thereby providing a fixed reference position. In an analogous manner, CR is chosen for complete denture fabrication or removable partial denture construction, where there is no stable occlusal contact to provide a point of reference.

A CR record may also be contemplated where the tooth being restored by means of an indirect restoration is the first point of tooth contact in CR, either to copy this onto the definitive restoration or as a means of evaluating a possible change in RCP on a tooth that may be suboptimal for the process of further occlusal loading.

## Procedures

For a dentate patient where the occlusal surfaces inter-relate in a manner where the intercuspal position is readily determined, an intercuspal record may be attained by placing a suitable quantity of recording material such as polyvinyl siloxane (PVS) bite-registration paste onto a dried occlusal surface (such as a tooth preparation), or bilaterally across the posterior occluding surfaces. Other materials such as cold-cured acrylic resin may also be used.

Place the chosen material evenly onto your patient's occlusal surface, and ask your patient to bring their teeth together into the position of 'best fit'[3] – this can be difficult for some patients. Once the material is set, carefully remove it and use it to mount your casts. The accuracy of the mounting can be determined by using ultra-thin foil articulating paper. Holding contacts identified intra-orally should be congruent with those on the dental casts. If not, this may be indicative of an error. Be mindful to check your casts for any casting nodules or incorrectly trimmed models, especially in the heel areas. For partially dentate patients, there may be a need to fabricate a wax occlusal rim, ideally supported by an acrylic base plate.

If you are planning on attaining a CR record, prior to the actual recording stage practise manipulating your patient into this position. Position your patient in the dental chair at an approximately 45° angle. Commence with manual manipulation of the condyles into the desired position. Be careful to avoid a forceful action, which will push the mandible backwards in a downward transalatory movement, culminating in an erroneous record.

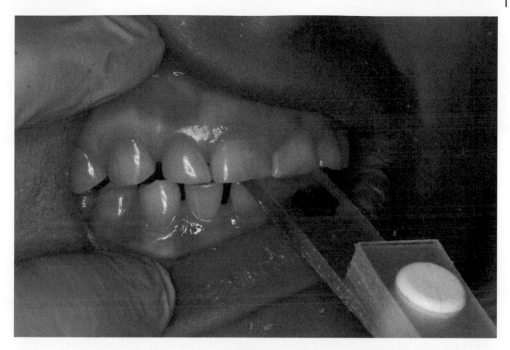

Figure 3.3.1 Leaf gauge (Huffman Dental Products LLC, South Vienna, OH, USA)

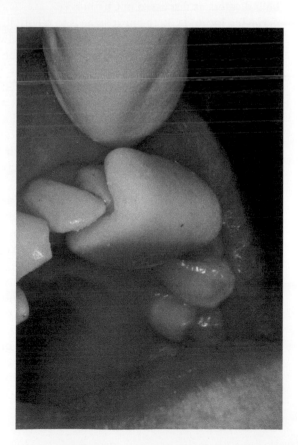

Figure 3.3.2 The use of a Lucia Jig (Great Lakes Orthodontics, Ltd, Tonawanda, NY, USA)

The technique of bimanual manipulation, as described by Dawson,[4] is often advocated and is shown in the video on the accompanying website. With experience, if you have managed to position the condyles in the correct position, the mandible will be hinged along its retruded arc of closure and you may be able to palpate this portion of the condyle by placing your finger in your patient's external auditory meatus.

However, due to the presence of protective neuro-muscular reflexes, which may be encountered in patients with parafunctional habits, finding CR may prove difficult. To assist with such cases, the use of an **anterior de-programming device** is helpful. This aims to overcome the neuro-muscular reflexes, which are initiated by tooth contact, by causing tooth separation. For this purpose, you may request your patient to bite on some cotton wool rolls, ensuring that all of the teeth are separated for a period of 5 minutes. Commercially available products for this purpose include devices such as a **leaf gauge**. An example is depicted in Figure 3.3.1, whereby thin plastic strips of 0.1 mm width are placed in the anterior region, and further layers sequentially added until there is evidence of posterior tooth separation when the patient bites down lightly.

However, you may find that for some patients this will prove insufficient. Under such circumstances it is appropriate to fabricate an anterior de-programming device, such as a **Lucia Jig**. As depicted in Figure 3.3.2, this is an anterior bite plane traditionally constructed using cold-cured acrylic resin. You may consider improving the efficacy of the device in determining CR by carrying out a gothic-arch tracing.

For patients who fail to permit manipulation of the mandible after having placed the jig in situ for more than 30 minutes, the use of an appropriate form of occlusal splint will be indicated, as discussed in Chapter 3.6.

Having located CR, the next stage is to record it. Commonly used materials are PVS-based bite-registration paste or extra-hard dental wax such as Moyco beauty wax.

If you are planning the use of a wax record, the outline of the record should extend approximately 5 mm beyond the buccal cusp tips. If you have prepared a Lucia Jig, simply cut a relief into the anterior portion of the record to permit concurrent placement of both the record and the jig. Re-soften the wax record and place it over the maxillary occluding surfaces. Lightly press the wax record against the cusp tips to produce shallow indentations and guide your patient into CR, such that the mandibular teeth form shallow indentations. Cool the record using an air gun. Remove the record and verify it for any signs of perforation. Chill the record using cold water, and re-position it to verify its accuracy.

An obvious drawback to the use of a thermoplastic material such as wax is distortion on cooling. Check the fit of the record on the dental casts. You may choose to apply a strip of zinc oxide eugenol paste, such as Temp-Bond, across a portion of the record, as shown in Figure 3.3.3. Cracking of this in due course may be indicative of unwanted distortion.

For a patient who is partially dentate or edentulous, wax rims mounted on a stable (ideally rigid) base plate will be needed, which should locate accurately onto the casts.

Finally, should you wish to programme your articulator's condylar guides (as opposed to using average value settings of 30° and 15° for condylar and Bennet angles, respectively), then you will need to produce lateral or protrusive inter-occlusal records. This process is demonstrated in the video on the companion website. Programming of the semi-adjustable articulator is discussed further in Chapter 3.4.

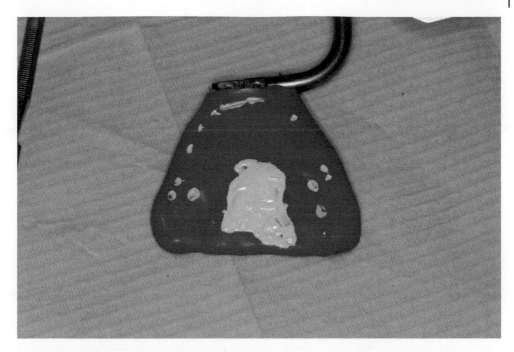

**Figure 3.3.3** Facebow record in pink beauty wax. Temp-Bond (Kerr Corporation, Orange, CA, USA) has been placed across a portion of the record; cracking of the set paste may be indicative of unwanted distortion

## Tips

- Finding CR can be challenging, even for an experienced operator. Develop competence and confidence with the different techniques described in this chapter.
- Allocate your appointments appropriately to allow sufficient time.

## References

1 Rosensteil S, Land M, Fujimoto J. *Contemporary fixed prosthodontics*. 4th ed. St Louis, MO: Mosby; 2006.
2 Mehta SB, Banerji S, Millar BJ, Suarez-Feito J-M. Current concepts on the management of tooth wear: part 1. Assessment, treatment planning and strategies for the prevention and passive management of tooth wear. *Br Dent J*. 2012;212:17–27.
3 Shillingburg HT, Sather DA, Wilson EL, et al. *Fundamentals of fixed prosthodontics*. 4th ed. Chicago, IL: Quintessence, 2012.
4 Dawson PE. Temporomandibular joint pain dysfunction problems can be solved. *J Prosthet Dent*. 1973;29:100.

## 3.4

# Semi-adjustable Articulators

*Bill Sharpling*

*Video: Semi-adjustable Articulators*
*Presented by Bill Sharpling*

## Principles

This chapter and the associated video aim to assist with understanding the procedure of mounting models into a semi-adjustable articulator, which takes place most often in the dental laboratory, following on from a facebow recording and intra-occlusal records being made.

### Preparing the Bite Fork, Records and Models for Despatch to the Laboratory

The bite-fork assembly should have had all the locking screws checked for tightness prior to being removed from the facebow.

The dental technician mounting the models will need to be confident that the bite fork has remained in the same position during transportation. It can be helpful to place the bite-fork assembly in padded material such as bubblewrap prior to placing it in the laboratory workbox.

The bite fork and occlusal records should have been disinfected prior to passing them onto the laboratory. If the records have been tried on any working models, then the models should also be disinfected.

## Procedures

The bite fork will be carefully removed from any packaging and a check will be made that the maxillary model to be mounted into the articulator sits in the bite-registration material in a stable manner. Bite-registration material is very accurate and will capture the occlusal anatomy in great detail. However, the occlusal surface of some study models produced from alginate impressions can show positive discrepancies such as small airblows. If so, these will be removed, as they can interfere with the fit into the registration material.

The registration material may also be trimmed to a minimal amount to check that the model is fully seated.

*Practical Procedures in Aesthetic Dentistry*, First Edition. Edited by Subir Banerji, Shamir B. Mehta and Christopher C.K. Ho. © 2017 John Wiley & Sons, Ltd. Published 2017 by John Wiley & Sons, Ltd.
Companion website: www.wiley.com/go/banerji/aestheticdentistry

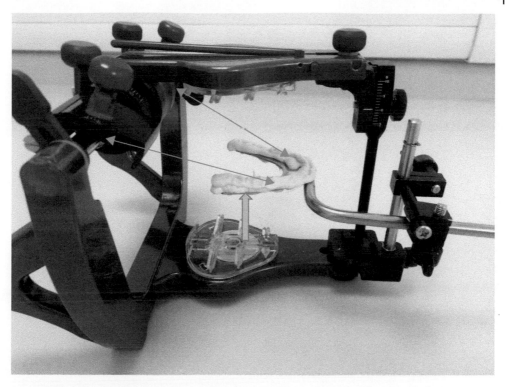

Figure 3.4.1 The relationship of the bite fork to the condylar head elements of the articulator, which relates the incisal edge of the maxillary teeth in the correct three-dimensional position to the condyles in the patient's head

The bite-fork assembly is then secured in the bite-fork assembly holder. This holder is then placed in the lower member of the articulator in the same slot where the incisal table, which has previously been removed, is normally housed.

The bite fork will now be sitting centrally above the lower mounting plate and should be in the same position in relation to the condylar elements of the mandible as the occlusal plane is in the patient (see Figure 3.4.1).

A bite-fork support is sometimes used (shown by the orange arrow in Figure 3.4.1) when a large and/or heavy upper model is being mounted, as this will ensure that the bite fork does not move/flex during the mounting procedure.

The maxillary model is then placed into the bite fork and is attached to the upper element of the articular via a mix of mounting plaster.

The lower model is then mounted against the upper model. If it is prescribed to have the models mounted in a retruded arc of closure, then the lower model will be mounted against the upper using the relevant intra-occlusal record supplied to the laboratory.

### Setting the Articulator Controls

A semi-adjustable articulator will have certain programmable elements. Most commonly it will be the condylar guidance angle and Bennett angle that can be adjusted. These can be set to average value readings or can be customised by the use of intra-occlusal records.

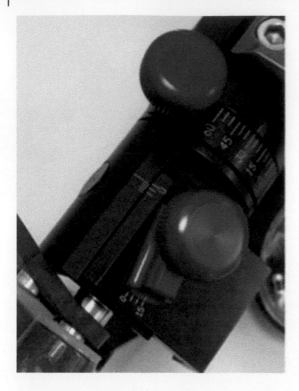

Figure 3.4.2 The condylar guidance angle set at 30°, immediate side shift at 0.5 mm and Bennett angle (progressive side shift) at 15°

## Condylar Guidance Angle

If setting to average values (assuming a Denar articulator), the condylar guidance angle would be set at 30°.

The condylar guidance angle determines the inclination of the element along which the condyle head travels in a protrusive movement. This is adjusted by loosening the protrusive adjustment thumbscrew. The scale is below the adjustment screw. The protrusive condylar path inclination scale is below the protrusive adjustment thumbscrew and is calibrated in increments of 5° (Figure 3.4.2). The protrusive adjustment range is 0–60°.

## Immediate Side Shift

The medial fossa wall can be displaced straight medially by means of the immediate side shift adjustment. The scale for the immediate side shift adjustment is lateral to the protrusive adjustment thumbscrew on top of the fossa. The scale is calibrated in 0.5 mm increments on the upper scale and 1 mm increments on the lower scale. To set the immediate side shift, loosen the thumbscrew below the scale and align the marks of the lower scale with either the long mark of the upper scale for shifts of 1 or 2 mm, or with the smaller marks for shifts of 0.5 or 1.5 mm.[1] Figure 3.4.2 shows an immediate side shift setting of 0.5 mm. The immediate side shift range is 0–2 mm.

## Bennett Angle (Progressive Side Shift)

This is the angle along which the head of the orbiting condyle will travel compared to the protrusive or sagittal line, when carrying out an excursive movement. This angle can be adjusted by loosening the same thumbscrew as with the immediate side shift and moving from 0° to 15°. The scale is underneath the screw and has 5° markings.

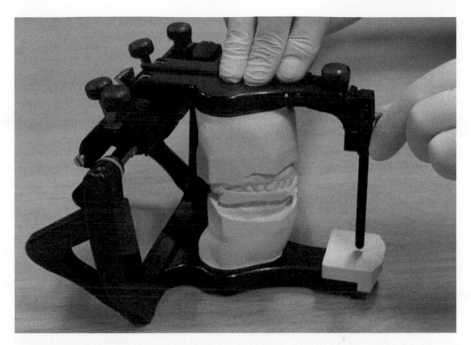

**Figure 3.4.3** The upper and lower casts correctly related by a jaw relationship record, with the incised pin prior to it being adjusted to offer extra support before the programming sequence

To custom set the condylar guidance angle and Bennett angle (as opposed to using average value settings), the dental laboratory will need to have been provided with protrusive and left and right lateral intra-occlusal records.

### Using the Lateral Records to Set the Bennett Angle

Simulating the orbiting condylar path is carried out by loosening both thumbscrews on either side of the upper arm of the articulator. Set the condylar guidance angle to 0° and move the medial walls as far inwards as they go on both sides.

Separate the upper and lower elements and seat the right lateral record within the casts. Firm pressure is used to ensure that the model is seated and that the incisal pin, which will now be raised off the incisal table, can be loosened and allowed to drop and rest on the table. This will provide extra stability during the lateral (and protrusive) programming sequence (see Figure 3.4.3).

With the right lateral record in place, the left condyle will now be positioned downwards and forwards from its starting position of centric relation. The left condylar element is rotated downwards from 0° until it touches the condyle. The thumbscrew is now tightened. The left medial wall is moved outwards laterally until it contacts the condyle. The Bennett angle thumbscrew is then tightened.

At this time the left condyle is positioned inwards, downwards and forwards from its centric-related position. Increase the inclination of the left protrusive condylar path until the superior wall of the fossa contacts the top of the condyle. Secure the protrusive condylar path in this position by tightening the thumbscrew. Record the settings on the patient's records/laboratory form.

The same procedure is then carried out using the left lateral check record to capture the orbiting path and Bennett angle of the right condyle.

The thumbscrews that allow rotation of the condylar guidance angle elements are loosened and the condylar guidance angle is set to 0°.

The protrusive record is set onto the lower model and the upper model is seated into the record. Firm pressure is again used to ensure that the model is seated and the incisal pin, which will now again be raised off the incisal table, can be loosened and allowed to drop and rest on the table. This will provide extra stability during the lateral (and protrusive) programming sequence, as shown in Figure 3.4.3.

The condyles now sit below and away from the fossa walls above them (see Figure 3.4.4).

The angle of inclination of the fossa walls is increased on both sides by rotating down (direction of orange arrow in Figure 3.4.4) until they touch their respective condyle. Increase the inclination of the protrusive condylar path on both fossae until the superior fossa walls contact their respective condyle. The thumbscrew is now locked at this position and the condylar guidance angle has been set. This should be noted and recorded on the laboratory records.

## Producing a Custom-Made Incisal Guidance Table

Once the models have been mounted and the articulator programmed using the intra-occlusal records, a custom-made incisal guidance table can be formed to capture

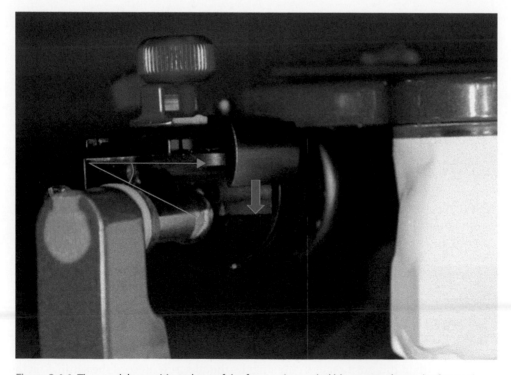

Figure 3.4.4 The condyles positioned out of the fossa – the angled blue arrow shows the forward and downward path of movement away from horizontal that the condyle has travelled during the protrusive movement

the existing anterior elements of the occlusal scheme. It is assumed that the existing anterior occlusal scheme is 'working' and is either formed in the provisional restorations that are being worn or is being copied from the existing dentition.

To produce the custom-made incisal table, the following procedure is carried out:

- Apply model hardener to incisal and occlusal edges of all teeth.
- Set incisal pin 1 mm high of incisal guidance table.
- Apply thin layer of separating medium to incisal guidance table and to tip of incisal pin.
- Mix Duralay/trim to dough consistency and place on incisal guidance table.
- Ensure centric latch is 'off' and both ends of spring are located on their 'keepers'.
- Move articulator through all eccentric movements; keep doing this until Duralay has set. Duralay can be trimmed with scissors to eliminate any overhang or flash.
- Remove pre-op model and re-articulate with the working model. The incisal scheme that has been captured in the Duralay can be used to determine the scheme for the restorations that are being made (see Figure 3.4.5).

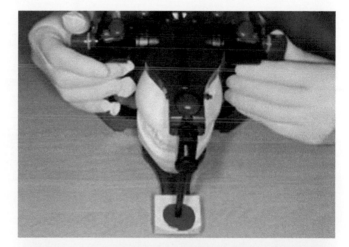

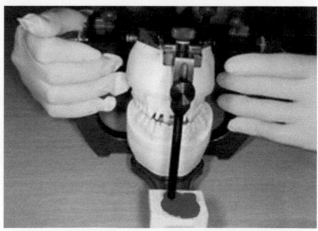

Figure 3.4.5 Forming the Duralay pattern resin capturing the incised scheme during all eccentric movements

## Tips

- It is good practice to communicate with your laboratory technician so that you are both familiar with the articulator being used.
- You may choose to take your preliminary impressions and have your study casts fabricated prior to the appointment when you will be taking your facebow and intra-occlusal records.

## Reference

1 Denar Mark 300 Series Articulator System Instruction Manual. Whip Mix Corporation, Fort Collins, CO, USA. www.whipmix.com.

## 3.5

# Functional Diagnostic Waxing Up

*Il Ki Ricky Lee*

## Principles

Wax is an excellent material that is widely used in dentistry. It can be transformed into many other materials, so its role is to connect one material to another. It can be transformed into a metal, zirconia, lithium disilicate, acrylic or resin-based restoration or coping. Moreover, it can be an excellent learning tool for understanding or reproducing tooth or gum shapes, because it is simple to apply, remove and shape.

It is essential for the dental team to understand the anatomy of teeth and the oral cavity before performing any prosthetic treatments on the patient. Wax-ups can provide a blueprint and a prescription for the final prosthetics for the dentist, dental technician and patient. This diagnostic wax-up becomes a vital communication tool for the dental team involved.

Therefore, a diagnostic wax-up can be used for temporary or provisional crowns, to guide the preparation of the teeth as well as to frame the outline of ceramic build-ups.

However, many dentists and dental technicians forgo this step and sometimes ignore the importance of a diagnostic wax-up due to the costs involved to produce this stage. By doing so they are ignoring the overall time saved in the treatment of the case.

This chapter explains how to fabricate prosthetics by using wax. The most difficult task is to mimic the natural teeth, not only to resemble their colour or internal structure, but also to reproduce the shapes and balanced contours within biological and functional limitations.

To mimic nature's complicated shapes and colours, first of all we have to have knowledge of the anatomical features and their biological and functional correlations. Furthermore, we need to observe precisely the relationships with the surrounding adjacent teeth to achieve the contact points, the height of the ridge, the bucco-lingual limits and the opposing tooth for occlusion and functionality, with reference to the contralateral side to reproduce a mirror image.

To reproduce the natural appearance and replace prosthetics on an abutment or tooth preparation means that there are anatomical starting points such as cervical margins

*Practical Procedures in Aesthetic Dentistry*, First Edition. Edited by Subir Banerji, Shamir B. Mehta and Christopher C.K. Ho. © 2017 John Wiley & Sons, Ltd. Published 2017 by John Wiley & Sons, Ltd.
Companion website: www.wiley.com/go/banerji/aestheticdentistry

or contact areas, and ending points such as incisal edges or marginal ridges. The final shapes are created by joining together these points of reference.

To achieve the correct form and contour it is important to identify these reference starting and ending points in each situation and then to merge these points with the wax to produce the final contour.

## Procedures

The stages in a wax-up are shown in Figure 3.5.1. The reference points are as follows:

- **Embrasures**. These not only provide an escape channel for food to escape during chewing, but also outline the shape for the final restorations. Embrasures exist in buccal, lingual, occlusal, incisal and cervical areas and determine the size of the tooth in length, height and thickness.
- **Emergence profile**. This is taken from the actual margin of the tooth preparation or abutment that the dentist has prepared (Figure 3.5.2). Emergence profiles are closely related to the surrounding soft tissues and form an important aesthetic area. The emergence profile should be designed to support the soft tissues passively, so as not to create undue pressure that may then lead to undesirable soft-tissue migration.

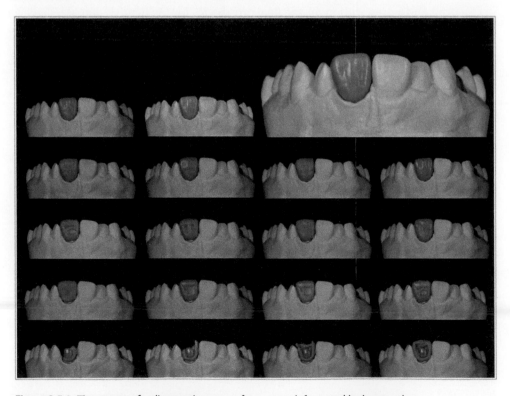

Figure 3.5.1 The stages of a diagnostic wax-up for a upper left central incisor tooth

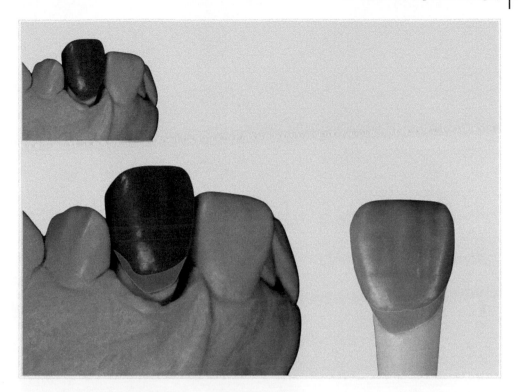

Figure 3.5.2 Development of the correct emergence profile

- **Contact points**. These offer stability and also have a role to play in determining the final shape of the tooth. Contact points should be designed three-dimensionally along the axis and angle of the teeth (Figure 3.5.3). A correctly contoured midline contact is critical for an aesthetic appearance. It is important to observe this area carefully, in all dimensions, to ensure development of the correct outline with respect to the embrasures both cervically and incisally, as well as the depth from the bucco-lingual aspects.
- **Prominent areas**. These are the shapes determined by three factors: margin at cervical region, contact area at mesial/distal region and incisal edge. These features influence the perception of the total size and inclination of the tooth. These areas can be placed widely or narrowly to match the target size, even when there are different spatial requirements. Prominent areas complete the three-dimensional form of the tooth shape and may help in many situations; the dental technician can solve problems relating to dimensional and space issues by positioning these features accordingly to produce a sense of aesthetic illusion.
- **Details**. These are textures, lustre, thickness and height of ridges, depth of pit and line angles of incisal edges from labial to lingual.

We always aim to mimic nature, and knowledge of the natural anatomy and its correlations, along with an understanding of the definitive restorations that we can use, enables a successful treatment outcome. Observing how light and optical characteristics reflect on teeth and supporting structures may allow us to come close to natural teeth both functionally and aesthetically.

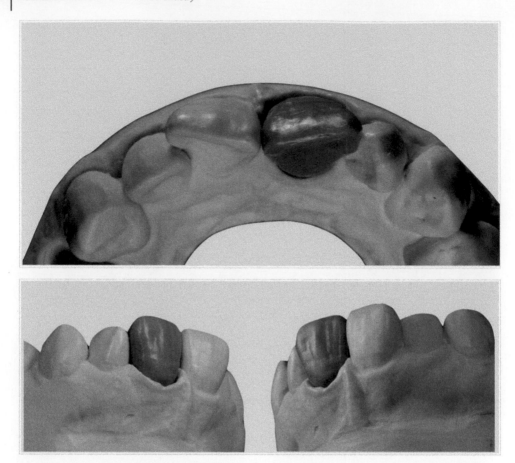

Figure 3.5.3 The three-dimensional nature of the contact area between the upper left and right central incisors and left lateral incisor

## Tips

- Always observe teeth, restorations and the wax-up from many different aspects: incisally, mesially, distally and buccally.
- Heat the die in a hot plate and dip it into a dipping wax during fabrication of wax copings or a full-contour wax-up. This prevents a double layer of wax forming inside the fitting area.
- Slightly over-contouring the wax-up allows space for polishing, especially when you make a lithium disilicate restoration to get rid of the reaction layers.

# 3.6

# Occlusal Stabilisation Splints

*Subir Banerji and Shamir B. Mehta*

*Video: Occlusal Stabilisation Splints*
*Presented by Subir Banerji and Shamir B. Mehta*

## Principles

An occlusal splint may be defined as a 'removable appliance covering some or all of the occlusal surfaces of the teeth in either the maxillary or mandibular arches'.[1]

Splints may be classified according to their **level of coverage** (full versus partial), their **consistency** (hard or soft), the **arch** to which they may be applied or whether they **reposition the mandible** into a pre-determined position or are flat, thus of the stabilisation variety.

The use of a splint may be considered in the following circumstances:

- Attempting to locate (and/or reposition a patient into) centric relation
- Management of temporomandibular joint disorders
- Diagnosis of occlusal pathology
- Stabilisation of the occlusal scheme prior to complex restorative care provision, including the assessment of patient tolerance to an occlusal scheme, with an altered vertical occlusal dimension
- Providing passive (preventative) management for cases of pathological tooth wear
- Attempting to create intra-occlusal clearance by the process of relative axial movement (occlusal adaptation) for cases such as those displaying tooth wear
- Protection of the natural and/or restored dentition during parafunctional (bruxist) activity

The ability to prescribe and construct a **stabilisation splint** has many merits for the restorative dentist. Stabilisation splints may be used for each of the above indications, and will be discussed further in this chapter.

The stabilisation splint essentially provides the patient with a removable 'ideal occlusal scheme' according to the principals of the **mutually protected occlusal scheme**. The use of a resilient material such as heat-cured acrylic culminates in a durable appliance that may be suitably contoured to the desired prescription, can be readily adjusted and will be minimally abrasive to antagonistic surfaces.

The maxillary stabilisation splint is commonly referred to as a **Michigan splint**, while the mandibular stabilisation splint is often termed a **Tanner appliance**. Examples are depicted in Figures 3.6.1 and 3.6.2, respectively. Although both offer analogous

*Practical Procedures in Aesthetic Dentistry*, First Edition. Edited by Subir Banerji, Shamir B. Mehta and Christopher C.K. Ho. © 2017 John Wiley & Sons, Ltd. Published 2017 by John Wiley & Sons, Ltd.
Companion website: www.wiley.com/go/banerji/aestheticdentistry

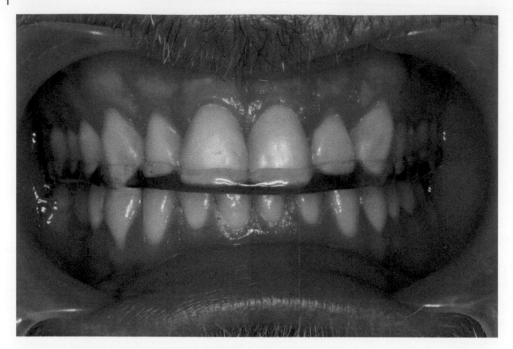

Figure 3.6.1  A maxillary, hard full-coverage acrylic Michigan splint

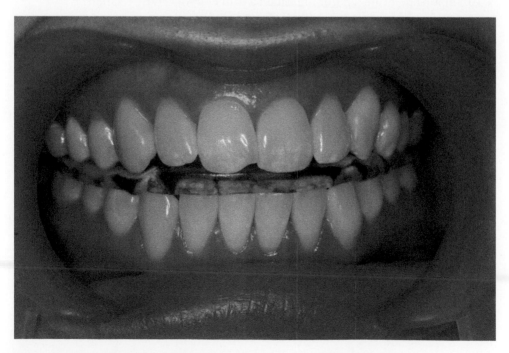

Figure 3.6.2  A mandibular, hard full-coverage acrylic Tanner appliance

outcomes, the latter are perhaps more suitable for patients displaying a Class 3 incisor relationship (as it may prove easier to develop the desired occlusal scheme) or where tolerance of a maxillary appliance may be of concern.

## Procedures

The account provided here relates to the construction of a Michigan splint, but the same principles apply to a mandibular stabilisation splint.

Accurate impressions and occlusal records are imperative. The use of custom trays with appropriate impression materials is optimal. However, the use of metal rim-lock impression trays with a silicone based impression material for the working arch and an alginate based impression material for the opposing arch can be used which are then cast in a suitable dimensionally stable material. The occlusal surfaces should be clean and dried prior to impression making. Carefully inspect the impression and trim the borders. Once the impressions have been cast, they should be permitted to dry for 24 hours after pouring prior to anatomical articulation, so as to provide the desired level of abrasion resistance.

You will also need to provide your laboratory with a facebow and an intra-occlusal record, to permit mounting on a semi-adjustable articulator.

Your technician will need a prescription relating to the thickness of the appliance. Usually such splints are fabricated to provide a minimal thickness (inter-occlusal clearance) of 1.5–2 mm. In a patient displaying pathological tooth wear, the thickness of the appliance will be dictated by the space requirements being proposed for the rehabilitation.

The outline of the splint is scribed onto the maxillary cast. It should ideally extend approximately 3–4 mm onto the palate and 3 mm onto the buccal cusps of the posterior teeth, as well as offering 2 mm of overlap of the incisal edges of the anterior teeth. Unnecessary blocking-out of undercuts on the proximal, buccal and palatal surfaces is to be avoided, as engagement of acrylic-based materials in these interstitial areas will provide the necessary mechanical retention to retain the splint in situ. Where retention form may be a concern, the addition of Adam Cribs to engage the first molar teeth can be considered.

Adapt sheets of softened pink base-plate wax to an adequately dampened maxillary cast, to conform to the outline already described. The articulator is then closed, such that the incisal pin is in contact with the incisal table, and this contact is verified by a positive tugging action on a piece of thin, 8 μm articulating foil interposed between the pin and table. This will result in indentations in the wax base, thereby forming the centric stops. Excess wax is then cut away. The occluding surface should be relatively flat so that there is no potential for the cusps of the opposing dentition to be locked and they are able to move freely across the splints' occluding surface. A minimum of one centric stop should be present per opposing tooth. This may be verified using articulating paper.

Wax is added in the canine areas, anterior to the established centric stops (so as to avoid an alteration in the occlusal prescription established so far), at an approximate angle of 45° to the occlusal surface. The **canine rise** formed should provide guidance to the mandible on protrusive and excursive movements, ensuring separation of all other teeth. The canine risers are then connected by the further addition of wax in the anterior segment, to form a shallow concave ramp that should provide immediate disclusion of the posterior teeth on mandibular protrusion, with anterior guidance being shared equally between the anterior teeth.

You may choose to try-in the wax pattern. However, more often than not the wax pattern is processed and finished using a transparent, heat-cured acrylic. You may also want to use a duplicate cast for processing, so that the splint may be repositioned on the mounted casts for verification and final adjustments.

On receipt of the processed splint from the laboratory, carefully inspect it. Next, attempt to insert the splint onto your patient's maxillary arch. If the splint is tight and the area of tightness is readily identifiable, carefully relieve the splint using an acrylic trimming bur. You may wish to apply an occlusal indicator medium such as Occlude aerosol indicator marking spray (Pascal Company, Inc., Bellevue, WA, USA) to identify any areas of interference.

If you are able to seat the splint with signs of minor instability, you may choose to reline your splint in this area.

Once the splint has been seated and deemed to be adequately retentive, use a suitable form of articulating paper such as GHM occlusion foil 12 μm (Hanel, Coltène/Whaledent, Langenau, Germany) and mark up the centric stops. If you are right-handed, support the articulating paper using a pair of Millers forceps in your left hand, ask your patient to close their mouth, then using your right hand positioned on your patient's chin, gently guide their mandible into position. With their opposing teeth contacting the splint, ask them to rub slightly back and forth on the splint in partial protrusive and excursive movements of the mandible. Remove the splint from your patient's mouth and, using a sharp pencil, mark up any desired areas of contact. Ideally a minimum of one contact should exist between opposing functional cusps. Use an acrylic trimming bur or a wheel to carefully remove any unnecessary occlusal contacts. Avoid creating any unwanted indentations in the occluding surface, while also checking the thickness of the splint at regular intervals using an Ivanson's calliper.

The splint should not reach any less than a minimum thickness of 0.5 mm in any area, otherwise it will not be sufficiently robust to withstand occlusal loading. Where an obvious lack of occlusal contact exists, there will be a need to add suitable increments of cold-cured acrylic on the occluding surface of the splint, making sure that your patient is carefully manipulated into position and maintaining the established vertical dimension.

Once the presence of centric stops has been identified between each occluding pair using articulating paper, verify these again using an 8 μm articulating foil. Contacts should be lighter between opposing anterior teeth.

Now, using a different colour of articulating paper (for the purpose of visual clarity), confirm the presence of a suitable canine rise that permits posterior disclusion on protrusion and lateral excursive movements. If this is inadequate, cold-cure resin may need to be added. Avoid a very steep rise, as this may be poorly tolerated.

Finally, using a third colour of articulating paper, establish the presence of evenly shared anterior guidance on protrusion and amend accordingly if initially suboptimal. Figure 3.6.3 provides an example of a splint at the end point of initial appraisal, with contacts marked up in both static and dynamic occlusal positions.

If you are providing the splint to evaluate tolerance to a new occlusal scheme, instruct your patient to wear the appliance continually (other than when eating) for a period of 1–3 months. For cases where it has been prescribed for the control of nocturnal bruxism, instruct the patient to wear the splint every night until the recall appointment.

The patient should be reviewed after 2 weeks. Comfort, compliance with wear and occlusal contacts are verified at this appointment. It is likely that at this visit a discrepancy may be noted due to mandibular repositioning, as muscle relaxation may

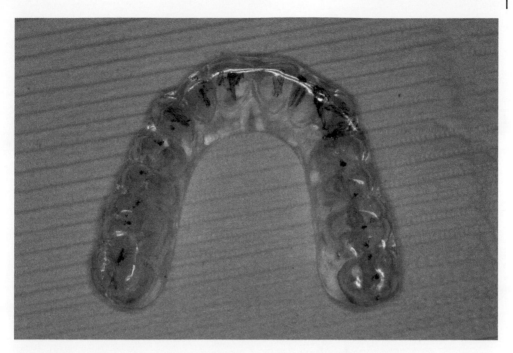

**Figure 3.6.3** A hard, full-coverage acrylic appliance with the end-point occlusal contacts marked in articulating paper

be taking place. A further review is recommended after another 2 weeks. Adjustments are made to the occlusal form until the stage where occlusal contacts are consistent between consecutive visits and the patient is comfortable.

## Tips

- Encourage the patient to bring their splint in during their regular check-ups for you to check compliance with wear and to make adjustments if necessary.
- If you do have to make an indirect restoration for a tooth in the arch where the splint is worn, then sending the splint to the laboratory along with the working impression enables any adjustments to be made efficiently.

## Reference

1 Capp NJ. Occlusion and splint therapy. In: Ibbetson R, Eder A, editors. *Tooth surface loss*. London: BDJ Books; 2000. p. 15–20.

Part IV

**Periodontology in Relation to Aesthetic Practice**

## 4.1

# Clinical Assessment of Periodontal Tissues

*Jorge André Cardoso*

## Principles

Periodontal tissues play an important role in the appearance of a smile (Figure 4.1.1). While teeth contribute to the 'white' aesthetics, the periodontal soft and supporting hard tissues form an important tridimensional architecture that can be referred to as the 'pink' aesthetics.

The periodontal assessment is fundamental for disease diagnosis as well as for recognising some parameters that will largely influence the aesthetic possibilities and treatment plan. A specific appointment for an initial examination that includes periodontal parameters is essential for patient assessment.

Although the main cause of periodontal disease is the presence of dental plaque, several risk factors have been recognised, such as smoking, diabetes and stress.[1] Any genetic or systemic condition that affects the host immunological response can also increase a patient´s risk.[2] A possible link between periodontal disease and cardiovascular disease has been considered, although this correlation is not entirely clear.[3] For all of these reasons, a detailed clinical history is important for a correct assessment.

Additionally to the traditional periodontal assessment, in aesthetic practice the position of pink tissues needs be carefully examined. Since the periodontal tissues surround the dental tissues, any change in soft tissues will have a significant impact on the patient's smile. The appearance of a tooth's length is largely dependent on the correct position of soft tissue. If gingival recession is present it can cause a tooth to appear longer. In the same way, if too much soft tissue is covering a tooth, it will appear shorter.

### Gingival Exposure during Smile

One of the first parameters to consider in periodontal aesthetics is the overall amount of gingival tissue showing above upper anterior teeth while the patient smiles (Figure 4.1.2). Kokich et al.[4] suggest that 1–3 mm of gingival exposure should be present during smile. The gingival level of upper centrals and canines should be approximately the same, while laterals should be about 1 mm shorter. The premolar margin is usually 1 mm shorter than the canine margin and this level is maintained through the posterior maxillary teeth.

*Practical Procedures in Aesthetic Dentistry*, First Edition. Edited by Subir Banerji, Shamir B. Mehta and Christopher C.K. Ho. © 2017 John Wiley & Sons, Ltd. Published 2017 by John Wiley & Sons, Ltd.
Companion website: www.wiley.com/go/banerji/aestheticdentistry

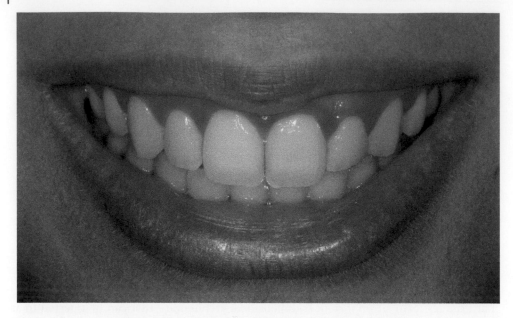

Figure 4.1.1  The periodontal tissues play a major role in the aesthetics of the smile

### Gingival Margins and Zenith Points

It may seem obvious, but it is worth remembering that the gingival margins set the tooth´s appearance and size in the apical zone. The gingival zenith can be defined as the most apical position of the gingiva in a tooth. Therefore, it sets the tooth's apical limits and greatly influences the perceived shape of the tooth. This position should not

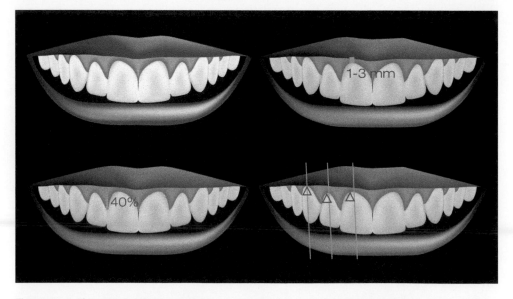

Figure 4.1.2  The main aesthetic parameters in periodontics: gingival exposure during smile, papillae proportions and location of gingival zenith

be the same in every anterior tooth. If we divide each anterior upper tooth in half at its long axis (and these axes are not vertical), the zenith is about 1 mm distal to that line in centrals, 0.5 mm distal in laterals and more or less coincident in canines. This soft-tissue configuration seems to provide a natural and aesthetically pleasing situation.[5]

### Gingival Papillae

According to Chu et al.,[6] the papillae tissue occupies 40% of the distance between the zenith and the incisal edge of a tooth. The biological factors that determine the presence of the papillae are directly related to the underlying interproximal bone level.

It is also important to evaluate the relation between the periodontal tissue and any future restorative procedures that are planned. This is usually called the perio-restorative interface and is key for the successful aesthetic and biological integration of any restorative work to be carried out.

## Dentogingival Complex (Biologic Width and Gingival Sulcus)

Biologic width is the human body interface that separates the alveolar bone from the oral cavity.[7] It is an important area where internal tissues defend themselves from external aggression, just like in every mucosa of the body. Together with the gingival sulcus, it forms the dentogingival complex. Although there are significant variations, the average proportion of this complex is 3 mm,[8–10] distributed according to the parameters in Table 4.1.1 and Figure 4.1.3.

Although these values can be good reference points, the dentogingival complex is variable both intra- and inter-individually.[8,9] Moreover, these variations are affected by tooth type and site, inflammation of tissues, periodontal disease and surgeries performed.[10] Clinicians should have an idea of the dentogingival complex composition in teeth to be intervened in so that aesthetic and restorative procedures can have a predictable outcome.

### Periodontal Biotype and Keratinised Tissue

Morphology of periodontal tissues was first classified by Maynard and Wilson,[11] but the term 'periodontal biotype' was introduced by Seibert and Lindhe in 1989[12] and is still widely used today. It represents a clinical reference to the dimensions and architecture of periodontal tissues over teeth and also to the resistance and stability of these tissues to restorative and implant procedures. Two types of periodontal biotypes are usually considered: thin with high scalloped form and thick with flat scalloped form (Table 4.1.2 and Figure 4.1.4).

Table 4.1.1 Dentogingival complex dimensions in a healthy individual (no presence of periodontal disease)

|  |  | Average | Range |
|---|---|---|---|
| Biologic width | Connective tissue | 1 mm | 0.5–4 mm |
|  | Junctional epithelium | 1 mm |  |
| Gingival sulcus | 1 mm | 0.5–2 mm |  |

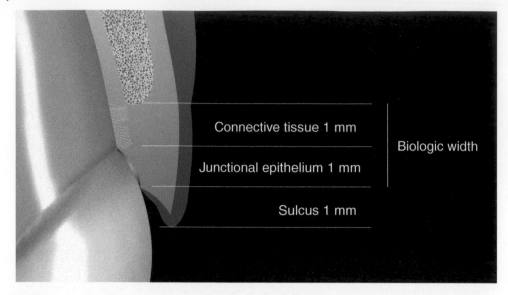

Figure 4.1.3 Average dimensions of different areas of the dentogingival complex

The periodontal biotype can influence several aspects of restorative procedures:

- Placement of the finishing margin[13]
- Tissue retraction technique for impressions[14,15]
- Emergence profile[16]
- Light transmission in the cervical area[17]
- Tissue stability and resistance to retraction and impression procedures.[18]

The presence of thick keratinised tissue or thin mucosa around teeth provides no significant differences in recession risk[19] or the aesthetic appearance of the gingiva if underlying teeth are healthy, non-restored and non-discoloured. However, if teeth are discoloured, restored with subgingival opaque materials or if there are replacement implants with metallic abutments, then the thin soft tissues may transmit the

Table 4.1.2 Periodontal biotype: Main differences

| Thin Biotype | Thick Biotype |
| --- | --- |
| Less keratinised tissue present | More keratinised tissue present |
| Metallic substructures visible if placed subgingivally | Metallic substructures non-visible if placed subgingivally |
| Less favourable tissue stability following implant placement | More favourable tissue stability |
| Associated with high scalloped form, more triangular tooth form | Associated with flat scalloped form, more square tooth form |
| Less stable and difficult to handle during retraction procedures for impressions | More stable and easier to handle during retraction procedures for impressions |

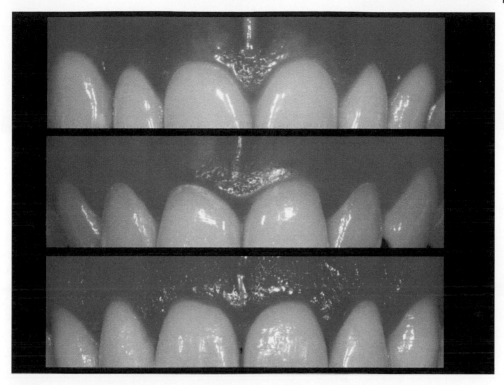

Figure 4.1.4 From thinner to thicker biotypes

underlying darkish colour. Even more important than light transmission is that thin marginal tissues are more prone to recession if subgingival restorations are performed.[20]

## Procedures

The Basic Periodontal Examination (BPE)[21] is helpful and efficient for evaluating the patient's periodontal needs. Any active periodontal disease should be controlled or, if indicated, specialist referral considered.

For aesthetic evaluation the following are useful considerations.

### Photography

Take facial, smile and intra-oral photographs. The photographs you take on your regular aesthetic evaluation should provide the information needed to assess periodontal aesthetic parameters. Refer to Chapter 2.2 for more on photography.

For periodontal aesthetic analysis, photographs of lip position and gingival exposure during smile are essential. Additionally, any soft-tissue defect such as recession, papillae loss or lack of keratinised tissue should be photographed per sextant and individually.

### Video

The smile dynamics and the relationship of the lips to the exposure of the teeth and gums are better evaluated with a video rather a photograph.

## Probing

The use of probes is important not only to evaluate sulcus and pocket depth during basic examination, but also to measure soft-tissue conditions such as recession and amount of keratinised tissue (Figure 4.1.5). Probing can also be used to evaluate the periodontal biotype. A thin biotype will allow the dark colour of a probe to be easily noticed through the marginal tissues. Sometimes bone probing also needs to be performed.

## Tips

- Intra-oral reversible mock-ups are very useful in determining and assessing your patient's expectations.
- Consider applying composites to the gingival margin to give an idea to the patient of the effect of crown lengthening or, in the case of a recession defect, pink composite can be used to simulate root coverage.
- Remember that age, ethnicity and in some cases peer and media pressure may also influence the patient's choice.
- Make sure that your patient's expectations are realistic.
- If the margin needs to be hidden subgingivally, it should remain limited to this sulcus and not violate biologic width.
- Supra- or equigingival restorative margins are always easier to control and keep clean.

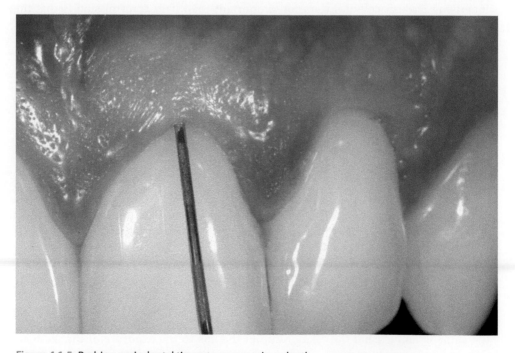

Figure 4.1.5 Probing periodontal tissue to assess sulcus depth

# References

1 AlJehani YA. Risk factors of periodontal disease: review of the literature. *Int J Dent.* 2014 Jan;2014:182513.

2 Rettori E, De Laurentiis A, Dees WL, Endruhn A, Rettori V. Host neuro-immuno-endocrine responses in periodontal disease. *Curr Pharm Des.* 2014 Jan;20(29):4749–59.

3 Hajishengallis G. Periodontitis: from microbial immune subversion to systemic inflammation. *Nat Rev Immunol.* 2014 Dec 23;15(1):30–44.

4 Kokich VO, Kiyak HA, Shapiro PA. Comparing the perception of dentists and lay people to altered dental esthetics. *J Esthet Dent.* 1999 Jan;11(6):311–24.

5 Chu SJ, Tan JH-P, Stappert CFJ, Tarnow DP. Gingival zenith positions and levels of the maxillary anterior dentition. *J Esthet Restor Dent.* 2009 Jan;21(2):113–20.

6 Chu SJ, Tarnow DP, Tan JHP, Stappert CFJ. Papilla proportions in the maxillary anterior dentition. *Int J Periodontics Restorative Dent.* 2009 Aug;29(4):385–93.

7 Ingber JS, Rose LF, Coslet JG. The 'biologic width': a concept in periodontics and restorative dentistry. *Alpha Omegan.* 1977 Dec;70(3):62–5.

8 Gargiulo AW, Wentz FM, Orban B. Dimensions and relations of the dentogingival junction in humans. *J Periodontol.* 1961;32:261–7.

9 Vacek JS, Gher ME, Assad DA, Richardson AC, Giambarresi LI. The dimensions of the human dentogingival junction. *Int J Periodontics Restorative Dent.* 1994 Apr;14(2):154–65.

10 Alpiste-Illueca F. Morphology and dimensions of the dentogingival unit in the altered passive eruption. *Med Oral Patol Oral Cir Bucal.* 2012 Jan;17(5):e814–20.

11 Maynard JG, Wilson RD. Physiologic dimensions of the periodontium significant to the restorative dentist. *J Periodontol.* 1979 Apr;50(4):170–4.

12 Seibert J LJ. Esthetics and periodontal therapy. In: LindheJ, editor. *Textbook of clinical periodontology.* 2nd ed. Copenhagen: Munksgaard; 1989. p. 477–514.

13 Kois JC. New paradigms for anterior tooth preparation. Rationale and technique. *Oral Health.* 1998 Apr;88(4):19–30.

14 Kois JC, Vakay RT. Relationship of the periodontium to impression procedures. *Compend Contin Educ Dent.* 2000 Aug;21(8):684–90.

15 Vakay RT, Kois JC. Universal paradigms for predictable final impressions. *Compend Contin Educ Dent.* 2005 Mar;26(3):199–209.

16 Bichacho N. Achieving optimal gingival esthetics around restored natural teeth and implants. Rationale, concepts, and techniques. *Dent Clin North Am.* 1998 Oct;42(4):763–80.

17 Magne P, Magne M, Belser U. The esthetic width in fixed prosthodontics. *J Prosthodont.* 1999 Jun;8(2): 106–18.

18 Koke U, Sander C, Heinecke A, Müller H-P. A possible influence of gingival dimensions on attachment loss and gingival recession following placement of artificial crowns. *Int J Periodontics Restorative Dent.* 2003 Oct;23(5):439–45.

19 Wennström JL. Lack of association between width of attached gingiva and development of soft tissue recession. A 5-year longitudinal study. *J Clin Periodontol.* 1987 Mar;14(3):181–4.

20 Nevins M. Periodontal considerations in prosthodontic treatment. *Curr Opin Periodontol.* 1993 Jan;151–6.

21 Dowell P, Chapple ILC. The British Society of Periodontology referral policy and parameters of care. *Dent Update.* 2002 Sep;29(7):352–3.

## 4.2

# Crown Lengthening without Osseous Reduction: Gingivectomy and Lasers

*Jorge André Cardoso*

*Video: Crown Lengthening without Osseous Reduction*
*Presented by Jorge André Cardoso*

## Principles

Aesthetic situations that can benefit from crown lengthening are very common. Any gingival margin that could aesthetically benefit from being in a more apical position can be considered for crown lengthening after a correct diagnosis of the cause has been carried out. Many of these situations, where the gingiva has excessive aesthetic exposure, are commonly described as a 'gummy smile', especially when it is evident in anterior teeth (Figure 4.2.1). Table 4.2.1 describes the common causes of excessive gingival display.

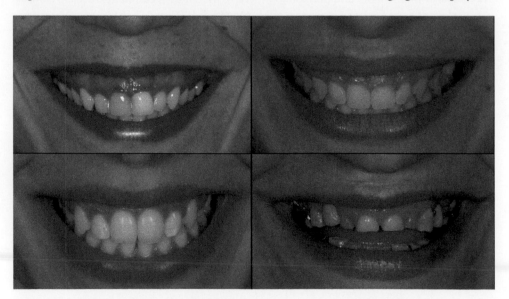

Figure 4.2.1 Examples of gummy smiles where the main causes are maxillary vertical excess (upper left), altered eruption (upper right), short lateral incisor teeth (lower left) and secondary eruption due to wear (lower right)

*Practical Procedures in Aesthetic Dentistry*, First Edition. Edited by Subir Banerji, Shamir B. Mehta and Christopher C.K. Ho. © 2017 John Wiley & Sons, Ltd. Published 2017 by John Wiley & Sons, Ltd.
Companion website: www.wiley.com/go/banerji/aestheticdentistry

Table 4.2.1 Common causes of excessive gingival display and main treatments to be considered for aesthetic improvements

| Causes | Main treatments to be considered (may not be exclusive and different or combined approaches may be considered) |
| --- | --- |
| Altered active eruption (bone level coronally positioned, causing excessive coverage of crown) | Crown lengthening with osseous reduction |
| Altered passive eruption (bone levels correct, but soft tissue coronally positioned, causing excessive coverage of the crown) | Crown lengthening without osseous reduction |
| Gingival overgrowth | Crown lengthening without osseous reduction and treat underlying cause |
| Maxillary vertical excess | Orthodontics and orthognathic surgery |
| Wear and secondary eruption | Intrusion with orthodontics and/or Dahl concept<br>Restorations<br>A new occlusal vertical dimension may be needed |
| Overjet during growth causing overbite | Orthodontics |
| Proclined anterior teeth causing excessive lip displacement during smile | Orthodontics |
| Short teeth | Orthodontics and/or restorations<br>A new occlusal vertical dimension may be needed |
| Short upper lip | Referral to plastic surgery may be considered |
| Hypermobile upper lip | Referral to plastic surgery may be considered |

Variation in the normal morphology of the dentogingival complex where the periodontum is comprised of a different configuration being located at a more coronal zone has been described as altered eruption, making reference to a possible alteration during the tooth eruption process.[1] Table 4.2.2 describes the differential diagnosis and treatment of altered eruption.

Altered eruption has been subcategorised into two different groups according to the problem that is causing the excessive coronal position of tissues[2] (Figure 4.2.2):

- Bone correct and excessive soft tissues failed to recede, causing the margin to be too coronal – altered passive eruption
- Bone failed to recede, causing the gingival margin to be too coronal – altered active eruption

A cone beam computerised tomography (CBCT) scan[3] will provide the most accurate diagnosis in terms of bone position and cemento-enamel junction (CEJ). However,

Table 4.2.2 Altered eruption: Differential diagnosis and treatment

| Diagnosis | | Amount of keratinised tissue | Treatment |
|---|---|---|---|
| Altered passive eruption | Bone level in normal position, 2 mm or more to the CEJ | More than 2 mm of keratinised tissue band | Gingivectomy leaving at least 2 mm of keratinised tissue band in place |
| | | 2 mm or less of keratinised tissue band | Apically repositioned flap |
| Altered active eruption | Bone too close to the CEJ, 1 mm or less | More than 2 mm of keratinised tissue band | Osseous reduction and gingivectomy leaving at least 2 mm of keratinised tissue band in place |
| | | | Apical repositioned flap may also be considered if more reduction of the keratinised tissue is needed |
| | | 2 mm or less of keratinised tissue band | Osseous reduction and apically repositioned flap |

*Note*: CEJ = cemento-enamel junction.

probing the bone, the sulcus and periapical X-rays will be sufficient in most cases. Careful observation of the tooth shape to try to understand the amount of anatomical crown that is still covered is also important. For bone probing, a stiff metallic probe is needed and the area should be anaesthetised. The pressure used to reach the bone is much higher than regular sulcus probing. In a short-appearing tooth, if the bone level is 4 mm or more distant from the gingival margin, an altered passive eruption can be suspected.

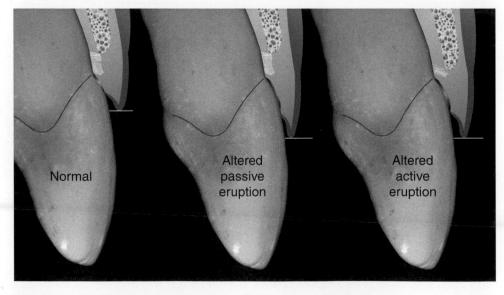

Figure 4.2.2 Normal dentogingival complex and altered eruption types

On the other hand, if the bone is present within a 3 mm distance from the margin, then a tooth of this appearance probably has an altered active eruption. In this case the bone is too close to the CEJ.

Once the diagnosis has been made that no osseous reduction will be needed, it will have to be decided how the soft-tissue reduction will be made:

- Gingivectomy – tissues are removed.
- Apically repositioned flap – tissues are replaced in a more apical position.

A simple gingivectomy will be possible if, after it is performed, a minimum amount of 2 mm of keratinised tissue height will be left at the site. This is considered a reasonable band of attached mucosa to maintain stability of soft tissues to allow comfortable hygiene procedures and provide some protection to aggression such as excessive brushing and eventual restorative procedures. If this minimum height of keratinised mucosa will not be guaranteed after a gingivectomy, then an apically repositioned flap should be preferred.[4]

## Procedures

The gingivectomy design depends on the final shape planned for the soft-tissue margin. Figure 4.2.3 shows a typical incision design for a gingivectomy in the aesthetic area of maxillary teeth. Correct zenith positions should be re-established into the new contour. It is always better to remove less and then re-contour to avoid excessive tissue

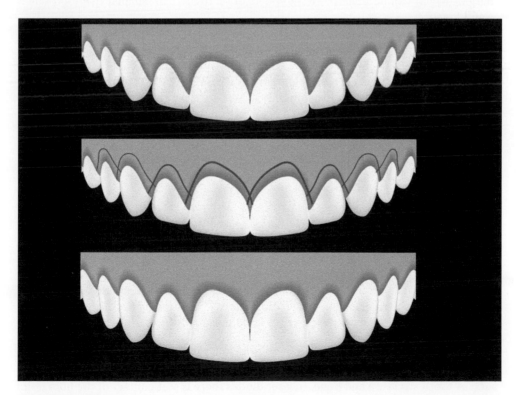

Figure 4.2.3 Typical incision design for gingivectomy

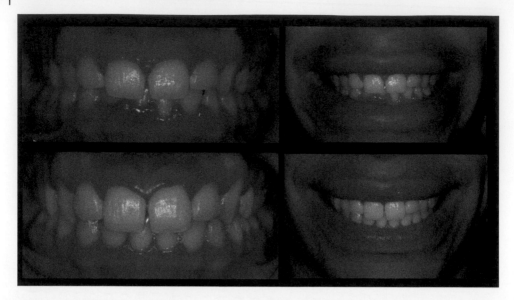

**Figure 4.2.4** Gingivectomy performed in a case of altered passive eruption and gingival overgrowth

reduction. Margins should be bevelled after tissue removal to avoid thick tissue in the margin, which can be unaesthetic. A spherical or rugby ball–shaped diamond bur is useful for this.

This simple procedure can have a very positive impact on a patient´s smile (Figure 4.2.4).

Gingivectomy can be performed with a traditional scalpel, electrosurgery or lasers. Although a scalpel is easily available, achieving a smooth tissue contour is not always easy and will imply some degree of bleeding. Electrosurgery, which uses high-frequency electrical current in tissues, is commonly available in dental offices and provides an effective and fast method to perform a gingivectomy. A thin single-pointed tip used in 'Cut' (higher-voltage) mode enables the operator to have good control of the contours of the incisions with minimal pressure and 'brush-like' movements. 'Cut/Coag' mode can also be used to reduce bleeding, although it is usually not needed.

### Lasers

The use of lasers for periodontal aesthetic surgery has been noted as having several advantages, including reduced bleeding and favourable tissue healing. One of the most important features of lasers is increased coagulation, which yields a dry surgical field with improved visualisation.[5,6]

Several authors have also pointed out the strong antibacterial activity, and reduced post-operative scarring, oedema and discomfort.[7-9] Appearing to be less traumatic than a scalpel and being perceived as a technological advance, lasers tend to be more accepted by patients.[10]

A laser diode has been recommended as the ideal laser for soft-tissue procedures.[11] This type of laser is specific for soft tissue, with less chance of damage to the hard tissue such as tooth structure and bone. In laser diodes there is soft contact of the fibre point with the tissues, providing good tactile feedback for the operator (Figure 4.2.5).

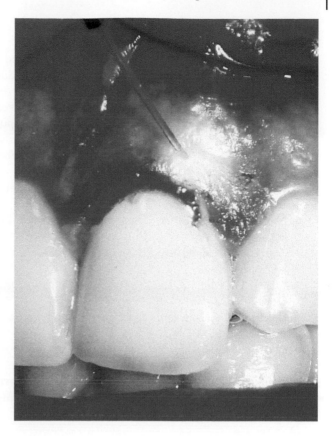

Figure 4.2.5 Using a laser for a gingivectomy *Source*: Reproduced with permission from Dr João Mouzinho.

## Tips

- Diagnosing the causes of a 'gummy smile' is essential for a successful treatment strategy.
- Use opaque composite on top of gingiva for mock-ups of crown-lengthening procedures so that patients can preview the desired outcome.
- From the mock-up, the laboratory can provide you with a template to guide you through the procedure.
- You can also use small perforations on the soft tissue to mark the incision.
- A periodontal curette is very helpful to remove the incised tissue.
- If a simple gingivectomy is done in case of altered active eruption (excessive bone on a coronal level), it will regrow to the original position. In these cases an osseous reduction needs to be performed.
- Always use profound local anaesthetics when employing electrosurgery.
- Post-operative healing is usually very good. Chlorhexidine mouthrinses for a week and gentle but efficient oral hygiene as soon as possible will help to reduce plaque accumulation, avoid infections and promote healing. In case of pain, non-steroidal anti-inflammatory drugs can be prescribed.
- Final maturation of tissues takes about 4 weeks if the final gingival margin is correctly placed according to bone position.

## References

1 Goldman HM, Cohn DW. *Periodontal therapy*. 4th ed. St Louis, MO: Mosby; 1968.

2 Chu SJ, Karabin S, Mistry S. Short tooth syndrome: diagnosis, etiology, and treatment management. *J Calif Dent Assoc.* 2004 Feb;32(2):143–52.

3 Batista EL, Moreira CC, Batista FC, de Oliveira RR, Pereira KKY. Altered passive eruption diagnosis and treatment: a cone beam computed tomography-based reappraisal of the condition. *J Clin Periodontol.* 2012 Nov;39(11):1089–96.

4 Alpiste-Illueca F. Altered passive eruption (APE): a little-known clinical situation. *Med Oral Patol Oral Cir Bucal.* 2011 Jan;16(1):e100–4.

5 Cobb CM. Lasers in periodontics: a review of the literature. *J Periodontol.* 2006 Apr;77(4):545–64.

6 Asnaashari M, Zadsirjan S. Application of laser in oral surgery. *J Lasers Med Sci.* 2014 Jan;5(3):97–107.

7 Convissar RA, Goldstein EE. An overview of lasers in dentistry. *Gen Dent.* Jan;51(5):436–40.

8 Adams TC, Pang PK. Lasers in aesthetic dentistry. *Dent Clin North Am.* 2004 Oct;48(4):833–60.

9 Coleton S. Lasers in surgical periodontics and oral medicine. *Dent Clin North Am.* 2004 Oct;48(4):937–62.

10 Dederich DN, Bushick RD. Lasers in dentistry: separating science from hype. *J Am Dent Assoc.* 2004 Feb;135(2):204–12.

11 Shankar BS, Ramedevi T, Neetha MS, Reddy PSK, Saritha G, Reddy JM. Chronic inflammatory gingival overgrowths: laser gingivectomy & gingivoplasty. *J Int Oral Health.* 2013 Feb;5(1):83–7.

## 4.3

# Crown Lengthening with Osseous Reduction

*Jorge André Cardoso*

*Video: Crown Lengthening with Osseous Reduction*
*Presented by Jorge André Cardoso*

## Principles

### Determining the New Bone Level

According to the principles outlined in Chapters 4.1 and 4.2, osseous reduction is needed when there is an altered active eruption, where the bone level is coronally positioned too close to the cemento-enamel junction (CEJ), making the soft tissue excessively cover the crown. In these cases, once the correct amount of bone and soft tissue is repositioned in a more coronal position, the appearance of the tooth will be more aesthetic, with a more pleasant length/width ratio, and no root exposure will result. The fundamental notion that clinicians must have is that, in an average dentogingival complex, the gingival margin will be established 3 mm apical from the bone margin after healing from an osseous reduction – 2 mm of biologic width plus 1 mm of gingival sulcus.[1,2] This is critical for predictable results.

In other situations when aesthetic crown lengthening is desired, the clinician has to consider the possibility of root exposure after healing. This means that the CEJ should always be the most apical limit of the final gingival margin. Again, the critical rule that the gingival margin will heal, on average, 3 mm apical to the bone level needs to be remembered. So the final bone position should never be more than 3 mm of the CEJ if the tooth is not to be restored. However, root exposure after healing from osseous reduction can be acceptable if restorations such as crowns are planned to cover the exposed root.

There are limits to the amount of crown lengthening with bone reduction that can be performed:

- The final crown/root ratio should not be unfavourable bio-mechanically.[3]
- The root diameter gets smaller in an apical position. If excessively performed, crown lengthening can result in a rectangular-shaped tooth and papillae loss.
- While a crown has a retentive form and can be cemented, veneers need to be bonded. If veneers are planned, root exposure is not recommended, as the apical limit of the veneer should be kept in enamel and avoid bonding to the cementum/dentin of the root, which is less predictable in the long term.[4-6]

*Practical Procedures in Aesthetic Dentistry*, First Edition. Edited by Subir Banerji, Shamir B. Mehta and Christopher C.K. Ho. © 2017 John Wiley & Sons, Ltd. Published 2017 by John Wiley & Sons, Ltd.
Companion website: www.wiley.com/go/banerji/aestheticdentistry

Once the bone-reduction level is chosen, the second decision will be whether the soft tissue should simply be removed or placed in a more apical position. As stated in Chapter 4.2, a minimum amount of 2 mm of keratinised tissue height will be left at the site to provide an efficient biological seal that is more stable to potential aggression such as subgingival margins or excessive brushing.[7] Therefore, a gingivectomy can be performed only if the remaining keratinised tissue will be at least 2 mm. If this is not the case, then the keratinised tissue must be kept and, ideally, repositioned apically.[8]

## Procedures

There are five essential factors to be considered in the process: final incisal edge position, final desired gingival margin, bone level, CEJ and attached gingiva.

### Final Incisal Edge and Gingival Position

These factors are concerned with treatment planning and smile design. Once the incisal edge is determined, the final gingival position is established according to the desired length of the teeth involved. The key is to understand that a gummy smile look is a proportion between white and pink.[9] Sometimes only lengthening the incisal edges may have a significant impact and solve the aesthetic problems without changing the soft tissues. In other cases, combined incisal edge lengthening with soft-tissue removal can allow a more conservative alteration at the gingival margins. The desired final outcome should be previewed with a mock-up, as suggested in Chapter 4.1, and recorded in photographs (Figure 4.3.1). Impressions and models should be made of the original

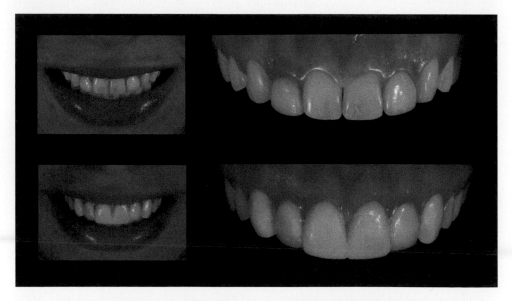

Figure 4.3.1 Initial situation (top) with unpleasing gingival levels, short teeth and incorrect relative widths of anterior teeth. With an additive direct mock-up (bottom), the potential aesthetic benefits can be visualised intra-orally. The lengthening of incisal edges and their better width distribution gives an improved gingival appearance

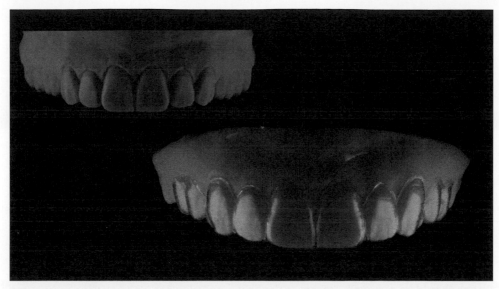

Figure 4.3.2 Wax-up made by improving the shape and contours of a direct mock-up. From this wax-up a surgical guide was constructed

situation and the mock-up in place. This way references will be kept during surgery and a template can be used to guide the necessary reduction (Figure 4.3.2).

Bone Level and CEJ

Although bone probing and CEJ detection can be performed beforehand at the treatment planning stage, they are not always reliable.[10] Only after the flap is raised can the bone level and CEJ positions actually be confirmed (Figure 4.3.3). This means that

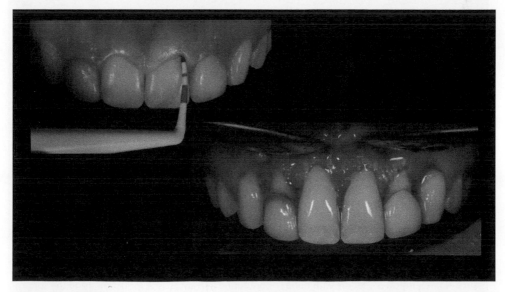

Figure 4.3.3 Although probing soft tissues and bone can be helpful, only after raising the flap can the bone levels be correctly assessed

there can be a change in the planned procedure if the bone level and CEJ positions are different from those previously thought. If, for example, after raising the flap the bone is already at 3 mm of the CEJ, then in most cases only the soft tissue will need to be altered and the bone will be left untouched.

A sharp, full-thickness dissection, starting with intra-sulcular incisions, is essential for correct exposure of the site and good healing.[11] The papillae is raised in the buccal area, included in the flap, but the interproximal soft tissues remain in place to minimise papillae loss.

The bone should be removed with an electric handpiece with a tungsten carbide bur. A piezosurgery instrument can provide better control, but it is usually slower to remove bone.[12] The final 0.5 mm to be reduced and the final contours should be done with a small bone chisel to avoid touching the root surface, which can potentially cause root resorptions (Figure 4.3.4). Soft-tissue fibre insertions need to be removed in the areas where bone is to be re-contoured.

If the concern is only aesthetic, the bone reduction should be limited to the buccal area. Zeniths should be re-established at their correct position according to the mock-up and guide. Final bone anatomy should be smooth and sharp edges or abrupt transitions should be removed, otherwise the final gingival appearance may look unnatural. The surface depressions in interproximal areas should also be re-established, but the bone height in these zones should never be touched, as this can cause loss of the papillae.

### Attached Gingiva

Although in the traditional approach removing the soft tissue is performed before raising the flap, in the author´s perspective this should only be performed after the flap has

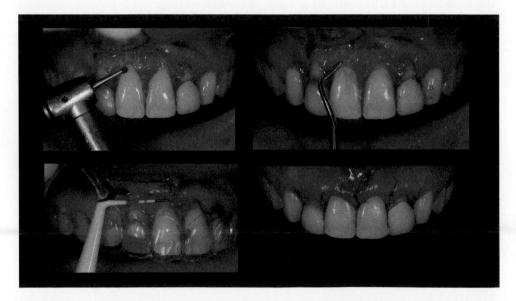

**Figure 4.3.4** Surgical procedure with bone re-contouring and soft-tissue reduction using the surgical guide as a reference

been raised and bone and CEJ levels accessed, as these may condition the final position of the gingival margin (Figure 4.3.4).

### Suturing and Healing

Suturing with a 4-0 to 6-0 monofilament is recommended for reduced inflammatory response during healing.[11] Simple sutures are usually effective. In the case of apically re-positioning the flap, vertical releasing incisions may need to be performed about 1 or 2 teeth distal to the re-contoured areas. These will help to stabilise the flap in a more apical position, but will also result in more post-operative discomfort.

The flap should ideally be positioned 3 mm coronal to the bone level. The closer it is to this level, the sooner tissues will heal and mature:

- If the flap is sutured just at the bone level, it might take up to 6 months to regain the dentogingival complex maturation. If a subgingival finishing margin is placed before maturation, it will probably be invading the biologic width.
- If the flap is sutured too coronal (more than 3 mm) to the bone level, any subgingival finishing margin before maturation will probably become supragingival with healing.

Probing the bone (after at least 4 weeks) will provide information about the maturation process and the establishment of biologic width and sulcus. Only after complete maturation takes place should the final restorative procedures be performed (Figure 4.3.5). After maturation it is also common to occur some degree of relapse (soft tissue regrowth), especially in the first year. Simple and localised gingivectomies may be needed to maintain the desired margin levels (Figure 4.3.6).[13]

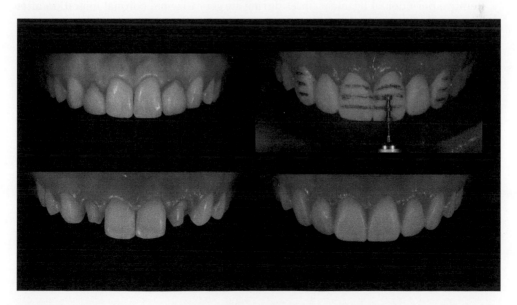

Figure 4.3.5 Restorative procedures after healing – preparations and provisionals

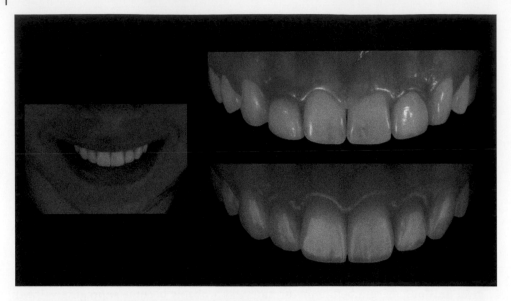

Figure 4.3.6  Final result after restorative procedures

## Tips

- Mock-ups, templates and guides are very helpful during the procedure.
- Avoid reducing bone height at the papillae. It is rarely needed and may result in papillae loss.
- Gingival appearance will be a result of the bone contours, so make sure that you respect zenith positions and the tridimensional anatomy.
- Remove periodontal ligament fibres during surgery to avoid coronal migration after healing. Coronal migration is the main complication, occurring especially in the first year.
- The contour of a provisional restoration may help, placing the apically repositioned flap at the correct position. However, the final restorations should only be placed after complete maturation.
- Bone is difficult to probe and after raising the flap you may find that your previous bone probing was incorrect and change plans during surgery. A cone beam computerised tomography (CBCT) scan will give you the accurate position of bone and CEJ before surgery.
- Post-operative discomfort and swelling are proportional to bone reduction and surgical time. Chlorhexidine mouthrinses for a week and gentle but efficient oral hygiene are essential. Ice packs to avoid swelling in extensive cases and non-steroidal anti-inflammatory drugs in case of pain should be prescribed. Antibiotics are usually not needed.
- Always inform the patient that soft tissue re-touches may be needed after healing.

# References

1  Vacek JS, Gher ME, Assad DA, Richardson AC, Giambarresi LI. The dimensions of the human dentogingival junction. *Int J Periodontics Restorative Dent.* 1994 Apr;14(2):154–65.

2  Gargiulo AW, Wentz FM, Orban B. Dimensions and relations of the dentogingival junction in humans. *J Periodontol.* 1961;32:261–7.

3  Grossmann Y, Sadan A. The prosthodontic concept of crown-to-root ratio: a review of the literature. *J Prosthet Dent.* 2005 Jun;93(6):559–62.

4  Oztürk E, Bolay S. Survival of porcelain laminate veneers with different degrees of dentin exposure: 2-year clinical results. *J Adhes Dent.* 2014 Oct;16(5):481–9.

5  Burke FJT. Survival rates for porcelain laminate veneers with special reference to the effect of preparation in dentin: a literature review. *J Esthet Restorative Dent.* 2012 Aug;24(4):257–65.

6  Gurel G, Sesma N, Calamita MA, Coachman C, Morimoto S. Influence of enamel preservation on failure rates of porcelain laminate veneers. *Int J Periodontics Restorative Dent.* Jan;33(1):31–9.

7  Wennström JL. Lack of association between width of attached gingiva and development of soft tissue recession. A 5-year longitudinal study. *J Clin Periodontol.* 1987 Mar;14(3):181–4.

8  Oh S-L. Attached gingiva: histology and surgical augmentation. *Gen Dent.* Jan;57(4):381–5.

9  Chu SJ, Karabin S, Mistry S. Short tooth syndrome: diagnosis, etiology, and treatment management. *J Calif Dent Assoc.* 2004 Feb;32(2):143–52.

10  Batista EL, Moreira CC, Batista FC, de Oliveira RR, Pereira KKY. Altered passive eruption diagnosis and treatment: a cone beam computed tomography-based reappraisal of the condition. *J Clin Periodontol.* 2012 Nov;39(11):1089–96.

11  Burkhardt R, Lang NP. Fundamental principles in periodontal plastic surgery and mucosal augmentation: a narrative review. *J Clin Periodontol.* 2014 Apr;41 Suppl 1:S98–107.

12  Agarwal E, Masamatti SS, Kumar A. Escalating role of piezosurgery in dental therapeutics. *J Clin Diagn Res.* 2014 Oct;8(10):ZE08–11.

13  Deas DE, Moritz AJ, McDonnell HT, Powell CA, Mealey BL. Osseous surgery for crown lengthening: a 6-month clinical study. *J Periodontol.* 2004 Sep;75(9):1288–94.

## 4.4

# Management of Gingival Recession and Graft Harvesting

*Jorge André Cardoso*

*Video: Management of Gingival Recession and Graft Harvesting*
Presented by Jorge André Cardoso

## Principles

Gingival recession is defined as the displacement of the gingival margin above the cemento-enamel junction (CEJ).[1] It has been estimated that above 60% of the population has gingival recession. Its causes and contributing factors include[2]:

- Poor oral hygiene and periodontitis
- External trauma like excessive brushing, piercings etc.
- Thin alveolar bone, thin periodontal biotype and thin band of attached (keratinised) gingiva
- Anatomically unfavourable tooth form or position such as orthodontic movement to far from alveolar bone
- Strong or long muscle attachments
- Occlusal trauma, although it is non-consensual
- Secondary factors such as age and systemic diseases.

Non-carious cervical lesions' aetiological factors, such as chemical erosion, are also frequently associated with gingival recession. It is important to realise that factors act in combination in most cases.

The most used categorisation of gingival recession is Miller´s classification, expressed in Table 4.4.1.

Gingival recession does not always require treatment. With adequate oral hygiene, reduced or absent attached gingiva does not place the tooth at higher risk of periodontitis or further recession. Treatment should be considered in the following cases:

- Hypersensitivity due to root exposure
- Aesthetic concerns
- Orthodontic treatment, because tooth movements might worsen the condition and there will be increased plaque accumulation
- Discomfort of difficulties in performing correct hygiene in the area due to the limited amount of attached gingiva
- Planned subgingival restorations, since restorative procedures can worsen the condition.

*Practical Procedures in Aesthetic Dentistry*, First Edition. Edited by Subir Banerji, Shamir B. Mehta and Christopher C.K. Ho. © 2017 John Wiley & Sons, Ltd. Published 2017 by John Wiley & Sons, Ltd.
Companion website: www.wiley.com/go/banerji/aestheticdentistry

Table 4.4.1 Gingival recession classification according to Miller[1] and possibility of root coverage

| | Level of recession | Level of interproximal tissues | Possibilities of root coverage |
|---|---|---|---|
| Class I | Recession not extending to the mucogingival junction | No loss | Complete root coverage might be possible |
| Class II | Recession extending into or more apical to the mucogingival junction | No loss | Complete root coverage might be possible |
| Class III | Recession extending into or more apical to the mucogingival junction | Loss of interproximal bone or soft tissue apical to the CEJ but coronal to the apical extent of the recession | Partial root coverage might be possible, depending on the level of interproximal soft tissues |
| Class IV | Recession extending into or more apical to the mucogingival junction | Loss of interproximal bone or soft tissue apical to the apical extent of the recession | No possible root coverage |

Additional to periodontal surgical treatment, aetiological factors should be controlled. For example, excessive tooth brushing should be eliminated with proper hygiene instructions and evident occlusal trauma should be removed. The combination of different treatment strategies is also advised according to each situation. For example, periodontal root coverage procedures are often combined with restoration of sensitive areas that could not be completely covered; orthodontic movement to a more favourable position within the alveolar bone increases the bone and soft-tissue thickness; and frenectomies and other procedures are used to remove or improve other causative factors.

As described in Table 4.4.1, the predictability of root coverage procedures is dependent on the level of bone and papillae height in the interproximal areas. This knowledge should be used to provide clear communication for managing patients' expectations and also for medico-legal reasons.

Periodontal plastic surgery is an active field of research, with several new microsurgical techniques appearing every year. Despite many variations, the use of a connective tissue graft combined with a coronally advanced flap is still the most effective procedure for root coverage.[3] The technique uses an autologous subepithelial connective tissue graft that is trimmed to the receptor site and is then covered as much as possible with a coronally advanced flap, providing vascularity so that good healing integration of grafted tissues can take place.

## Procedures

### Graft Harvesting

There are two types of soft-tissue grafts: subepithelial connective tissue grafts and free full-thickness connective tissue grafts, where the connective tissue is collected without the epithelium or with the epithelium, respectively. The hard palate, maxillary tuberosity and mandibular retromolar areas have been used as donor sites. The most used donor site area referred to in the literature is the hard palate.[4] The palate has the same histological components as the periodontal keratinised mucosa, it is surgically accessible and it provides a significant volume of tissue.

The connective tissue graft is usually harvested from the premolar area with one or two access incisions parallel to the gingival margin.[5,6] After the access incisions, the graft is created with two incisions towards the midline, one just under the epithelium surface and other near the bone surface. While some authors suggest a full-thickness dissection in the bone surface to include the periosteum, others suggest that the periosteum should be left in the bone for better healing. The two incisions towards the midline are connected at the medial, distal and mesial so that the graft can be detached and removed. Suturing should attempt to close the access incisions completely (Figure 4.4.1). The palatine artery, which is located around 10 mm from the gingival margin in the premolar area in periodontally healthy patients, should be completely avoided.[7] Nevertheless, there is considerable bleeding from its branches during palatal harvesting.

The tuberosity provides excellent fibrous tissue, with less fat component than the palate, but it is not always present. If it is present with adequate volume, it can provide more tissue stability in the long term compared to palatal grafts, and has much better post-operative comfort for the patient (Figure 4.4.2).

### Receptor Area

The receptor area is created before harvesting so that the time for which the graft is left outside the tissues is minimal. The goal is to raise a partial thickness flap that can advance coronally and cover the graft as much as possible and without tension. Microsurgical, minimally invasive approaches, although technically more demanding, promote better graft vascularisation and healing.[8] Vertical releasing incisions and elevation of

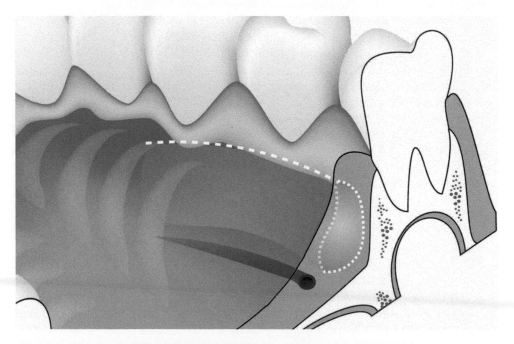

Figure 4.4.1 A subepithelial connective tissue graft is harvested in the premolar area. The access is through an incision near the gingival margin and the graft is detached through internal incisions towards the midline, but avoiding the palatine artery.

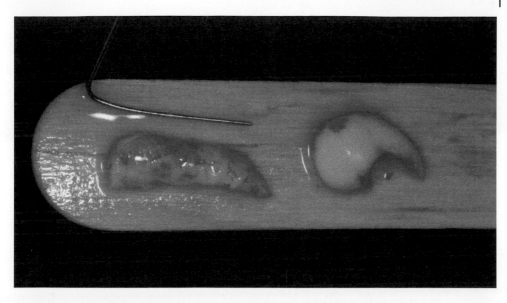

Figure 4.4.2 Palatal (left) and tuberosity (right) grafts. Tuberosity grafts are more fibrous with less fat

papillae should be avoided, as they reduce flap vascularity and can potentially cause scar-like texture in the mucosa. Intra-sulcular tunnel approaches and loosening of the papillae without elevation should be preferred, but in some cases they are not possible (Figures 4.4.3 and 4.4.4).[9] Contrary to vertical releasing incisions, horizontal internal incisions on the periosteum are almost always needed so that tension-free closure can be achieved. Other important concerns during the procedure include the following:

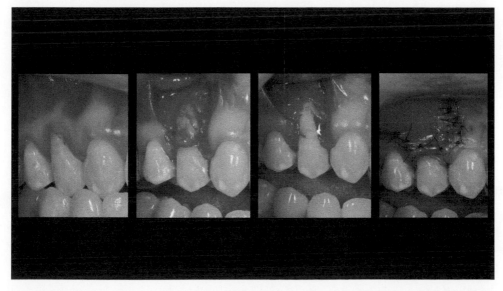

Figure 4.4.3 Root coverage: traditional approach using vertical releasing incisions, graft and coronally advanced flap

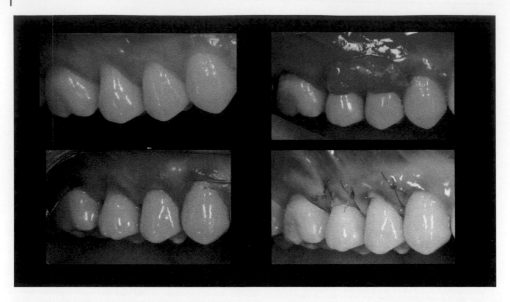

Figure 4.4.4  Root coverage with a less invasive approach. The graft is inserted through a tunnel technique. The flap is moved by internal releasing incisions on the periosteum, allowing the tissue to advance coronally without raising the papillae

- Any epithelial area of the graft should be removed to allow complete vascularisation and integration.
- Graft should be involved in saline-soaked sterile gauze while waiting to be placed.
- Immobilisation of the graft with sutures without tension on the flap is key to proper healing.
- Sutures should be the least amount needed for stability. Thin, monofilament suturing promotes less vascularisation disturbance and avoids bacterial growth. Sutures should be removed as soon as their stabilising function has ended (7–15 days).
- Post-operative care to avoid trauma and infection in the area is essential.

Root coverage with periodontal plastic surgery is a predictable procedure with stable, long-term results as long as correct techniques are used for the appropriate cases and aetiological factors are controlled (Figure 4.4.5).[8]

## Tips

- Remove existing restorations, and prepare the root surface at the receptor site to remove plaque and calculus. Then a convex root profile should be made flat or slightly concave to allow more space for the graft.
- During palatal graft harvesting, have your assistant place pressure at the emergence of the palatine artery around the second or third molar area. This will significantly reduce bleeding during the procedure.
- Before surgery, have a palatal stent made of a rigid material so that the patient can take it home and place it in case of post-operative bleeding.

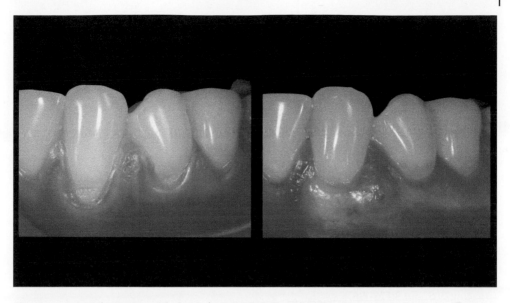

Figure 4.4.5 Initial situation with dentin hypersensitivity with Miller Class I gingival recession due to aggressive tooth brushing (left). After proper patient education concerning hygiene technique, a root coverage procedure was performed and tissues have remained stable for 5 years (right)

- Microsurgical techniques and instruments are very helpful: eye magnification; 15C and microsurgical blades; tunnelling instruments to raise the flap, avoiding releasing incisions; and 5-0 to 7-0 monofilament sutures.
- Use sharp blades and change them frequently during the procedure so that a maximum cutting ability is always present.
- Use frequent syringe irrigation with saline during the whole procedure to keep tissues moist, easy to manipulate and less prone to trauma.
- Allocate appropriate time, as these procedures are delicate and lengthy. Patient anxiety can be controlled in a calm atmosphere, and by providing proper pain control and sedative drugs if needed.
- Post-operative care includes regular hygiene as soon as possible while being very delicate with any movement or pressure at the receptor area. Chlorhexidine mouthrinses should be prescribed for at least one week. Antibiotics are usually not prescribed, but non-steroidal anti-inflammatory drugs should be prescribed for the first few days in cases of discomfort.
- While simple cases can be straightforward, some cases can be challenging and advanced training is required.

## References

1  Miller PD. A classification of marginal tissue recession. *Int J Periodontics Restorative Dent.* 1985 Jan;5(2):8–13.
2  Dominiak M, Gedrange T. New perspectives in the diagnostic of gingival recession. *Adv Clin Exp Med.* Jan;23(6):857–63.

3 Cairo F, Nieri M, Pagliaro U. Efficacy of periodontal plastic surgery procedures in the treatment of localized facial gingival recessions. A systematic review. *J Clin Periodontol.* 2014 Apr;41 Suppl 1:S44–62.

4 Studer SP, Allen EP, Rees TC, Kouba A. The thickness of masticatory mucosa in the human hard palate and tuberosity as potential donor sites for ridge augmentation procedures. *J Periodontol.* 1997 Feb;68(2):145–51.

5 Hürzeler MB, Weng D. A single-incision technique to harvest subepithelial connective tissue grafts from the palate. *Int J Periodontics Restorative Dent.* 1999 Jun;19(3):279–87.

6 Langer B, Calagna LJ. The subepithelial connective tissue graft. A new approach to the enhancement of anterior cosmetics. *Int J Periodontics Restorative Dent.* 1982 Jan;2(2):22–33.

7 Reiser GM, Bruno JF, Mahan PE, Larkin LH. The subepithelial connective tissue graft palatal donor site: anatomic considerations for surgeons. *Int J Periodontics Restorative Dent.* 1996 Apr;16(2):130–7.

8 Roccuzzo M, Bunino M, Needleman I, Sanz M. Periodontal plastic surgery for treatment of localized gingival recessions: a systematic review. *J Clin Periodontol.* 2002 Jan;29 Suppl 3:178–96.

9 Burkhardt R, Lang NP. Fundamental principles in periodontal plastic surgery and mucosal augmentation: a narrative review. *J Clin Periodontol.* 2014 Apr;41 Suppl 1:S98–107.

Part V

Direct Aesthetic Restorations

# 5.1

# Adhesive Dentistry

*Subir Banerji and Shamir B. Mehta*

## Principles

The term **adhesion** may be defined as the 'force that binds two dissimilar molecules together when they are brought into intimate contact'.[1] Contemporary advances in the field of adhesive dentistry have now made it possible to *predictably* bond a variety of different materials (namely resin-based and glass ionomer cements) to the dental hard tissues (notably where there is copious enamel of a desirable quality available). This can take place without the need to prepare a significant mechanical retention or resistance form to the involved/affected tooth surface, with concomitant biological conservation.

Glass ionomer cements do not offer the aesthetic and mechanical merits of resin composite materials. They do, however, offer the potential for direct, inherent dynamic chemical adhesion to enamel and dentine without the need for an adhesive bonding agent.

This chapter will focus on the use of adhesive systems in conjunction with resin composite restoration placement and also discuss the difficulty of bonding to 'living' dentine tissue, which appears to be less predictable than enamel bonding, primarily on account of its higher water content, the structural heterogeneity of dentinal tissues (with the presence of a tubular arrangement and a higher organic content as opposed to the heavily mineralised, prismatic, hydrophobic nature of enamel), as well as the long-term stability of the bond developed.[2] Histological variations in dentine, such as those that occur with the process of ageing (culminating in a hypermineralised substrate, by the process of sclerosis of dentine as well as the formation of reparative and reactionary dentine) or those that occur as dentine approaches the pulp (resulting in a 'wetter' bonding surface with a concomitant increase in the number of tubules), also compound the predictability of the adhesion of resin composite to dentine.

There are a large number of adhesive bonding systems in the marketplace. For the purposes of simplicity, it is perhaps easier to consider any commercial dentine bonding agent by virtue of its chemical content, thus having a component that acts as a:

- Etchant
- Primer
- Bond
- Provider of management of the smear layer.[2]

*Practical Procedures in Aesthetic Dentistry*, First Edition. Edited by Subir Banerji, Shamir B. Mehta and Christopher C.K. Ho. © 2017 John Wiley & Sons, Ltd. Published 2017 by John Wiley & Sons, Ltd.
Companion website: www.wiley.com/go/banerji/aestheticdentistry

The **etchant** most commonly used is 37% orthophosphoric acid, which not only demineralises the hydroxyapatite structure in enamel (as well as in dentine, although with less uniformity), creating pores in the microstructure and thus allowing the permeation of resin of flowable consistency to enter these pores and form a micro-mechanical lock of **resin tags**, but also leading the modification of the **smear layer**. The latter is a thin layer comprised of debris formed by the process of cavity preparation. Typical shear bond strengths of resin composite to phosphoric acid–etched enamel are in the range of 20 MPa, which is considered to be sufficient to resist the stresses produced by polymerisation shrinkage of resin composites.[3]

**Primers** are adhesion-promoting agents with a bi-functional molecular structure comprising a monomer component with hydrophobic properties that will have an affinity to any exposed collagen present in the dentinal tubules and a hydrophobic monomer, which can form a chemical link with the resin present in the bond. This results in the formation of a **hybrid layer** between the tooth surface, primer and resin-bonding agent. Hydroxethyl methacrylate (HEMA) is generally present in most primers, as well as solvents such as ethanol or acetone to help displace water from the dentine surface. On solvent evaporation, porosities are left in the dentine substrate, which will enhance the adhesive bond.

Other bi-functional monomers used in commercially available bonding systems include 4- methacryloxydecyl trimelliate (4-META), 10-methacrlyoxydecyl dihydrogen phosphate and 2-methacryloxyethyl phenyl hydrogen phosphate (phenyl-P).

The **bonding resins** most commonly used are based on bisphenol A-glycidyl methacrylate (Bis-GMA) or urethane dimethacrylate (UDMA). As these monomers are inherently viscous as well as being hydrophobic, they are usually diluted in hydrophilic monomers of lower viscosity to improve their wettability. **Diluents** most commonly used include HEMA and TEG-DMA (triethylene-gycol dimethacylate).

Bonding resins will enter the porosities created by the removal of the smear layer and the demineralisation of the surface layer of the hydroxyapatite crystal by the process of acid etching, therefore creating resin tags that will provide micro-mechanical retention, as well as by penetration of the dentinal tubules and also by the formation of a chemical bond with the primer, resulting in the development of the 'hybrid layer'.

It is common to refer to bonding agents by their **generation of introduction**. The first three generations are perhaps best considered obsolete.

It is the **fourth generation** (also termed Type 1), based on a three-step total etch technique, which is regarded as the gold standard in contemporary dental practice.[2] This includes the stage of applying a separate etchant (37% orthophosphoric acid) to sound enamel for 20 seconds and dentine for 10–15 seconds (total etch technique), followed by complete rinsing away with water to remove the smear layer. This is followed by placement of a bespoke primer. Gentle drying of the primer is often advocated to permit solvent evaporation, followed by placement of the bonding resin.

Examples of commercially available Type 1, fourth-generation bonding systems include OptiBond FL (Kerr Corporation, Charlotte, NC, USA), All-Bond 2 (Bisco, Inc., Schaumburg, IL, USA) and Adper Scotchbond MP (3M, St Paul, MN, USA). Bonds attained with fourth-generation systems are longer lasting than those with successor products.

The **fifth-generation** (Type 2) systems are characterised by a two-bottle system, comprising a separate etchant that will also help to remove the smear layer and a combined prime and bond. Commonly used examples include OptiBond Solo Plus (Kerr), Prime and Bond NT (Denstply Detrey GmbH, Konstanz, Germany) and Excite (Ivoclar Vivadent AG, Schaan, Liechtenstein). The use of these agents carries the risk of desiccating the collagen layer after the process of rising and drying of the etchant. There is a need to avoid the collapse of the collagen scaffold (by the process of excessive drying) in order to produce adequate bond strength. There is therefore a need to **wet** or moisten dentine, which is typically achieved by blotting the dentine with a moistened cotton wool pledget. Variations in the latter by different clinicians may affect the efficacy of the bond strength developed, however.

The **sixth and seventh generations** (Types 3 and 4, respectively) differ in the way in which the smear layer is modified. While they aim to attain a similar type of bond to enamel, they do not remove the smear layer in the same manner as their predecessors, but rather penetrate the smear layer, dissolve it and incorporate it in the final adhesive interface.[2] The two generations differ in that the seventh generation of bonding agents has a single-bottle system, with combined etchant, primer and bond, while the sixth generation has a two-bottle arrangement with a combined etchant and primer and a separate bonding resin.

Commercial examples of sixth-generation agents include Clearfil SE (Kuraray Co. Ltd, Kurashiki, Japan) and One Coat SE Bond (Coltene Whaledent Ltd, Burgess Hill, UK), while popular seventh-generation agents include Adper L- Pop Prompt (3M), G Bond (GC Corporation, Alsip, IL, USA) and iBond (Heraeus Kultzer GmbH, Hanau, Germany). It has been shown, however, that the bond strengths developed with these agents are less than those of the fourth generation, thereby increasing the risk of restorative failure by the process of breakdown of the adhesive interface.

## Procedures

To help you attain a desirable bond between your resin composite materials and bonding agent, you may consider some of the following aspects:

- Ensure the removal of carious enamel and infected dentine, which will otherwise provide a poor substrate for adequate bonding. Dentine that has been affected by the carious process but not infected may be retained, provided there is a rim of peripheral, high-quality enamel.
- Careful cavity preparation may also include the use of air abrasion techniques to enhance micro-mechanical retention.
- Use of isolation techniques involving dental dam application provides a moisture- and saliva contaminant–free environment that is conducive to optimal resin bonding.
- Longer etching periods may be used for sclerotic dentine (as seen with older patients). Fluoridated, demineralised or stained enamel may also require further attention.
- Complete removal of etchant and dissolved calcium phosphates produces a clean etched field, making sure that air and water syringes are free of contaminants (especially compressor oil).
- Use optical magnification to make sure that agents are applied uniformly across the entire adhesive interface. Also avoid excessive pooling of bonding agents.
- The use of a 2% chlorhexidine digluconate after the etch and rinse step may potentially inhibit intrinsic MMP (matrix metalloproteinases), which are activated in an acidic environment created by the process of dental caries or during dentine bonding. MMP can degrade the hybrid layer.

## Tips

- Pay close attention to the timing and mode of application of various agents.
- Keep a close watch on your light-curing units, which may decline in function over time and will need regular testing.
- It is useful to hold the high-volume aspirator tip next to the tooth after the etch rinsing and drying process has taken place. This ensures that the surfaces remain dry prior to the application of the next step.
- While light curing, bring the light-curing tip close to the surface and then, holding it rigidly, start the activation process. This ensures that the materials receive the full recommended polymerisation process.
- While light curing, beware of undercut areas in the cavity, particularly during the replacement of an amalgam restoration. You may need to angle the light source to reach these areas effectively.

## References

1 Van Noort R. *An introduction to dental materials.* 3rd ed. London: Mosby Elsevier; 2007.
2 Green D, Banerjee A. Contemporary adhesive bonding: bridging the gap between research and clinical practice. *Dent Update.* 2011;38:439–50.
3 Gilpatrick R, Ross J, Simonsen R. Resin-to-enamel bond strengths with various etching times. *Quintessence Int* 1991;22:47–9.

## 5.2

# Teeth Isolation

*Subir Banerji and Shamir B. Mehta*

*Video: Teeth Isolation*
*Presented by Subir Banerji and Shamir B. Mehta*

## Principles

The effective isolation of the teeth from the soft tissues, the tongue and fluids in the oral cavity can prove pivotal to the safe and successful practice of restorative dentistry. It is commonly accepted that the use of a dental **dam** can provide a *complete* form of isolation. The use of a dental dam is considered mandatory during the undertaking of non-surgical endodontic therapy. Other means of attaining isolation include the use of **retraction devices** and/or the use of **high-volume suction techniques**; however, the level of isolation may be considered to be only *partial*. An example of a commonly used retraction device is one by Ivoclar Vivadent (Schaan, Liechtenstein), OptraGate.

Dental dam isolation offers a number of key benefits:

- **Protection of the patient**, especially against the accidental aspiration of dental instruments and chemical agents such as irrigating solutions and etchants. The dam will also confer some level of protection against rotary and hand instruments.[1]
- Effective **isolation against saliva and other oral fluids**. This may be required to provide the optimal environment for adhesive luting, to avoid adversely affecting the longer-term prognosis of chemically bonded dental restorations.[2]
- A barrier against cross-contamination, including aerosol sprays from dental handpieces and the air and water syringe.
- Enhanced visual access for the operator.
- Improved patient comfort, as patients need not fear the swallowing of chemicals, irrigants or instruments.[1]
- Avoidance of fogging of dental mirrors.
- Reduced chairside time by virtue of treatment being carried out in an uninterrupted manner.

While the use of a dental dam appears to be inconsistent in the dental profession, it is important for the contemporary operator to be competent and proficient with the placement technique, as described in this chapter.

*Practical Procedures in Aesthetic Dentistry*, First Edition. Edited by Subir Banerji, Shamir B. Mehta and Christopher C.K. Ho. © 2017 John Wiley & Sons, Ltd. Published 2017 by John Wiley & Sons, Ltd.
Companion website: www.wiley.com/go/banerji/aestheticdentistry

## Procedures

Dental dams are commercially available in a range of different **colours**, **consistencies** and **materials**. The selection of colour is largely operator dependent. However, try to select one that provides an effective contrast with the teeth. If your patient has a latex allergy, non-latex dams must be used. The selection of a dam by virtue of its thickness (light, medium, heavy or extra heavy) is also based on personal preference. In general, lighter dams place less tension on the clamp and are easier to pass between inter-proximal contact areas. However, lighter dams may be difficult to invert and are more susceptible to tearing, so they may not offer the desired level of isolation. Medium-weight dams can provide a good balance between ease of application, fit at the gingival margin and soft-tissue retraction. Some operators choose to place an absorbent tissue napkin between the patient's face and the underside of the dam to improve comfort.

A **dental dam punch** is used to create a hole in the dam. The position of the hole may be determined by the use of a template or stamp. The maxillary central incisors should be placed about 2–3 cm away from the top of the dam to avoid covering the nasal apertures. Alternatively, place the dam in your patient's mouth (or on a study cast) and use a market to mark the middle of the incisal edge, cusp tips for premolar teeth or the buccal groove for molar teeth. The holes can be punched in varying sizes and the appropriate diameter according to the tooth needs to be selected to ensure good isolation at the base of the tooth or teeth to be isolated.

There are also a variety of **dental dam frames** available. These may be metallic, such as the Young's frame, or plastic. Metallic frames are less bulky and more robust, but plastic frames, by virtue of not being radio-opaque, permit the taking of radiographs without having to be removed. However, plastic frames are more susceptible to deterioration through the process of repeated heat sterilisation. Some frames are better placed on the underside of the dam, while others, such as the Young's frame, are placed over the top of the dam to avoid contact with the patient's face. Rubber dams with built-in frames such as Optradam (Ivoclar Vivadent) may also be useful.

Similarly, there are a large number of **clamps** available. They may be metallic or plastic, be winged or have a non-winged design. Winged clamps allow the dam to be fitted to the clamp prior to insertion into the patient's mouth. Clamps with smaller, deeper-reaching beaks (commonly known as 'butterfly' clamps) are useful for anterior and premolar teeth.

Clamps are usually placed on the distal-most teeth that you are planning to isolate. Select a clamp that has four points. You may also choose to use elastic cord, a strip of rubber dam or dental floss to help retain the dam in situ.

Having selected the band and marked up the hole positions, tie a ligature to the bow of the clamp using dental floss. This will help to retrieve the clamp in the event of inadvertent misplacement.

Floss the interdental contacts to verify the presence of tight contacts.

There are a number of techniques for dam placement. When placing the dam over the clamp, using a set of rubber dam forceps expand the clamp to allow it to pass over the crown of a tooth; over-expansion should be avoided, or you risk damaging the clamp. Check the stability of the clamp once placed on the tooth. If it is unstable, you may choose to re-position it or select a different design of clamp. Some clinicians prefer to lubricate the dam to ease placement.

By placing a finger on either side of the hole, stretch the hole and place the dam over the bow and jaws of the clamp. Where multiple teeth are being isolated, two clamps may be required. Adapt the dam to the last hole at the end of the sequence and pass the dam material past the contact areas. Complete the process with the other teeth, using dental tape to help pass the material past the contact areas. If the latter is not completely successful, double the tape on itself, repeat the action and pull the tape out from a buccal direction.

When using a winged clamp, you may attach the clamp to the dam, position the frame and place the entire assembly as a single unit.

If you are planning to use a butterfly clamp for anterior tooth isolation, you will need to place the dam over the tooth first, followed by the clamp.

When using a napkin, it should be placed under the dam prior to the attachment of the frame.

The dam should be inverted, so as to tuck in the edge gingivally. Inversion may be achieved using air from a three-in-one syringe, a flat plastic instrument or dental floss. The latter may be tied to the cervical aspect of anterior teeth to maintain the dam in an inverted position. Figures 5.2.1 and 5.2.2 depict the use of a a plastic clamp to retain a rubber dam in situ, providing isolation for the restoration of the lower first molar tooth using direct resin composite. A ligature has been applied using dental floss to aid inversion.

If you note signs of seepage with the dam in situ, special silicone sealants such as Oraseal (Ultradent Products, Inc., South Jordan, UT, USA) may be used.

Once you have completed your dental procedure, remove the dam by first removing any ligatures. Then stretch the interproximal septa. With a pair of scissors directed away from the soft tissues, cut the septa. This is followed by removal of the clamp using the rubber dam forceps. The dam and frame should be lifted off and the patient's mouth inspected for any remnant of the dam between the teeth.

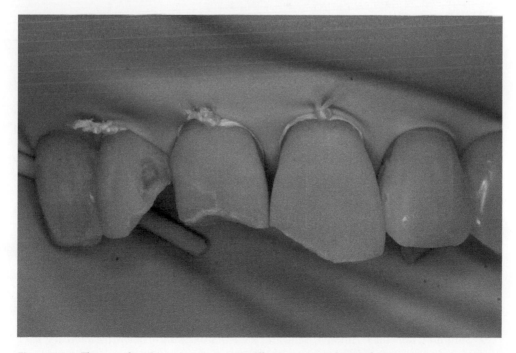

Figure 5.2.1 The use of a rubber dam to provide effective moisture control

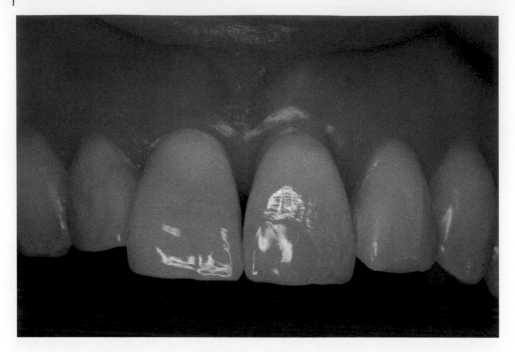

Figure 5.2.2 Completed resin composite restoration, where good moisture control is paramount to success

## Tips

- For effective colour contrast, avoid the use of ivory-coloured dams.
- There is a large number of clamps available in the marketplace. You usually will not need more than a set of five or six different clamps. You may wish to try a selection to ascertain which types of dam, frame and clamp work best for you.
- Where your patient has a ceramic crown on the tooth to be clamped, employ caution as there may be a risk of ceramic fracture. You may wish to use a plastic clamp or an alternative form of retainer, or consider fitting the clamp on a different tooth.
- In the presence of a fixed bridge, periodontal splint or orthodontic appliance, you may choose to cut a slit in the dam between two holes, followed by the use of a sealant to avoid seepage.
- In the presence of severe tooth loss, consider the use of a deep-reaching clamp with a short beak, or clamp adjacent teeth.
- When cementing veneers, a modified dam technique may prove highly beneficial.

## References

1  Walton R, Torabinejad M. *Principles and practice of endodontics*. 3rd ed. St Louis, MO: WB Saunders; 2002.
2  Summit J, Robbins J, Hilton T, Schwartz RS. *Fundamentals of operative dentistry: a contemporary approach*. 3rd ed. Chicago, IL: Quintessence; 2006.

## 5.3

# Cavity Preparation

*Subir Banerji and Shamir B. Mehta*

## Principles

For an adhesively retained restoration, cavity preparation is usually limited to access to the defect, removal of diseased/compromised tissue (and/or failed restorative material) and development of a convenience form to facilitate matrix placement and application of the restorative material. All peripheral stain should also be removed to avoid poor aesthetics and to optimise adhesion.

There are a variety of burs available for the preparation and placement of plastic restorations. For a Class 3 restoration, access to the carious lesion is perhaps best approached from a lingual direction (where possible), using a small diamond bur to gain initial access in a high-speed handpiece (such as a No. 2 round bur). Cavity preparation for a posterior carious lesion may be commenced using a flat-fissure bur. The use of round, water-cooled burs of progressively increasing sizes in a contra-angled handpiece can then be used to remove carious dentine.

It is imperative to preserve as much enamel at the cavity margins as possible, particularly at the cervical floors of the boxes, as bonding to enamel is considerably more effective and significantly more predictable in the longer term than that to dentine or cementum. Cavity walls and floors should be finished with rounded internal line angles. For posterior resin restorations, interproximal boxes should be finished just beneath the contact point to permit caries removal and matrix application. It has also been shown that the preparation of a conservative concave cavity with a 4° taper not only lends itself to a minimally invasive design, but significantly improves the strength of the resin composite restoration, regardless of the type of material used.[1]

The **bevelling** of enamel margins (by 0.5–1.0 mm) has been advocated for proximal surfaces, as it exposes enamel rods transversely, thereby presenting a greater surface area for etching and bonding; it is also thought to provide a more effective etching pattern. Bevelling is best achieved using a flame-shaped finishing bur or a fine diamond bur.

In the case of a posterior cavity, the gingival cavosurface margin should only be bevelled if it is well above the cemento-enamel junction and if there remains a thin band of

*Practical Procedures in Aesthetic Dentistry*, First Edition. Edited by Subir Banerji, Shamir B. Mehta and Christopher C.K. Ho. © 2017 John Wiley & Sons, Ltd. Published 2017 by John Wiley & Sons, Ltd.
Companion website: www.wiley.com/go/banerji/aestheticdentistry

enamel after cavity preparation. However, bevelling is not generally recommended for use on occlusal cavosurface margins, because:

- It increases the loss of sound tooth tissue.
- It increases the surface area of the final restorations, increasing predisposition to wear.
- It can result in the formation of a thin area of composite resin that may be vulnerable to fracture.
- A less well-defined peripheral outline is developed, which may not be conducive to attaining a precise finish.[2]

Thus, a butt-joint margin is preferred occlusally for posterior cavities.

For anterior teeth, there appears to be a variation in opinion as to the size and form of the bevel, with some operators advocating the use of a two-part bevel: an initial, smaller bevel (perhaps less than 1.0 mm) at 45° followed by a wider, diffused scalloped bevel that is less steep but slightly longer in width to further enhance the transition between the resin composite material and the tooth. On the palatal surface, as aesthetics are less critical, the use of a longer bevel has little merit. However, should the placement of a bevel result in the loss of enamel tissue at the cervical margin, then bevel placement in this area should be avoided so as not to compromise the marginal seal (which will be inferior in the absence of enamel tissue). Figures 5.3.1, 5.3.2 and 5.3.3 show the restoration of two central incisors with direct composite restorations using a bevel cavity preparation to achieve an acceptable transition in colour at the margins of the cavity.

The use of air abrasion following cavity preparation is beneficial as it may help with the removal of peripheral stain in a minimally invasive manner, as well as assisting with the provision of micro-mechanical retention.

Brown silicone rubber points, discs or ultrasonic instrumentation can also be used to finish the cavity margins to remove any unsupported enamel prisms.

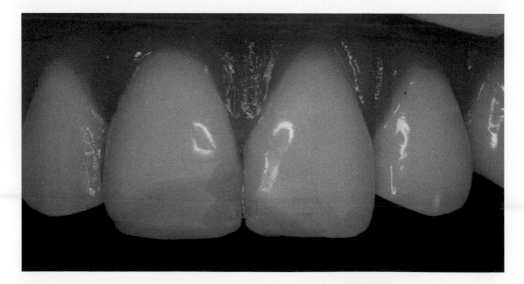

Figure 5.3.1 The patient is unhappy about the appearance of the anterior composites

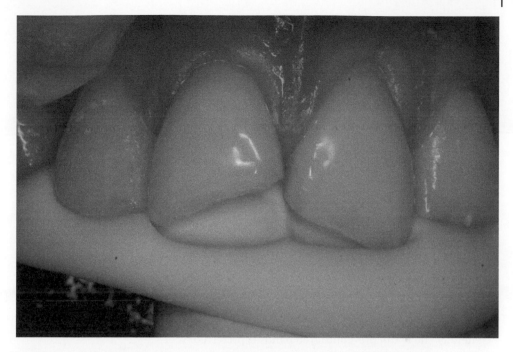

Figure 5.3.2 The old composites have been removed and the cavity has been bevelled to create a smooth transition of colour

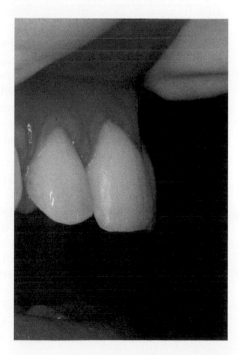

Figure 5.3.3 The new composite is seen from the distal aspect on the upper right central incisor to show the transition of colour across the labial surface

In some cases there may be no need to provide any cavity form, such as the additive management of worn or fractured surfaces, or diastema closure. Under such circumstances, the adhesive interface may simply require cleaning and augmentation to enhance its micro-mechanical and adhesive retention form by using an abrasive strip, pumice or air abrasion.

Prior to the application of an appropriate matrix system with lesions that extend to involve the interproximal area, the operator may give consideration to the process of **pre-preparation wedging**, whereby a suitable wedge is placed interproximally for a period of a few minutes to open patent contact areas.

Pre-preparation wedging may also be useful at this stage with the following aims:

- Protecting the interdental papillae and rubber dam intraproximally.
- Prevention of bleeding, which could otherwise compromise bonding.
- Promotion of a slight separation between the teeth, thus favouring matrix application and the achievement of adequate proximal contact.

For lesions where there may be uncertainty about the extent of the lesion into the interproximal region, pre-wedging may also allow the clinician direct visual access to this area.

One of the greatest technical challenges when placing direct posterior resin composites is the formation of an ideal interproximal contact point. Open contact points will result in continual food impaction.[3]

The **matrix bands** used may be fabricated from either transparent plastic or metal. Generally, the use of pre-contoured bands is preferred.

**Transparent plastic matrices** are commonly employed in the anterior regions and are normally based on cellulose acetate-based materials. They are available in a variety of shapes and forms, ranging from pre-formed crowns to strips (both of flat and curved varieties) or specially formed sectional matrices designed to restore the complex three-dimensional anatomy of the anterior interproximal region.

Plastic matrix bands are less commonly used to restore posterior teeth. When used with transparent light-reflecting wedges, they offer the ability to light cure from more than just the occlusal approach. However, when compared to metal matrix bands they tend to be thicker, less easy to apply, do not hold their shape very well and do not offer the potential to be burnished against adjacent teeth, thereby increasing the risk of overhang formation and an open contact area.

The use of PTFE (polytetrafluoroethylene) tape is commonly described for the restoration of anterior teeth. It is an inert, non-stick and relatively cheap material that can be wrapped around adjacent teeth to prevent unwanted bonding.

**Metal matrix bands** can be subdivided into sectional systems or circumferential systems:

- **Sectional matrix systems** are reported to produce the best proximal contact points, particularly for narrower box preparations. Sectional systems typically comprise a metal ring that is placed between teeth adjacent to the box preparation, following placement of the matrix band. The engaged ring is thought to exert a continuous separating force on the two adjacent teeth, thereby leading to the formation of a small space that will help promote the formation of a patent contact. The tines of the ring also help to ensure good adaptation of the band and thus reduce the need for proximal finishing. However, the removal of sectional matrices can be problematic, especially if very tight contact points have been formed.
- **Circumferential matrix systems** tend to be indicated for use with larger cavities with wider box preparations. However, their use is associated with the formation of poor-quality contact points, flat proximal contours and 'high/coronal' contact point areas (often very

close to the marginal ridge). Care should also be taken during the tightening of circumferential band systems, as this may apply considerable tension to the remaining walls.

## Procedures

- The technique for matrix placement and customisation where there is a need to restore an anterior surface is described at length in Chapter 5.4.
- For a posterior tooth, following the principles described for cavity preparation the use of a sectional matrix system is advocated.
- Measure the size of the interproximal box using a calibrated periodontal probe. Select an appropriate size of sectional matrix.
- When pre-wedging, place your chosen wedges in the interproximal areas and leave them in situ for a few minutes.
- Otherwise, using a pair of tweezers place your matrix in the interproximal area. When using a curved matrix, ensure that the concave surface is coronal. Secure the matrix with wedges, which can be customised with a scalpel.
- Using a set of forceps, having selected the metal ring, open the beaks of the ring to allow it to be placed over the maximum bulbosity of the teeth. The ring should contact the outer surface of the band and be seated over the wedge.
- Check the adaptation of the matrix to the tooth and to the adjacent tooth, making sure that there are no openings that will result in overhanging margins. You may wish to use a burnisher or an interproximal carver to further amend the desired shape of the interproximal contact area. However, heavy burnishing will lead to the formation of indentations in the matrix, which will then be duplicated in the restoration, culminating in rough contact areas.
- The coronal surface of the matrix should end at the level where the marginal ridge is desired. The matrix may need to be adjusted.

## Tips

- Often the selection of a matrix will depend on the level of support offered by the residual tooth structure. The use of sectional matrices is challenging where one of the axial walls is heavily undermined (unless augmented first).
- The use of Teflon-coated rings avoids adhesion between the matrix and resin-based materials.

## References

1  Anand S, Kavitha C, Subbarao C. Effect of cavity design on the strength of direct posterior composite restorations: an empirical FEM analysis. *Int Jour Dent*. 2011;2011:1–5.
2  van der Vyver P, Bridges P. Posterior composite resin restorations: part 2 cavity preparation. *SADJ* 2002;57:174–180.
3  van der Vyver P. Posterior composite resin restorations: part 3 matrix systems. *SADJ* 2002;57:211–26.

## Further Reading

Mackenzie L, Shortall A, Burke F. Direct posterior composites: a practical guide. *Dental Update*. 2009 Mar;71–94.

## 5.4

## Anterior Restorations

*Subir Banerji and Shamir B. Mehta*

*Video: Anterior Restorations*
*Presented by Subir Banerji and Shamir B. Mehta*

## Principles

Of the direct aesthetic materials available in today's marketplace, few clinicians would dispute the role of resin composite as the most suitable form of product for the restoration of anterior teeth. It has the ability to almost mimic lost or damaged natural tooth tissue (being available in an array of shades, textures and opacities), adequate mechanical properties, stability and predictability in the oral environment, the provision of a good marginal seal, relative ease of use and repair, time and cost efficiency.

However, in order for the clinician to provide patients with a desirable result when planning anterior restorations, there is a need to understand several key principles. These include the following:

- The macro- and micro-anatomical variations that exist in the anterior dentition, including morphological variations of the whole tooth when viewed in differing planes, as well as surface textural changes and variations in the anatomy of the incisal edge.
- The fluctuations that exist in shade and colour between different patients as well as in different regions of a tooth for the same patient.
- The effects of ageing on the properties of the enamel and dentine as well as aesthetic issues.
- A good working knowledge of the available materials as well as their respective techniques of handling and application.
- The fundamentals of adhesion and clinical occlusion.

This chapter will focus on Class IV restoration.

## Procedures

In order to gain predictability with form when planning and preparing anterior Class IV restorations, many clinicians choose to use a **silicone key** to 'copy' a given occlusal morphology.

*Practical Procedures in Aesthetic Dentistry*, First Edition. Edited by Subir Banerji, Shamir B. Mehta and Christopher C.K. Ho. © 2017 John Wiley & Sons, Ltd. Published 2017 by John Wiley & Sons, Ltd.
Companion website: www.wiley.com/go/banerji/aestheticdentistry

The silicone key is usually fabricated in polyvinyl siloxane (PVS). It is imperative that the key is extended to the premolar occlusal surfaces and has an adequate level of thickness to ensure stability and rigidity in the oral cavity. The index should be extended to the incisal edge.

Commence with shade selection prior to the application of an etchant, ideally while the tooth is moist and under appropriate lighting conditions. You may wish to use a proprietary shade guide or apply a selection of trial shades (sometimes in a layered manner) to the patient's tooth. It is good practice to attain a pre-operative photograph of the adjacent tooth/teeth. When the latter is reduced in contrast by a factor of three, it is possible to visualise the morphological and physiological colour variations that exist in your patient's anterior teeth, including features detailing the appearance of the incisal edge, such as the presence (or indeed absence) of mamelons, lobes, grooves, minor fractures and surface stains that you may choose to imitate. You may consider creating a sketch noting these variations, additionally documenting any macro- and microscopic variations you wish to impart into the restoration.

Following the marking of centric stops using articulating paper as well as the recording of occlusal contacts during dynamic mandibular movements, apply your chosen form of isolation. Following cavity preparation (if required), place a bevel along the entire cavity margin, facially, interproximally and palatally. The use of a chisel may prove helpful for finalisation of this stage.

Micro-mechanical retention form as well as the removal of stains may be enhanced by the use of air abrasion. With a matrix (such as a metal or cellulose acetate strip) or polytetrafluoroethylene (PTFE) tape (as shown in the video on the accompanying website), isolate the adjacent teeth prior to tooth conditioning, to avoid unwanted adhesion to these surfaces.

Condition the teeth using your chosen form of bonding system. With your silicone key in situ, apply a quantity of your chosen enamel shade to the matrix. The use of warmed resin can prove helpful at this stage with the process of material adaptation. Take care to avoid excessive material. The objective is to develop a thin **palatal shelf**. Using a commercially available resin application brush or a titanium nitride–coated interproximal carver, closely adapt the material between the matrix and the tooth, making sure that the material extends to the incisal edge but is still slightly short of the full width of the tooth, thus leaving the interproximal contact area 'open'. Light cure the material as per the manufacturer's instructions. The use of coated instruments renders them almost 'non-stick' in use.

Try to remember that resin composites do not have the same optical properties as their physiological analogues. Consequently, if you try to apply increments to reflect the anatomical dimensions, your final result may not be what you might have desired at the outset. As a note of caution, the final enamel layer should be approximately half the thickness of the physiological counterpart, otherwise you will end up with a highly translucent restoration.

Carefully remove the silicone key. Check the palatal aspect and further light cure this palatal shelf after checking for any excess in the gingival areas. The next stage involves the development of the **interproximal pillar**. There are variations in the literature on how this critical area is best formed. It is not the authors' preference to use flowable resins for this area. Furthermore, the use of a flat strip matrix will not allow you to develop the three-dimensional form that this area usually requires, taking into account the curvatures present in this region of anterior teeth in both vertical and horizontal dimensions. The use of a curved matrix is therefore advocated. There are a number of pre-curved cellulose acetate matrices available in the marketplace, but a dead-soft metal matrix can be particularly useful, as it is able to be contoured (and retain the imparted form) and therefore can also be used to develop a tight contact with the adjacent surface (if desired).

Place your chosen contoured matrix in the interproximal area, making sure that it is adapted to the cavity margin. The use of a pre-formed wedge to support the matrix is common clinical practice. However, the latter can sometimes cause unwanted trauma, bleeding or flattening of the interproximal papilla. Hence, the authors advocate the use of a section of cotton wool, which can be tightly packed into the space between the outer surface of the matrix and the adjacent tooth surface. In the presence of a subgingival cavity, you may consider the use of a dry-retraction cord or surgical correction so as to create a supragingival surface, which is more conducive to optimal bonding.

Apply either an enamel shade or dentine shade according to your patient's requirements to the interproximal area. When using an enamel shade, take care to avoid excessive increments. With a resin application brush, adapt the material to the matrix and sculpt using a coated, small rounded condenser. The pillar should extend to the incisal edge in a vertical dimension and is formed to the level of the facial plane. Light cure to secure this section.

Carefully remove the matrix. If necessary, attend to the contralateral side. You will now have formed an **envelope** into which you can place your dentine shade. The latter should be applied to a thickness that will permit you space to place your final enamel layer and also develop the desired morphology of the incisal edge. Thus, if you wish to develop an edge that has well-defined mamelons, they can be sculpted into the dentine layer using a small rounded condenser, a PKT 2 burnisher instrument or a coated, fine-bladed instrument such as an interproximal carver. It is also at this stage that you may wish to apply resin tints to mimic colour variations such as stains or hypoplastic areas. The use of very fine resin applicator brushes can be particularly helpful here. Light cure.

Finally, apply the enamel shade. It should be finished to be flush with the bevel. The use of coated, paddle-shaped instruments can be helpful for this stage. The surface layer should be formed so as to mimic the three-dimensional gross variations in the anatomical form of the tooth being restored when viewed in frontal and lateral profiles. You may also choose to impart surface characteristics such as lobes on the incisal edge, a cervical bulge in the gingival third or craze lines, grooves or subtle perikymata (small surface striations formed by the enamel prisms) on the labial face. The use of a size 8 K flex file prior to light curing to produce craze lines can be quite effective.

Finally, cure and assess. You may sometimes choose to add minor quantities of a translucent shade of resin composite to enhance the optical property. Where possible, try to develop the desired anatomical form in an **additive** manner rather than by cutting material away, as doing so may affect the final shade.

The next stage will involve the processes of finishing and polishing, which are discussed in Chapter 5.6.

Figures 5.4.1, 5.4.2, 5.4.3 and 5.4.4 demonstrate many of these concepts.

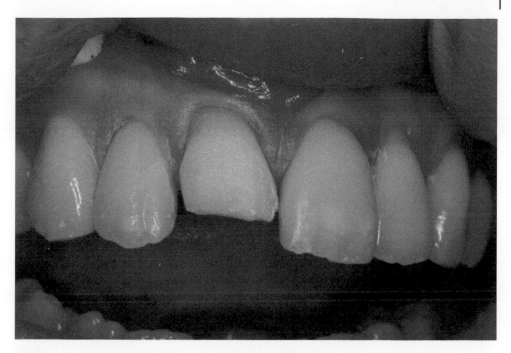

Figure 5.4.1 An example of an anterior tooth requiring a direct resin composite restoration

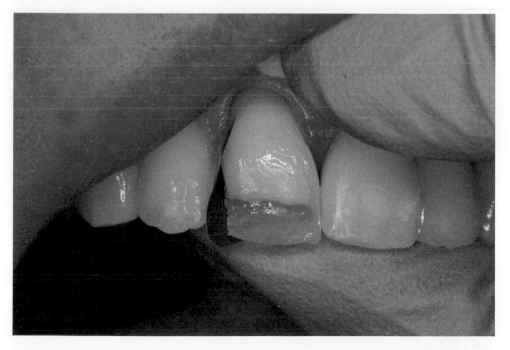

Figure 5.4.2 A palatal shelf has been formed using a silicone key. The figure shows the use of a Teflon-coated 'dead-soft' matrix to form an interproximal pillar, as seen on the lefthand side

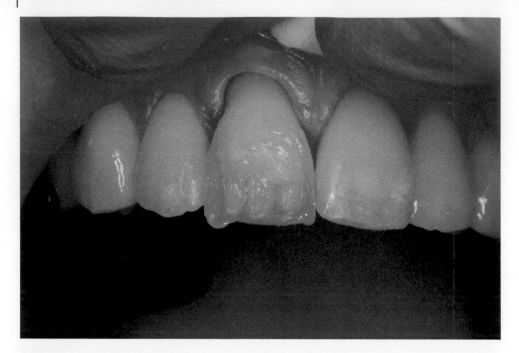

Figure 5.4.3  Dentine layer build-up

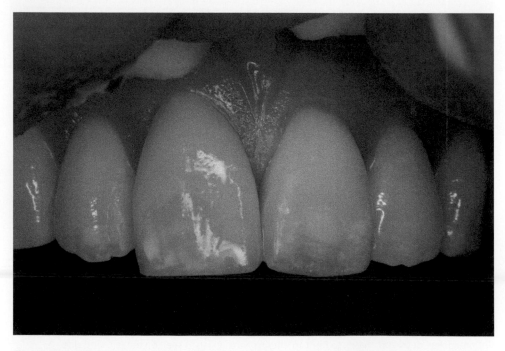

Figure 5.4.4  Completed restoration. Subsurface resin tints have been added to mimic physiological hypoplastic areas

## Tips

- It can take some time to develop confidence and competence with your chosen resin composite material, so be prepared to be patient! The layering of composite is an art form that requires practise to develop.
- Learn to critically evaluate your restorations; take post-operative photographs.
- Remember that the tooth will need to rehydrate in order for both the clinician and the patient to appreciate the colour and aesthetics of the restoration.

## Further Reading

Mackenzie L, Parmar D, Shortall C, Burke T. Direct anterior composites: a practical guide. *Dental Update.* 2013;40:2–16.

## 5.5

# Posterior Restorations

*Subir Banerji and Shamir B. Mehta*

*Video: Posterior Restorations*
*Presented by Subir Banerji and Shamir B. Mehta*

## Principles

Concerns with the use of dental amalgam have paved the way for alternative dental materials for the direct restoration of posterior teeth.[1] **Resin composite** is one such material. The advantages and disadvantages of resin composite in this application have been summarised in Table 5.5.1.

The **indications** of directly bonded posterior composite restorations include the following:

- The treatment of small to moderately sized restorations
- Where aesthetics are of prime importance
- Where an occlusal prescription is being developed or monitored in cases of tooth wear.

However, caution is advised where:

- The centric occlusal stops are likely to be placed on the restorative material, due to concerns with material wear
- The patient exhibits signs of excessive occlusal wear or loading
- It is not possible to achieve good moisture control
- The patient is allergic or sensitive to resin-based materials

Table 5.5.1 The merits and drawbacks of resin composite as a posterior restorative material

| Merits | Drawbacks |
| --- | --- |
| Aesthetics | Polymerisation shrinkage |
| Conservation of dental hard tissues | Post-operative sensitivity |
| Reduced thermal conductivity | Secondary caries |
| Potential for repair | Decreased wear resistance and bulk fracture |
| Adhesion to tooth tissue | Technique sensitivity |
| Lack of galvanic conduction | Water sorption |

*Practical Procedures in Aesthetic Dentistry*, First Edition. Edited by Subir Banerji, Shamir B. Mehta and Christopher C.K. Ho. © 2017 John Wiley & Sons, Ltd. Published 2017 by John Wiley & Sons, Ltd.
Companion website: www.wiley.com/go/banerji/aestheticdentistry

- The patient has a poor standard of oral hygiene/plaque control with high caries pre-disposition
- The gingival cavosurface margin is not located on intact enamel, as the bonding of resin composite to dentine is less effective.

## Procedures

Pre-operative shade selection must be accomplished (with the aid of a proprietary shade guide) prior to the application of rubber dam, as dehydration and isolation may alter shade. It is advisable to undertake shade selection following the completion of cavity preparation to enable you to gain a better insight into the colour variations that may be present in the dentinal layer. It is important to be aware that most available composite resin shade guides are based on acrylic materials (rather than the actual composite resin). Hence, it is prudent to compose a customised shade guide. With the availability of opaque shades, it is also possible to mask residual discoloration at the base of a cavity.

Pre-operative centric stops should be marked with articulating paper. Eccentric contacts should also be identified. Ideally, occlusal contacts should be maintained on tooth tissue where possible; if not, they should be reproduced in the anatomy of the restoration (when undertaking 'conformative procedures').

Complete moisture control is mandatory for clinical success with posterior resin composites, as outlined in Chapter 5.2.

For details about adhesive cavity preparation and matrix application for a posterior resin restoration, refer to Chapter 5.3. For some restorations, especially where they are in close proximity to the pulp chamber, there may be a need to consider the use of a **base/liner**. Commonly used materials include glass ionomer cements, auto-cured and flowable resins, as well as 'bioactive dentine substitutes'.

The use of **RMGICs** (resin-modified glass ionomer cements) as base materials is preferred to the use of conventional GICs (glass ionomer cements), as they offer the benefits of higher tensile strength, higher bond strength to resin composites and the potential to be light cured. The rationale for the use of GICs as bases for posterior composite restorations includes the following:

- Potential to bond to both tooth tissue and overlying resin restorative
- Reduced overall polymerisation shrinkage, as less bulk of resin composite will be used
- Reduced post-operative sensitivity
- Avoidance of a rise in pulpal temperature, often seen when curing resin-based materials
- Sustained fluoride release.

However, GICs have a comparatively lower elastic modulus, which may reduce the overall fracture resistance of the final restoration. The use of a glass ionomer base may also impart a more opacious, less life-like appearance to the completed restoration. GICs may be applied prior to etchant application in the form of either:

- **an open sandwich**, whereby material is applied over the pulpal dentine; or
- **a closed sandwich** ('bonded-base technique'), which is for use with Class II cavities where the gingival cavosurface finishing margin is in enamel (but within 1 mm of the cemento-enamel junction) or in dentine.

An RMGIC is placed as an initial increment into the proximal box (apical to the proximal contact point, due to the heightened wear characteristics versus resin composite) and light cured.

**Flowable composites** offer reduced viscosity and have the potential for better adaptation to the cavity walls (as opposed to regular resins). They also have a reduced elastic modulus, conferring a 'stress-breaker role' in helping to absorb forces. However, due to their higher resin content, they can display as much as three times the amount of polymerisation shrinkage.

**Biodentine** (Septodont, Saint-Maur-des-fossés, France) is a material based on tricalcium silicate, which has been suggested to have good sealing properties, biocompatibility and high compressive strength. It may be used as a bio-compatible dentine substitute in order to attain pulpal healing, where evaluation of pulpal healing is required prior to the placement of a definitive restoration.[2]

The walls of the preparation should prepared for adhesive bonding, as described in Chapter 5.1. Clinical studies have suggested that post-operative sensitivity (POS) is encountered in approximately 30% of posterior composite restorations. This may be related to the inability of the adhesive system to seal patent dentinal tubules and also due to the effect of cuspal flexion, which occurs as a result of polymerisation shrinkage. Bacterial presence in the smear layer with further ingress due to micro-leakage may also account for the occurrence of delayed POS.

**Hybrid, visible light-cured resins** are the most commonly used materials in contemporary practice. It is advocated that such materials are applied in successive, **laminated increments**, as they have limited depth of light cure; the depth of cure of darker shades is less than lighter shades as they do not absorb light as effectively.

The so-called **incremental technique** offers the following advantages:

- Uniform, effective polymerisation
- Prevention of excessive polymerisation shrinkage (as less bulk material is cured per increment), thereby helping to enhance marginal adaptation, reduction in post-operative sensitivity and reduced risks of cuspal contraction and increased resistance to fracture
- A reduction in the **C-factor** (ratio of bonded to unbounded surfaces), thereby increasing bond strength
- Development of a more pleasing anatomical form and reduced risk of overhang formation.

Composite resin may be dispensed directly from a compule using a 'wiping motion' or applied directly to the tooth with hand instruments. A range of instruments have been developed to facilitate the handling, placement and contouring of resin composite materials, which are often titanium nitrite coated. However, this is also largely dependent on operator preference. The use of proprietary brushes to assist in the manipulation and sculpting of increments of resin composite (particularly when pre-warmed) may prove helpful. Pre-warming resin will help to improve the flowability of your material.

Careful placement of the **first increment** is vital to ensure effective adaptation. This should be no greater than **1 mm in thickness** to allow for effective light curing (particularly as it will be the layer that will be the farthest away from the light source).

For a Class II cavity, develop your proximal wall first in your chosen enamel shade. You may choose to form this in two separate sections; this will help establish an optimal contour in this area of the restoration and will also help reduce the C-factor. Take caution to avoid excessive enamel shades, as your restoration may appear highly translucent otherwise.

Where a clear matrix and light-reflecting wedge have been used for a Class II cavity, initial irradiation should be directed through the flat end of the wedge (gingivally). Where metal matrices have been used, proximal areas should receive additional curing after the removal of the matrix.

You will now have created a Class I cavity. Subsequent increments should be no greater than 2 mm in thickness, placed in **oblique layers**. With each increment, contact should only be made with one wall of the cavity (to create a more favourable C-factor) and light cured accordingly. The C-factor can be further reduced by the application of an initial 'triangular wedge' of material, as contact would only be made by one cavity wall.

Two methods have been described to replace occlusal anatomy:

- **Successive cusp build-up technique**, whereby oblique layering is stopped at a point judged to be the base of the pit and fissure anatomy of the final restoration. Increments of resin are then positioned and adapted to replace cuspal inclines (one cusp at a time), analogous to the PK Thomas technique describing the formation of wax occlusal patterns. Dentine shade resins are applied to the level of the enamel-dentine, followed by sloping increments of 'enamel' shade. Stains (resin tints) may be applied prior to the application of the final layer.
- **Use of an occlusal index**, fabricated in PVS silicone material. This method can produce a very close reproduction of the occlusal anatomy with little need for adjustment and polishing.

The temptation to use bonding resins to lubricate instruments should be avoided, as they contain agents such as HEMA (2-hydroxyethyl methacrylate) that can lead to discoloration.

The importance of the role of the **light-curing unit** is often overlooked. It is important to make sure that the light source is kept rigid and as close to the restoration as possible and that curing units are periodically checked for optimal output using radiometers. Care should also be taken to ensure that the material receives the full time recommended by the manufacturer.

Figures 5.5.1, 5.5.2 and 5.5.3 provide an example of a posterior resin composite restoration.

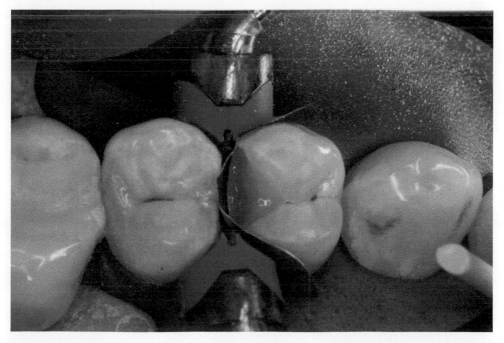

Figure 5.5.1 A disto-occlusal cavity; a sectional matrix has been applied supported by a metal ring, which can permit the insertion of a proprietary wedge under the beaks of the jaws

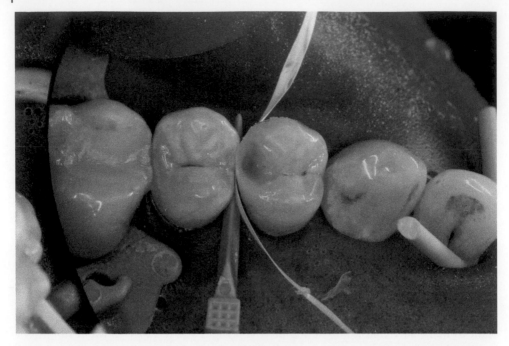

Figure 5.5.2  The interproximal wall has been formed; the matrix and ring can be removed having 'formed' an occlusal, Class 1 cavity. The wedge is retained in situ to avoid unwanted bleeding

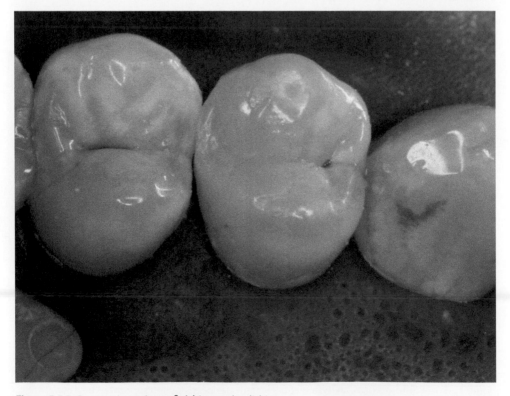

Figure 5.5.3  Restoration prior to finishing and polishing

## Tips

- Open proximal contacts can be a major problem in posterior resin composite restorations – the use of a sectional matrix can be highly beneficial in this context.
- Try to develop form during placement, as opposed to carving it in the set material.
- Avoid making your fissure pattern too deep as this will result in plaque retention.

## References

1 Burke F, Mackenzie L, Sands P. Dental materials – what goes where? Class I and class II cavities. *Dental Update.* 2013;40:260–74.
2 Koubi G, Colon P, Franquin J, et al. Clinical evaluation and safety of a new dentine substitute, biodentine in the restoration of posterior teeth – a prospective study. *Clin Oral Invest.* 2013;17:243–9.

## Further Reading

Mackenzie L, Shortall A, Burke F. Direct posterior composites: a practical guide. *Dental Update.* 2009 Mar;71–94.
Mjor I. The reasons for replacement and the age of failed restorations in general dental practice. *Acta Odotol Scand.* 1997;55:58–63.
Opdam N, Bronkhorst E, Loomans B, Huysmans M. 12 year survival of composite vs amalgam restorations. *J Dent Res.* 2010;89:1063–7.

## 5.6

# The Finishing and Polishing of Resin Composite Restorations

*Subir Banerji and Shamir B. Mehta*

*Video: The Finishing and Polishing of Resin Composite Restorations*
*Presented by Subir Banerji and Shamir B. Mehta*

## Principles

The process of **finishing** a resin composite restoration should aim to attain the **desired form and gross texture**, while the **polishing** phase should aim to impart the required **lustre**, such that the restoration is ultimately unnoticeable by the patient. The importance of finishing and polishing is often overlooked in general dentistry, but they are critical when trying to provide the patient with a restoration that is functionally conducive to the prescribed occlusal scheme, in helping to sustain good oral health by permitting and maintaining effective plaque control, as well as fulfilling the aesthetic expectations of all parties concerned.

Finishing and polishing should ideally be delayed for at least 10–15 minutes following the final phase of light curing so as to permit some **dark polymerisation** to take place. Premature finishing may otherwise result in an increased risk of initiating micro-cracks and possibly accelerated surface wear.

There is a variety of materials and instruments available to assist with finishing and polishing. The choice of a system or indeed a protocol very much depends on operator preference. The use of non-flexible abrasive discs and strips should be undertaken with caution, however, as there is a risk of 'flattening' anatomical contours developed during the process of resin application, which may result in suboptimal functional and aesthetic form.

A sound knowledge of dental anatomy is helpful, especially when concerning the location of fissures, ridges, fossae, cones, lobes and grooves, as well as attention to the surface texture. It is also good practice to make detailed observations of adjacent and contralateral teeth when planning aesthetic resin composite restorations.

## Procedures

Following resin application, initially aim to establish the correct static occlusal form. When conforming, adjust your restoration using a fine (red-banded 30–40 micron) diamond bur, such that the pre-restorative centric stops coincide with those following restoration placement in maximum intercuspation. Confirm the presence of centric stops

*Practical Procedures in Aesthetic Dentistry*, First Edition. Edited by Subir Banerji, Shamir B. Mehta and Christopher C.K. Ho. © 2017 John Wiley & Sons, Ltd. Published 2017 by John Wiley & Sons, Ltd.
Companion website: www.wiley.com/go/banerji/aestheticdentistry

on the tooth being restored (if present pre-operatively) using articulating foil. The use of a rugby ball–shaped bur is very helpful for this process. Copious water cooling will avoid the inadvertent overheating of the restoration.

Now assess your restoration when your patient makes dynamic mandibular movements. This may require the addition of further material, which if done in the same session may necessitate the use of a coat of unfilled or lightly filled flowable resin to permit re-bonding. If this is to take place at a subsequent visit, the use of abrasion as well as the application of etchant should also be given due consideration.

The use of a number 12 scalpel can be helpful to remove gross flash from the margins, especially in the gingival areas and interproximal regions. Place the tip of the blade on the tooth tissues and direct movements towards the restoration, taking care to avoid iatrogenic damage to the soft tissues.

Using a set of tungsten carbide (TC) burs starts to develop the desired macro-texture. Burs with more than 12 flutes should be avoided (as should coarser diamond burs), as they will increase the risk of causing damage to the surface layer of the restoration. The use of a proximal bur is very valuable for gingival and proximal finishing. A conical bur may be employed to finish occluding surfaces for both anterior and posterior restorations.

An 8–12-fluted, needle-shaped TC bur is particularly useful for developing macro-texture with anterior resin restorations. **Macro-texturing** will affect the surface light properties of your restoration, such as **reflection** and **light dispersion**. TC burs may be used to place 'valleys and peaks' on the labial surface, which in turn will help to create shadows that can give a sensation of depth and light reflection, resulting in 'prominence'. Lines of both horizontal and vertical direction may also be placed to create an illusion of widening and lengthening anterior teeth in these respective dimensions.

Embrasure spaces can be grossly contoured, with the aim of developing symmetry. Placing the labial embrasure further apically will have the effect of making the tooth appear narrower. Flattened areas may be developed on the labial face to mimic the shape of adjacent or contralateral teeth. You may also choose to contour the incisal edge with (or without) grooves according to the patient's age and wear pattern.

The inattentive use of non-flexible abrasive discs will help to remove the macro-textural form. However, flexible discs are sometimes helpful for the definition of the incisal edge as well as the refinement of the embrasure space.

You will most likely have a variety of finishing strips at your disposal to contour and polish the proximal surfaces. The use of coarse strips carries the risk of opening up patent contact areas as well as unwanted damage to the dental hard tissues. Plastic strips ranging from medium to extra-fine grit are ideal when employed in an 'S'-shaped motion (as opposed to developing a 'U'-shaped form) so as to avoid flattening or indeed opening up of contact areas.

A set of green and white dental stones can then be used for further gross finishing and to commence the polishing phase. Pointed burs are helpful in finishing marginal areas.

Re-assess your restorations. For some anterior resin restorations, you may choose to place some resin tints to impart stains or opacities, which may be overlaid by a very thick layer of translucent resin composite. You may sometimes elect to use a sterile pencil to mark the positions of accessory grooves and flattened surfaces to assist you with this stage.

Having determined the gross form and macro-characterisation, commence the process of polishing with a series of impregnated rubber points. A variety of shapes of burs are available to suit your needs. Burs should be used with light pressure and with copious coolant. Rubber points are employed to polish the surface, including macro-textural surface undulations such as the lobes and ridges that you have formed, as well as to develop a shiny surface.

Finally, high shine can be achieved with impregnated bristle brushes and/or a proprietary diamond or aluminium oxide polishing paste system on a felt or goat's-hair wheel.

Re-polymerise your restoration for a further 60 seconds.

Apply a final surface glaze of unfilled composite resin to seal off any micro-defects. This will help to improve the aesthetic outcome, improve wear resistance and marginal integrity, as well as possibly avoid crack propagation. Some clinicians also choose to use a layer of glycerine over the restoration followed by subsequent light curing, to permit curing of the surface layer, which may otherwise remain uncured due to the effect of the oxygen inhibition phenomenon.

Appraise your restoration for occlusal form, aesthetics, patency of the contact area using dental floss and its ability to secure and maintain good oral health.

## Tips

- Avoid premature finishing and polishing.
- Use copious amounts of water coolant.
- Find a protocol that work best for you.
- Practise taking photographs. View these with a 'fresh set of eyes'. For aesthetically demanding cases, you may suggest that your patient re-attends for final refinement and polishing once you have made detailed notes from your photographic records.
- Avoid coating restorations with agents containing HEMA, as this will increase the risk of stain accumulation.
- Remember that composites do require long-term maintenance, so be prepared to re-polish the surface to enhance the aesthetic value.

## Further Reading

Chen RC, Chan DC, Chan KC. A quantitative study of finishing and polishing techniques for composite. *J Prosthet Dent.* 1988;59(3):292–7.

Sarac D, Sarac Y, Kulunk S, Ural C, Kulunk T. The effect of polishing techniques on the surface roughness and colour changes of composites. *J Prosthet Dent.* 2006;96(1):33–40.

## 5.7

## Direct Resin Veneers

*Subir Banerji and Shamir B. Mehta*

*Video: Direct Resin Veneers*
*Presented by Subir Banerji and Shamir B. Mehta*

## Principles

Direct resin veneer restorations offer the potential to apply changes to the colour and shape of a tooth in a minimally invasive manner when compared to the use of indirect restorations. There is evidence to suggest favourable, long-term success with ceramic laminate veneers. The use of resin composite offers an alternative to dental ceramic. Resin composite may be used either **indirectly** or in a **direct (chairside)** manner.

Direct resin veneers have a plethora of **indications** in restorative dentistry. These include:

- Management of fractured, discoloured and rotated teeth
- Treatment of tooth malformations (such as peg-shaped lateral incisors)
- Closure or narrowing of diastemata
- Management of congenital or acquired defects
- Management of palatally positioned teeth
- Treatment of worn anterior dentition
- Camouflaging of teeth, such as modification of a canine to mimic a lateral incisor
- Where an increase in tooth length or width may be indicated (as in Part 9).

Direct resin veneers offer a number of potential **advantages** over indirect veneers. Their primary merit is the lack of the need for any tooth preparation (or minimal preparation), thereby eliminating the need for the removal of healthy tooth tissue, as well as the ability to readily undertake intra-oral adjustments, repairs and polishing. Direct resin veneers may also be placed in a single visit, with the absence of associated laboratory costs, impressions or provisional restorations. The lack of the need for a cement interface is also beneficial. Direct resin veneers can allow for direct masking and chromatic customisation of the restoration without reliance on the dental technician, who without the benefit of the patient's presence will otherwise have to depend on photographic records and written instructions from the dental operator.

There are, however, some clear **drawbacks** to the prescription of direct resin veneers, such as a relatively lower resistance to wear, reduced lustre when compared to glazed porcelain, the tendency for discoloration, staining, chipping and fracture. However, there

*Practical Procedures in Aesthetic Dentistry*, First Edition. Edited by Subir Banerji, Shamir B. Mehta and Christopher C.K. Ho. © 2017 John Wiley & Sons, Ltd. Published 2017 by John Wiley & Sons, Ltd.
Companion website: www.wiley.com/go/banerji/aestheticdentistry

is evidence to suggest that patients will often be willing to accept these disadvantages in exchange for a less invasive approach, thus emphasising the importance of informed consent.

## Procedures

The need for tooth preparation may vary according to the desired outcome. Where there is a need to preserve the emergence profile or in the presence of a discoloured/darkened tooth, you may consider a labial reduction of up to 0.8 mm, following the principles of tooth preparation for ceramic veneers, as described in Chapter 7.2. It is imperative, however, that preparations are finished on enamel and are kept supragingival. The presence of dental caries, unaesthetic or failing dental restorations will need to be addressed beforehand.

For discoloured teeth, you may choose to see whether simply placing resin over an opacious material without any tooth preparation will suffice in a diagnostic manner. Figures 5.7.1 and 5.7.2 provide an example of such as case where no tooth preparation has been carried out.

Where there is a need to prescribe an increase in tooth length or width, you may choose to have a diagnostic wax-up at your disposal from which a silicone key can be fabricated. For cases involving a minor increase in length, you may elect to not use a key; however, it is important not to introduce an undesirable change to the occlusal scheme that may culminate in premature failure.

Prior to isolation, carry out a detailed exercise in **colour mapping**. Using an adjacent or contralateral tooth, determine the colour variations that you wish to introduce into your restoration. You can also add to the tooth itself prior to any etching or bonding

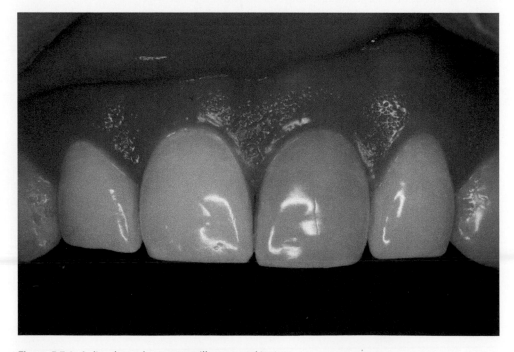

Figure 5.7.1  A discoloured upper maxillary central incisor

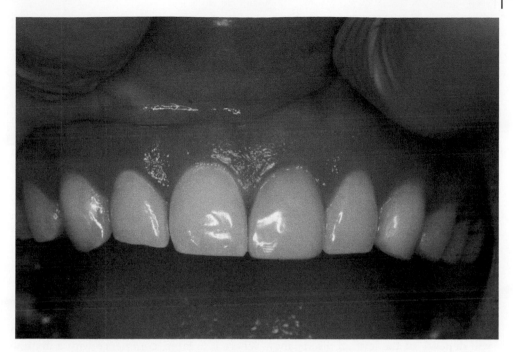

Figure 5.7.2 Completed direct resin veneer (3 years post-operative). Veneer was placed without any removal of tooth tissue

process. In the case of a stained tooth, this may require the placement of an opacious layer or indeed a white tint to mask out intrinsic stain prior to the opacious layer. Take note of any areas that may require further characterisation, such as craze lines, hypoplasia, translucency or the exposure of cervical dentine. It is worth noting these down in a diagrammatic format together with determining the shades you wish you use and their respective areas of placement.

Apply your chosen method of isolation. Rubber dam that has been inverted and retained in situ with ligatures is a gold standard, as in Chapter 5.2. The use of retraction cord will also help with the control of unwanted gingival crevicular fluid.

Using air abrasion, pumice or burs, roughen the surfaces where the resin is to be applied. Isolate adjacent teeth with an appropriate matrix such as PTFE (polytetrafluoroethylene) tape or a cellulose acetate strip. Condition the surfaces for resin bonding, as described in Chapter 5.1.

In the case of a deeply **discoloured tooth**, apply a thin layer of evenly distributed white resin tint over the labial face of the affected tooth, making sure that it is streak free. A thin layer of opacious dentine finished interdentally to an infinity margin should follow this. In the cervical area, you may choose to place some yellow tint to add body colour. In the incisal area, as the space to place restorative material may be too limited to allow the inclusion of mamelons, place some blue resin tint to mimic translucency and overlay with your chosen enamel shade. Finish and polish, as in Chapter 5.6.

For cases involving **diastema closure**, place a dead-soft sectional matrix band (as described in Chapter 5.3) into the interproximal area. The band should be gently slipped into the gingival crevice to avoid any overhanging margins developing. Contour your band using a burnisher, such that material may be applied to the desired horizontal dimension. The band may be additionally supported with the aid of a silicone key positioned palatally. Using a cotton wool pledget, form a custom wedge. Apply your chosen shade of material (which may be in enamel or dentine) as per your colour map. Form an interproximal pillar, as described in Chapter 5.4. Light cure according to the manufacturer's instructions. You may now remove the matrix. Apply further resin composite to complete the labial face. Repeat the procedure on the adjacent surface. Finish and polish accordingly, paying close attention to the embrasure space(s).

For cases involving an **increase in tooth length**, where the colour is acceptable (with or without the aid of a silicone key), place a thin layer of enamel shade across the entire labial face, finishing interproximally with an infinity margin. For resin veneers not involving an increase in tooth length, sculpt some mamelons and place some resin blue tint. Overlay with some enamel shade, finish and polish. Where an increase in length has been planned, you may choose to cut back palatally without breaching the labial face, and place some dentine shade into the areas of cut-back to characterise the incisal edge.

In the event of a **malformed tooth** such as a peg-shaped lateral incisor, resin augmentation would be carried out in a similar manner to a Class IV restoration, as described in Chapter 5.4.

For a **malpositioned tooth** such as a palatally placed tooth, the restorative approach will depend on the level of discrepancy. Where it is large, commence with a dentine shade of resin. The latter may be sculpted to account for the characterisation of the incisal edge, such as the presence of mamelons. Overlay with an enamel shade.

## Tips

- Resin composite veneers can provide a minimally invasive and desirable solution for the treatment of many problems in aesthetic restorative dentistry.
- The importance of informed consent should not be overlooked.
- Patients must be made aware of the maintenance requirements of resin veneers, including the need for regular polishing and possible repair.
- Allocate an appropriate amount of time when planning and making resin veneers; artistic efforts should not be rushed!

## Further Reading

Korkut B, Yanikoglu F, Gunday M. Direct composite laminate veneers. Three case reports. *J Dent Res Dent Clin Dent Prospects.* 2013;7(2):105–11.

Nalbandian S, Millar BJ. The effect of veneers on cosmetic improvement. *Br Dent Jour.* 2009;207(2):72–3.

## 5.8

# Repair and Refurbishment of Resin Composite Restorations

*Subir Banerji and Shamir B. Mehta*

*Video: Repair and Refurbishment of Resin Composite Restorations*
*Presented by Subir Banerji and Shamir B. Mehta*

## Principles

Very few clinicians would contest the notion of silver amalgam being a popular and successful restorative material. In recent years, however, particularly in light of the Minamata Treaty 2013 (which among several other objectives aims to phase down the use of dental amalgam), there has been an international shift concerning the placement of silver amalgam restorations, with countries such as Norway imposing a complete ban on the prescription of amalgam-based restorations by 2011 (primarily on account of environmental concerns).

In Australia, a government report published by a working group for the NHMRC (National Health and Medical Research Council) described a reduction in the provision of dental amalgam restorations by private general dental practitioners, from 57.9% in 1983–84 to 28.0% in 1997–98 (when considering the total number of dental restorations placed, inclusive of indirect restorations), thereby representing a reduction by almost 50%.[1]

This trend is most likely to be accounted for by the implementation of a more minimally invasive philosophy by dental practitioners, with a concomitant increase in the number of resin composite restorations, which *doubled* over the same time periods.

Directly bonded posterior resin composite restorations have indeed become increasingly popular for the conservative and aesthetic management of small to medium-sized cavities in posterior teeth. They may also potentially provide a means of strengthening and conserving the remaining tooth substrate in the longer term. However, direct resin restorations (of both the anterior and posterior varieties) are, as with most other dental materials, prone to failure or fracture. Many of the problems arise from inherent flaws relating to the physico-chemical properties of resin composite, such as polymerisation shrinkage, increased surface wear and bulk fracture.

Nevertheless, resin composite materials do offer the potential for **intra-oral repair** (which other materials such as metal alloys do not). Thus, in the case of a failed resin composite restoration, it has been advocated that the latter should be evaluated for possible repair instead of complete replacement and re-making, on the grounds of the need for reduced intervention.[2]

*Practical Procedures in Aesthetic Dentistry*, First Edition. Edited by Subir Banerji, Shamir B. Mehta and Christopher C.K. Ho. © 2017 John Wiley & Sons, Ltd. Published 2017 by John Wiley & Sons, Ltd.
Companion website: www.wiley.com/go/banerji/aestheticdentistry

There are a number of scenarios where **repair or refurbishment** of an existing resin composite restoration may be considered a suitable option:

- Loss of anatomical contour
- Marginal faults
- Surface roughness from wear
- Secondary caries when it is readily accessible
- Staining and reduced lustre.

There are also a number of more immediate considerations that may arise following the placement of a resin composite restoration that may require operator attention, such as the presence of voids, incorrect shade selection, suboptimal anatomical and occlusal form, inadequate proximal contact(s) or the presence of a white line or 'halo' at the restoration–tooth interface. The latter often results from traumatic finishing and polishing procedures, inadequate etching and bonding stages, or the use of a high-intensity light-curing source, which may result in excessive polymerisation shrinkage setting up stresses in the prismatic structure of the enamel.

For an immediately placed resin composite restoration that is yet to be contoured, further increments of resin composite may be predictably applied without any further intervention being required (such as abrasion or the addition of a bonding agent) due to the presence of an unpolymerised surface layer resulting from the oxygen inhibition phenomenon, which will permit successful chemical interaction with unpolymerised methacrylate groups.

For restorations that have been contoured, a number of different approaches have been described in the literature to permit **successful rebonding**. In each case, effective isolation, ideally with rubber dam, is optimal. The use of 50-micron diameter particles of aluminium oxide applied by **sandblasting** on the aged composite surface has been shown to enhance the shear bond strength of repaired dimethacrylate-based composites.[3] Abrasion will not only help to create **micro-mechanical retention**, but will also increase the surface energy to help wet the surface and will assist in removing any surface contamination.

Analogously, the application of a thin layer of bonding agent on aged composite restorations has been shown to enhance significantly the tensile strength of the repair procedure. The roughening of restoration surfaces associated with the application of a low-viscosity (flowable) resin also has the potential to enhance the repair bond strength.[3]

It is likely that surface roughening provides micro-mechanical retention, allowing monomer penetration into surface irregularities, as well as chemical adhesion promoted by solvents in the bonding system, which have been postulated to cause swelling and gelation of the surface layer, therefore allowing the monomer to penetrate the unconverted vinyl groups in the aged restoration. It is also possible that more recently placed resin composite restorations may offer slightly superior chances of successful re-bonding, as not only will the process of dark polymerisation possibly remain incomplete (resulting in the availability of unconverted monomers for chemical interaction), the material will also have been less contaminated by virtue of its presence in the oral environment over a relatively shorter time frame.

## Procedures

When carrying out a repair of an aged resin composite restoration, which may for instance have sustained a chip, commence by determining the appropriate shade. This may be challenging, as the aged restoration may have changed in colour following the absorption of chromogens and loss of lustre.

After isolation, **abrade** the fractured area using 50-micron aluminium oxide particles, or, if these are unavailable, use a coarse diamond bur. Cut back the existing material to expose fresh composite and bevel the fractured surface. You may choose to isolate the adjacent teeth with a suitable matrix to avoid unwanted adhesion.

Apply 37% phosphoric acid over the abraded surface for 15 seconds, rinse and air dry. This will help to provide a clean, contamination-free surface.

Apply either a lightly filled, low-viscosity resin (often referred to as a **surface sealer**) or an unfilled, very low-viscosity resin to the roughened surface. The lower the filler content, the better your material will penetrate the micro-mechanical areas created, as well as any interfacial crevices and cracks. Floss the interproximal contacts to remove any excess resin. Light cure for 40 seconds. This will also permit some polymerisation of the underlying resin composite, especially if it has been relatively recently placed.

When applying a viscous resin, use a sharp instrument to discard any excess resin.

Place your chosen resin composite and light cure.

Finish and polish, as described in Chapter 5.6, making sure to polish from the newly added material to the old – this will help to improve the marginal transition. Use a diamond or aluminium oxide polishing paste, and lightly glaze with a proprietary (solvent-free) glazing agent, such as Optraglaze (GC Corp., Tokyo, Japan). Light cure for 30 seconds.

In vitro evidence appears to suggest that for samples of material that have been aged in water and thermocycled to simulate oral conditions, the longer the period of time the material is soaked in water, or indeed if the material is subject to additional thermocycling, the lower the resultant shear bond strength will be. However, the use of a bonding agent to assist in the process of repair appears to improve the quality of the repair significantly.[4]

## Tips

- Consider the option of repair when dealing with failed resin composite restorations as part of attaining informed consent, as a possible minimally invasive alternative to replacement. Older restorations may offer lower prognostic outcomes. The use of abrasion and bonding resin is strongly advocated for restorations that have been previously finished and polished.
- Remember that the strength of the union between new and old materials may be less than 60% of the full strength of the material, as there will be limited methacrylate groups for reaction with the freshly placed material. Repair is therefore based primarily on micro-mechanical retention.

## References

1 Dental amalgam and mercury in dentistry. A report of a NHMRC working party. March 1999, Commonwealth of Australia. Available at www.nhmrc.gov.au.
2 Shawkat S, Shortall A, Addison O, Palin WM. Oxygen inhibition and incremental bond strengths of resin composites. *Dent Mater.* 2009;25(11):1338–46.
3 Hannig C, Laubach S, Hahn P, Attin T. Shear bond strength of repaired adhesive filling materials using different repair procedures. *J Adhes Dent.* 2006;8:35–40.
4 Staxrud F, Dahl J. Role of bonding agents in the repair of composite resin restorations. *Eur J Oral Sci.* 2011;119:316–22.

# Part VI

# Indirect Aesthetic Restorations

## 6.1

# Tooth Preparation for Full Coverage Restorations

*Christopher C.K. Ho*

*Video: Tooth Preparation for Full Coverage Restorations*
*Presented by Christopher C.K. Ho*

## Principles

The preparation of teeth for a full coverage restoration involves reduction of teeth to provide adequate mechanical and aesthetic properties in the restoration. This should be carried out atraumatically, with the conservation of tooth structures as an integral objective to minimise any pulpal or periodontal consequences from the procedures. Traditional preparation design for full coverage restorations has been based on retention and resistance form; however, the advent of adhesive dentistry has resulted in a paradigm shift towards less invasive preparations. There is increasing literature reporting on the ability to bond aesthetic materials adhesively with minimal or partial coverage preparations, although there is still concern in relation to a long-standing adhesive interface when dentine is the adhesive substrate.

Goodacre et al.[1] outline several scientific guidelines to ensure mechanical, biological and aesthetic success for tooth preparation in full coverage restorations.

### Taper or Total Occlusal Convergence (TOC)

This is the angle of convergence between opposing axial walls. The more parallel the opposing walls of the preparation, the greater the retention. Jorgensen described the inverse relationship between taper and retention and found a 6° taper to be ideal.[2] It is more common to see preparation TOC angles ranging from 12–27°. Goodacre et al. have proposed that the TOC ideally should range between 10° and 20°.[1]

### Occluso-cervical/Inciso-cervical Dimension

This dimension is an important factor for both retention and resisitance, with longer preparations possessing greater surface area and more retention. It is proposed that 3 mm is the minimal occluso-cervical (OC) dimension for premolars and anterior teeth, while 4 mm is suggested for molars when teeth are prepared within the TOC range of 10–20°.

*Practical Procedures in Aesthetic Dentistry*, First Edition. Edited by Subir Banerji, Shamir B. Mehta and Christopher C.K. Ho. © 2017 John Wiley & Sons, Ltd. Published 2017 by John Wiley & Sons, Ltd.
Companion website: www.wiley.com/go/banerji/aestheticdentistry

### Occluso-cervical/Inciso-cervical to Facio-lingual Dimensions

Masticatory function develops forces that are normally facio-lingual (FL) in direction. A critical factor is that adequate resistance is developed when the OC/FL dimension is 0.4 mm or higher for all teeth.

### Circumferential Morphology

Teeth that possess a round tooth morphology after preparation lack resistance and should be modified by the creation of grooves or boxes in axial surfaces.

### Margin Location

Subgingival margins are frequently required for retention and resistance form, to extend beyond caries, fractures or erosion/abrasion, to allow adequate ferrule or aesthetics. Orkin et al. have demonstrated the relationship of the position of crown margins and tissue health[3] and, despite research favouring supragingival margins, the majority of crown margins are placed subgingivally, which results in more recession, a higher plaque index, bleeding on probing and gingivitis. Biologic width is the distance established by the junctional epithelium and connective tissue attachment to the root surface of a tooth, or in simple terms it is the height between the deepest point of the gingival sulcus and the alveolar bone crest. Based on the 1961 paper by Gargiulio et al.,[4] the mean biologic width was determined to be 2.04 mm, of which 1.07 mm is occupied by the connective tissue attachment and another approximately 0.97 mm is occupied by the junctional epithelium. Placing crown margins that violate biologic width may lead to chronic inflammation of the gingiva, discomfort and loss of alveolar bone.

### Margin Design

Different margin designs include chamfer, knife-edge, shoulder and bevelled shoulder designs. Knife-edge preparations should be avoided, as they provide insufficient bulk at the margins and often over-contoured restorations result.

- **All-metal** – chamfer margins are recommended as they are distinct and well demarcated, providing sufficient bulk of material. This is recommended to be 0.5 mm in thickness.
- **Metal-ceramic** – different designs have historically been used, including chamfer, shoulder and bevelled shoulder. The selection of finish lines is based on personal preference, aesthetics and ease of fabrication (Figure 6.1.1). A recommended thickness of 1–1.7 mm has often been recommended for the porcelain veneered marginal area of metal-ceramic crowns.
- **All-ceramic** – either shoulder or chamfer finish lines can be selected for all-ceramic crowns bonded to prepared teeth, and margins of 0.8–1 mm are recommended.

### Reduction Depths

The required reduction depends on the position in the arch, aesthetic and occlusal considerations, as well as the different requirements of the materials used. Teeth that are

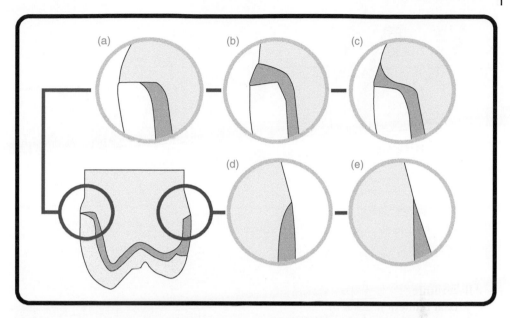

Figure 6.1.1 Marginal finish lines with marginal configuration for porcelain fused to metal restorations: (a) shoulder with porcelain butt margin, (b) deep chamfer with metal collar, (c) shoulder with bevel (metal collar), (d) knife edge with metal margin, (e) chamfer with metal margin

misaligned may require greater reduction to allow re-alignment to a satisfactory position. Sufficient reduction is required to allow for structural durability of the final restoration as well as ensuring that the final restoration is not over-contoured, endangering periodontal health (see Table 6.1.1 and Figure 6.1.2).

- **All-metal restoration**
  - Axial reduction: 0.5 mm
  - Occlusal reduction: 1.0 mm for non-functional cusps, 1.5 mm for functional cusps

- **Metal-ceramic restoration**
  - Axial reduction: a thickness of 1–1.7 mm has often been recommended for the porcelain veneered marginal area of metal-ceramic crowns
  - Incisal/occlusal reductions of 2.0–2.5 mm have been recommended for these restorations when restoring the surfaces with ceramic

Table 6.1.1 Preparation requrements for different materlals for crown and bridgework

| Crown type | Occlusal/incisal reduction | Axial reduction | Marginal design and depth |
|---|---|---|---|
| All metal | 1–1.5 mm | >0.5 mm | 0–1.0 mm Chamfer, knife-edge, shoulder or shoulder with bevel |
| Metal ceramic | 2–2.5 mm | 1–1.7 mm | 1.0 mm Shoulder or chamfer |
| All ceramic | 2–2.5 mm | 1.0 mm | 0.8–1.0 mm Rounded shoulder or chamfer |

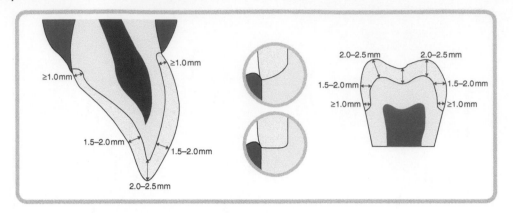

Figure 6.1.2 All-ceramic crown preparation requirements

- **All-ceramic**
  - ○ >Axial reduction: 1.0 mm
  - ○ Incisal/occlusal reduction: 2.0–2.5 mm recommeded to allow for correct occlusal morphology

### Line Angle Form

Internal line angles should be rounded to enhance strength, as sharp line angles create stress concentrations within all-ceramic restorations. In all-metal and metal-ceramic restorations, rounded line angles may allow simpler fabrication for technical procedures.

### Surface Roughness

In preparations with increased roughness there is improved crown retention for zinc phosphate cement. However, this does not appear to make any difference for adhesive cements.

### Auxillary Retention

In preparations where there may be limited retention and resistance form due to short axial walls, tapered preparations or circular geometric form, the use of mechanical grooves or boxes should be designed into the preparations. These grooves add near parallel-sided walls to prepare and assist with antirotation. Alternatively, surgical crown lengthening may be required to allow for adequate axial wall height. Consideration should also be given to using adhesive cementation to enhance the retention of the final restoration.

## Procedures

The preparation of teeth involves an understanding of the requirements of the different material properties for aesthetics and function, as well as balancing the need for conservative tooth preparation.

The amount of reduction can be controlled by the use of depth cuts. This should be with burs of known dimension, so for example if a 1 mm diameter bur is used to full depth, then understandably 1 mm of reduction has been achieved; if the bur is only taken to half the depth, then 0.5 mm has been prepared. Alternatively, preparation reduction matrices that are formed from diagnostic wax-ups can be used to gauge the required reduction to achieve the intended final tooth position.

The use of different bur designs can facilitate the required marginal finish line, from round-end flat cylinder diamonds to chamfered bur designs.

The author prefers a sequence that is systematically followed and allows predictability in preparation for crowns:

- **Depth cuts** – use the correct-sized bur for the amount of reduction, which allows depth cuts to be made to the correct depth.
- **Labial/buccal reduction** – preparation should remove enough tooth structure to remove the depth cuts. Care must be taken not to over-taper this axial wall, as it provides good retention with the lingual axial wall. Viewing the reduction from different viewpoints assists in ensuring that correct planes of adjustment have been carried out.
- **Lingual/palatal reduction** – the burs should be held parallel to the long axis of the tooth and the buccal prepared axial wall to allow relatively parallel preparations.
- **Occlusal/incisal reduction** – this reduction should follow the cuspal/incisal contours to allow adequate bulk of material. In posterior teeth adequate clearance should also be checked when patients move into lateral excursions.
- **Proximal reduction** – this can be difficult, as inadvertent damage to the adjacent tooth may take place. A fine tapered bur can be used for the preliminary reduction, keeping the bur within the tooth/core material and leaving a thin sliver that is eventually removed with subsequent burs.
- **Final preparation** – once the majority of the preparation has been undertaken in this sequence, investigate the taper of the preparation, reduction depth and lack of undercuts and adjust as necessary. The use of rubbers and polishing discs may help with the final stages of the preparation. Also assess adjacent teeth and ensure that adjacent restorations are smooth and free of overhangs. It may be necessary to modify the contact points so that a broad, flat contact is attained, in order that food does not get trapped between your new restoration and an old restoration. Assess whether additional retentive features may be required with the addition of grooves or boxes.

## Tips

- Closing one eye when assessing preparations will assist in checking the parallelism of the preparation and assessing for undercuts.
- Use of magnification with microscopes or loupes will aid in preparation as well as postural improvements.
- It can be difficult to gauge the amount of occlusal reduction for posterior teeth in certain patients. Asking a patient to bite into wax, then measuring the thickness with an Ivanson gauge (crown callipers), can ensure that sufficient reduction has been carried out.

- Ceramics are well able to withstand compressive stresses, but may fail catastrophically from tensile stresses. Non-axial forces produce the most stress occlusally and at the margins. Careful attention to occlusion to prevent shearing forces is advised, as well as the development of shallow cusp angles in the final restoration. Patients with severe parafunction should be provided with an occlusal splint.

## References

1 Goodacre CJ, Campagni WV, Aquilino SA. Tooth preparations for complete crowns: an art form based on scientific principles. *J Prosthetic Dent.* 2001 Apr;85(4):363–76.
2 Jorgensen KD. The relationship between retention and convergence angle in cemented veneer crowns. *Acta Odontol Scand.* 1955 Jun;13(1):35–40.
3 Orkin DA, Reddy J, Bradshaw D. The relationship of the position of crown margins to gingival health. *J Prosthet Dent.* 1987 Apr;57(4):421–4.
4 Gargiulo AW, Wenz FM, Orban B. Dimensions and relations of the dentogingival junction in humans. *J Periodontol.* 1961;32:261–7.

## Further Reading

Blair FM, Wassell RW, Steele JG. Crowns and other extra-coronal restorations: preparations for full veneer crowns. *Br Dent J.* 2002 May 25;192(10):561–71.
Owen CP. On form and function in all-ceramic restorations. *SADJ.* 2012;67(7):400–4.
Shillingberg HT, Hobo S, Whitsett L, Jacobi R, Brackett SE. *Fundamentals of fixed prosthodontics.* 3rd ed. Chicago, IL: Quintessenence; 1997.

## 6.2

# Tooth Preparation for Partial Coverage Restorations

*Christopher C.K. Ho*

## Principles

The development of adhesive dentistry has led to direct composite resin placement being the most conservative restoration. However, direct composite resin is subject to shrinkage as it is cured, which may lead to stresses within the material resulting in marginal failure, caries, marginal staining, tooth fracture and post-operative sensitivity. This shrinkage stress is increased with the size of the restoration. When the cavity preparation exceeds the limits recommended for direct application of composite resins, indirect full or partial coverage restorations are indicated. They can be superior to direct resins as they are fabricated indirectly, thereby optimising contour, anatomy, marginal and proximal finishing, with often better mechanical properties. Conventional full coverage preparation techniques provide the necessary mechanical retention for a restoration for conventional cementation; however, partial coverage all-ceramic restorations require bonding for retention.

The main principle of preparation is to maximise tissue preservation, with the cavity form depending on the decay present or previous restoration. There is a direct correlation of strength degradation with increased tooth structure removal.[1] Moreover, cusp stiffness is reduced significantly with increased tooth structure removal.[2] This increased tooth reduction may lead to catastrophic failure of the restoration and underlying tooth structure, hence preserving tooth structure may be critical for the longevity of the tooth and the restoration.

Deciding between use of a partial coverage onlay or a ceramic crown (whether fused to metal or not) can be difficult, but in general an onlay is preferred when sufficient tooth structure is present for predictable adhesion. With the onlay technique, adhesion between the etched ceramic and the tooth structure provides retention for the restoration, minimises marginal leakage and strengthens the tooth.

It is critical to conceptualise what is required in a partial coverage restoration preparation, and to be clear on the depth reduction in axial and occlusal/incisal planes, as well as the location of the margins to achieve the best clinical outcome.

A key to success with all-ceramic restorations is meticulous tooth preparation. The aims of tooth preparation are to provide the following:

- Sufficient thickness of the porcelain to ensure the necessary fracture resistance, without over-contouring of the final restoration.

*Practical Procedures in Aesthetic Dentistry*, First Edition. Edited by Subir Banerji, Shamir B. Mehta and Christopher C.K. Ho. © 2017 John Wiley & Sons, Ltd. Published 2017 by John Wiley & Sons, Ltd.
Companion website: www.wiley.com/go/banerji/aestheticdentistry

- A margin, so that the ceramist has a definite finishing line, allowing a normal emergence profile from the gingival margin.
- A finished preparation that, in addition to supporting and retaining the restoration, is smooth and free of any sharp line angles, which may cause stress concentrations within the ceramic.
- The creation of a passive seating pattern.

Before the preparation is initiated, removal of the failed restoration (with any carious tissue) is performed. There is often no need to eliminate internal undercuts, as these will be blocked by the technician before making the restoration. However, they can be filled with a base material to avoid destructive preparations. All line anges should be rounded to minimise stress. It is important that the required minimum thickness of material is ensured for the entire restoration. Insufficient tooth preparation, particularly in the areas of the central grooves or at the internal line angles (the ridge between the occlusal and interproximal box), may lead to fracture of the restoration. In cases where tooth structure is degraded due to caries, reconstruction is limited to removal of decay and establishment of a convenience form, as well as to provide ideal cavity form.

## Procedures

### Depth Reduction

- Occlusal isthmus width should be greater than 1.5 mm.
- Occlusal reduction needs to be at least 2 mm deep to allow sufficient thickness of ceramic. The occlusal plane constitutes an important reference with regard to tooth reduction. When the opposing dentition presents cusps that do not respect the occlusal plane, these should be re-contoured to avoid interference with the future restoration.

### Margin Design

- Butt joint preparations provide an acceptable finishing design on enamel, giving sufficient thickness and ease of preparation.
- A deep chamfer margin produces an alternative margin that simultaneously provides a better aesthetic transition between the restoration and the enamel. The use of a chamfer margin on occlusal margins is not recommended as the risk of marginal fracture is high, and thus it should only be used for marginal finishing lines on the axial walls.
- Margins should not coincide with occlusal contacts.

### Cavity Design and Configuration

- Adhesive resin bonding significantly increases retention, therefore a retentive preparation design is not a priority for bonded ceramic restorations.
- Due to the indirect nature of the restoration, there is a path of insertion/removal for the restoration and hence the walls are made divergent.
- This taper of divergence should be minimal for conservation; 10–15° of divergence has been advocated for ease of manipulation and cementation. Increasing the taper of divergence may simplify insertion and removal at the expense of removal of tooth structure, as well as weakening the overall structural integrity of the tooth.

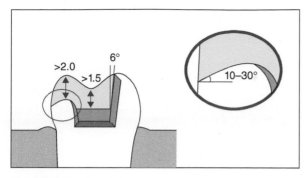 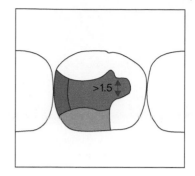

*Note:* Specifications in mm

Figure 6.2.1 Onlay and inlay preparation requirements

- Small undercuts are acceptable or may be blocked out with a base material such as a flowable composite liner or compomer restoration.
- All internal angles should be rounded and the cavosurface angle prepared to 90° with no bevels.

Onlay and inlay preparation requirements are summarised in Figure 6.2.1.

## Tips

- Mark occlusal contacts with articulating film when preparing for partial coverage restorations to avoid placing a margin in the occlusal contact areas.
- To assess that adequate depth of reduction is performed, depth grooves should be used within the preparation. If unsure, check adequate reduction by asking the patient to occlude into wax/bite-registration material and measure the thickness. Alternatively this can be assessed by measuring the provisional restoration.
- The use of a base is not always necessary, although it may help in removing undercuts. It may also aid in providing a more even thickness of ceramic, which minimises stresses within the ceramic during firing procedures.

## References

1 St-Georges AJ, Sturdevant JR, Swift EJ, Thompson JY. Fracture resistance of prepared teeth restored with bonded inlay restorations. *J Prosthet Dent* 2003;89:551–7.
2 Magne P, Knezevic A. Influence of overlay restorative materials and load cusps on the fatigue resistance of endodontically treated molars. *Quintessence Int* 2009;40:729–37.

## Further Reading

Dietschi D, Spreafico R. *Adhesive metal-free restorations: current concepts for the esthetic treatment of posterior teeth*. Berlin: Quintessence; 1997.
Magne P, Dietschi D, Holz J. Esthetic restorations for posterior teeth: practical and clinical considerations. *Int J Periodontics Restorative Dent*. 1996;16:104–19.

## 6.3

# Provisionalisation

*Christopher C.K. Ho*

## Principles

A provisional restoration is defined by the glossary of prosthodontic terms as a fixed or removable dental prosthesis designed to enhance aesthetics, stabilisation and/or function for a limited period of time, after which it is to be replaced by a definitive dental prosthesis. Often such prostheses are used to assist in determination of the therapeutic effectiveness of a specific treatment plan or confirming the form and function of the planned definitive prosthesis.

Provisionals serve the following functions:

- Pulpal protection from bacterial microleakage and thermal and chemical irritation, as well as providing a coronal seal for endodontically treated teeth.
- Maintenance and promotion of periodontal health. However, ensuring adequate contours and well-fitting margins is paramount in facilitating optimal oral hygiene. Moreover, a provisional restoration may also be used in clinical situations when the gingival margin may augment, such as after crown lengthening or following the removal of an overhanging restoration.
- Occlusion and positional stability. Inter-arch and intra-arch relationships are maintained through both proximal and occlusal contacts, preventing tipping, drifting and supra-eruption.
- Allowing adequate function. Patients should be able to function adequately, but should be cautioned on the temporary nature of the restoration.
- Providing adequate aesthetics. Acceptable aesthetics are required during the provisional phase as well as to assist in evaluating the planned intended changes.
- A diagnostic tool. Through duplication of the wax-up a preview of the intended aesthetic, occlusal and occlusal vertical dimension changes can be made (Figure 6.3.1). This allows adequate opportunity for the patient to receive a trial protoype to gain acceptance and approval. This is an important step when preparing multiple anterior restorations, as the patient may need time to adjust to the planned changes. It is the author's view that the patient should be left to assess changes over a few days before returning to assess any modifications that may be required, as the transformations

*Practical Procedures in Aesthetic Dentistry*, First Edition. Edited by Subir Banerji, Shamir B. Mehta and Christopher C.K. Ho. © 2017 John Wiley & Sons, Ltd. Published 2017 by John Wiley & Sons, Ltd.
Companion website: www.wiley.com/go/banerji/aestheticdentistry

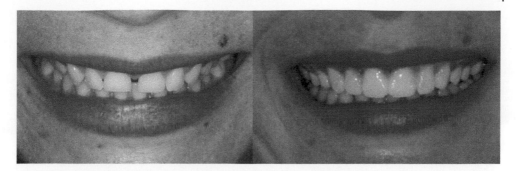

Figure 6.3.1 Diagnostic wax-up transferred to patient for mock-up to assess aesthetic changes with provisional materials for approval and consent

may take the patient some time to adjust to. Provisional restorations may also be used to measure the amount of reduction carried out by checking the thickness of the provisional restoration.

## Procedures

Provisional restorations can be fabricated directly chairside or indirectly in a laboratory. The majority of provisional restorations are fabricated chairside. However, for long-term provisionalisation or more complex and extensive rehabilitations, there are clear advantages to having them fabricated in a laboratory.

There is a diverse spectrum of materials that can be used for the fabrication of provisional restorations:

- Preformed crowns (resin, plastic or metal; Figure 6.3.2)
- Self-cured or light-cured resin
- Self-cured or heat-cured acrylic
- Metal, e.g. iso-form crowns of tin/silver alloy, stainless steel crowns of nickel chrome.

### Direct Techniques

The majority of provisional restorations are fabricated chairside, directly in the patient's mouth.

- **Shell crowns** – these can be made from custom or stock shells that are relined with resin, trimmed and polished.
- **Matrices** – these are the most common as they duplicate the external contours of teeth that are being prepared or from a diagnostic wax-up. They are usually formed by alginate, silicone or vacuum-formed thermoplastic materials (Figure 6.3.3).
- **Directly** – freehand build-up may be possible by adding material to the teeth, sculpting and trimming/polishing.

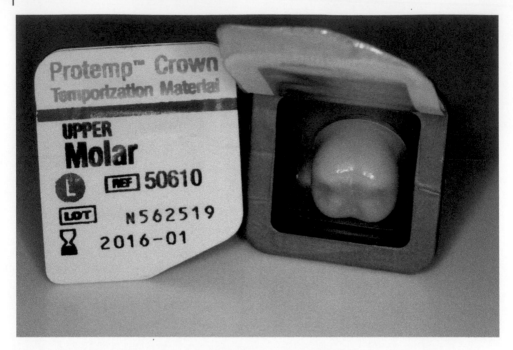

**Figure 6.3.2** Protemp crown (3M, St Paul, MN, USA) – malleable preformed crown that can be customised to size and adapted prior to curing

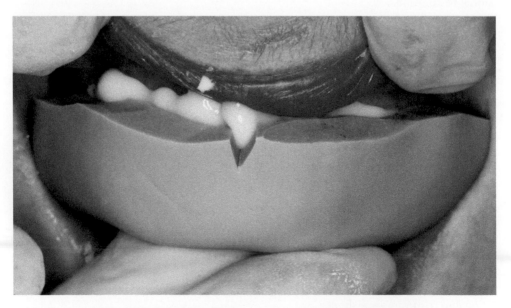

**Figure 6.3.3** Silicone key developed from diagnostic wax-up. Note that a notch has been made between the central incisors to allow easy placement on the teeth. The injection of the flowable tip should always be kept within the material in order not to incorporate voids

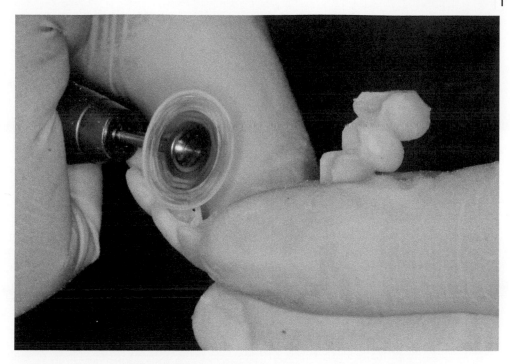

Figure 6.3.4 Trimming of multiple provisionals may be enhanced with the use of a disc that allows simpler adjustment of embrasure spaces

### Indirect Techniques

It is possible to make an impression and have a cast poured up in the laboratory, thereby making a provisional (Figure 6.3.4). This adds further cost, but it has several advantages, including using a material that may be stronger and more durable or reinforced with metal or fibres. It may be also used in multiple restorations and where an increase in vertical dimension or changes in occlusal scheme is planned.

### Provisionalisation of Adhesive Preparations

The development of adhesive dentistry has led to conservative preparations with partial coverage and minimal preparation. Consequently, this may lead to a lack of conventional retention, resulting in the temporary cement not being effective. In these situations no temporary may be necessary, for instance minimal preparation veneer preparations. Moreover, a harder cement such as polycarboxylate or zinc phosphate may be used temporarily, or the technique of spot etching and adhesively bonding the tooth may be helpful.

### Cementation

Provisional restorations are usually cemented with soft cements, such as TempBond, which allows ease of removal. The use of non-eugenol cements such as TempBond NE (non-eugenol) is recommended where the use of resin cements is anticipated, as euge-nol has a plasticising effect on resin cements and bonding agents.

There have been developments of resin temporary cements such as TempBond Clear, a translucent colourless temporary cement. This is useful for anterior provision-als where a conventional temporary cement may be opaque, rendering the temporary unaesthetic.

## Tips

- The use of provisional restorations when treating all anterior teeth in the arch is an opportunity to provide the patient with a 'trial smile'. Hence it is clinically significant to have a range of shades for your provisional material of choice, in order to demon-strate the shade selected for approval.
- Should there be a void or marginal deficiency, it is possible to add flowable composite resin to fill these areas.
- It is advisable to inform the patient of the correct 'flossing technique' around a provi-sional restoration. It is recommended to pull the floss through the embrasure rather than the contact point, to avoid possible decementation of the provisional restoration.

## 6.4

## Impressions and Soft Tissue Management

*Tom Giblin*

## Principles

When fabricating indirect restorations, the fit and accuracy are only as good as the impression that the clinician makes. The principles of making a good impression are the same whether performing traditional impressions or with the latest digital impression technologies: healthy tissues, sufficient tissue retraction, identifiable margins, a dry field, appropriate impression material and good impression technique.

### Tooth and Periodontal Health

Good periodontal health aids in restorative success by ensuring that the gingival levels are healthy and stable, the teeth are periodontally sound with minimal movement, and there is no bleeding when attempting to make impressions or cement the final prosthesis.

### Subgingival Margins

Traumatising the gingiva during tooth preparation should be avoided. A deep margin may also make it difficult to ensure complete excess cement removal.

Gargiulo et al. described the attachments of bone and soft tissues around teeth in 1961.[1] Placement of a subgingival margin may impinge on the biologic width. This has been addressed in Chapter 4.1. If the preparation violates the attachment of the tooth, a phenomenon called biologic width impingement occurs, a chronic inflammatory response that results in the soft tissues around the area being constantly red, inflamed and prone to bleeding. As a general rule, margins should be kept 3 mm from the bony crest to restorative margin, confirmed by bone sounding if necessary.

### High, Normal and Low Crest

When assessing periodontal tissues, it is important to establish how stable the tissues are. Kois described the stability of gingival tissues in relation to the underlying bone levels.[2] This is measured by bone sounding to the bony crest and measuring the distance to the

*Practical Procedures in Aesthetic Dentistry*, First Edition. Edited by Subir Banerji, Shamir B. Mehta and Christopher C.K. Ho. © 2017 John Wiley & Sons, Ltd. Published 2017 by John Wiley & Sons, Ltd.
Companion website: www.wiley.com/go/banerji/aestheticdentistry

gingival margin. Normal crest patients (3 mm from gingival margin to the crest of the bone) have normal biologic width, the bone levels are normal and the gingival margins should be stable. In high crest patients (<3 mm from gingival margin to bone), the alveolar bone sits very close to the cemento-enamel junction (CEJ) and may require crown-lengthening surgery to ensure that the biologic width is not invaded. In a low crest patient (>3 mm from gingival margin to bone), the alveolar bone is significantly below the CEJ, which may cause instability of the gingival tissues, and possibly recession even with the lightest of trauma, such as occurs when preparing teeth or placing retraction cord.

### Tissue Biotype

Thin tissues may be susceptible to recession associated with the trauma of preparations and impressions more than thicker tissue types. An easy determinant of this was described by Cook et al. and involves the placement of a periodontal probe into the sulcus and assessing whether or not it is visible through the tissues.[3]

### Retraction

The first requirement for a good impression is that the margin be free of soft tissue, blood and moisture. In order to achieve this, the dentist may either prepare the margin supragingivally, so that there is no tissue touching the margin, or use retraction cord or paste to reflect the tissues away from the margin of the tooth to achieve haemostasis and a patent sulcus (Figure 6.4.1).

Retraction cord is placed into the sulcus surrounding a tooth to displace the soft tissues physically out of the way. This produces a 'void' between the tooth and soft tissue in which the impression material can be placed to ensure capture of the preparation margin. Donovan states that a void of 0.2 mm is required to give an adequate amount of impression material bulk.[4] This not only ensures that the material does not tear on retraction due to being too thin, it also allows better definition of the margin in the laboratory, making trimming the die easier and more predictable for the laboratory technician.

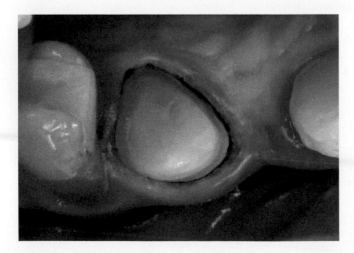

Figure 6.4.1 The aim of retraction is to displace tissues away from the margin and establish a moisture free sulcus to allow impression material to flow freely in

There are different types of cord available: twisted, knitted or braided cotton. However, the main characteristics required of them are to be easy to pack, to maintain their volume, not to stick to or tear the tissues and to act as a reservoir for astringent materials. There are different techniques and combinations of cord used depending on preference, but a common one is a two-cord technique.

Recently there has been an increase in the number of non-cord retraction methods. These are generally a clay-based material mixed with an astringent that is injected under some pressure into the sulcus, causing tissue retraction. The material then absorbs sulcular and oral fluids and swells, maintaining the retraction. After the required time, the material is rinsed out with water before impressions are made. A disadvantage is that the retraction may not be sufficient and uniform around the tooth, leading to problems with impression material tearing or difficulties reading the margins in the laboratory. In the author's experience, a combination of cord and retraction paste can work well, depending on the situation.

Surgical retraction using a tissue trimming bur, a laser, electrocautery or radio frequency device that physically 'troughs' around the tooth, leaving a void for the impression material to flow into, can also be effective. However, further tissue ablation may be needed to achieve haemostasis, or a haemostatic agent may be applied. These methods ensure good retraction of the tissues, but as they cause trauma to the gingiva, it may not return to the state or position it was in previously, leading to an unpredictable result.

### Chemical Astringents

These products are designed to stop blood and gingival crevicular fluids seeping into the gingival sulcus and affecting the impression material. Some of the products that are generally considered safe are ferric sulfate, aluminium chloride, zinc chloride and aluminium sulfate.

### Impression Materials

Three main types of impression materials are available.

Polyvinyl siloxane (PVS) is the current rubber material of choice for the majority of clinicians for final impressions. It is easy to dispense, comes in a variety of consistencies, set times and rigidities, and is quite stable. It can be mixed together with other PVS materials and may be added to if needed. The material is generally well tolerated, with the flavour not being too offensive to patients. The downside to PVS is that it is chemically a hydrophobic material. This is not desirable in a wet environment like the mouth. Most brands will add surfactants of some sort to the product to reduce the impact of this problem, but to limited effect (despite their vigorous marketing to the contrary!). Therefore, moisture and blood control is vital with this material, but in a dry environment it is very accurate and predictable.

Polyether is another material that is very popular. It is more hydrophilic than PVS and so tolerates a moist environment better. It does not come in as many set times or consistencies as PVS, but flows nicely, has good tear strength and is quite rigid. This can be a benefit when making implant and multiunit impressions, but can create problems in cases where there are large undercuts or existing bridges at the impression, which can get locked in easily.

Alginate is an excellent material for study models, opposing models and removable partial denture impressions. It is economical, fast setting and accurate. It can be mixed to different consistencies without affecting the final set accuracy and is generally well tolerated by patients. It does need to be poured within 10–15 minutes, as it undergoes significant dimensional change with water imbibition or syneresis (dehydration). For this reason it may be unsuitable for dentists without facilities to pour models immediately.

### Impression Trays

Impression trays are designed to contain the impression material during an impression and allow application of direct pressure when seating the impression. Ideally, the impression tray should fit as closely to the teeth and tissues as possible without touching or distorting them. Custom impression trays may be more desirable and more accurate, as they provide a universal spacing of the impression material.

Inaccuracies may occur if material separates from the tray when it is withdrawn from the mouth. Perforations and adhesives in the trays allow mechanical locking of the impression material to the tray. Rim-lock trays enable the impression material to be seated back into the same position without distortion if separation were to occur.

### Digital Impressions

As dentistry advances and new computer-aided design/computer-aided manufacturing (CAD/CAM) technologies have developed, there is more of a push to do away with traditional impression techniques and their mess and discomfort. With digital fabrication of restorations, it makes sense to dispense with many of the inaccuracies of the traditional workflow and acquire the impression digitally (Figure 6.4.2).

Most of the scanners on the market today are accurate for up to 4–5 units using either still image or video technology, with scanning accuracy down to 10–20 microns. The digital technology has been shown to be better than traditional impressions in numerous studies, and in comparison is accurate to around 35 microns. The role of CAD/CAM is covered in Chapter 6.9.

## Procedures

- Once contacts are broken and the margin is accessible around the entire tooth, a small cord soaked in a haemostatic agent should be placed to retract the tissue slightly. If in doubt about the bone levels, bone sounding can be done at this point.
- Once the preparation is finished, a second, larger haemostatic-soaked cord can be placed, or if minimal retraction is required an astringent paste may be used (e.g. Expasyl, Kerr Corporation, Orange, CA, USA).
- Light body material should be ready to do a wash and some heavier material should be loaded in the tray. If the gingiva is thick and might displace the light body, consider using a wash with monophase/medium viscosity or similar.
- When ready to pull the cord or remove the astringent, flush the area gently with water and remove the cord gently or rinse the paste away.
- Dry the mouth and preparations, being sure not to accidentally traumatise the site and cause bleeding. If there is bleeding, a quick application of pressure with a cotton pellet soaked in haemostatic agent usually suffices before carefully drying again.

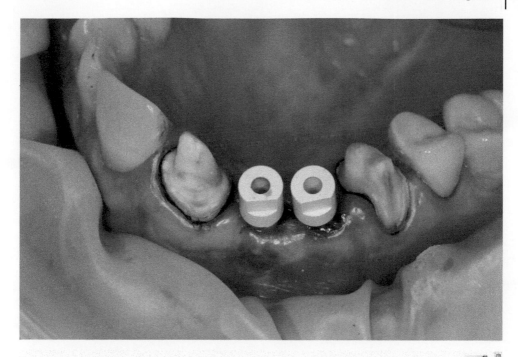

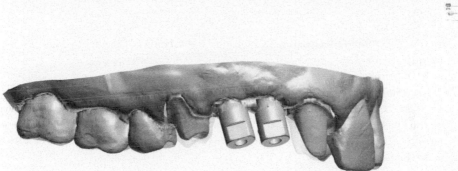

Figure 6.4.2 Intra-oral digital implant impressions can also be acquired using special abutments called scan bodies

- While applying the light body around the tooth using a fine mixing tip, care should be taken so as not to traumatise the sulcus. The tip should be kept buried in the material to avoid creating air bubbles. Once the tooth is covered, it can help to air thin the material gently using a triple syringe before re-applying more material. It also helps to flow light body into the fissures of the surrounding teeth to avoid occlusal air bubbles, and often into the embrasures and undercuts around the arch to stop the impression becoming locked in (the light body is less rigid and therefore is less likely to get stuck in an undercut, and it also makes the impression easier to remove).
- Gently seat the impression straight down on the teeth with even pressure. Ensure that you only seat the tray 80–90% so that you do not touch the teeth. At this point a timer may be useful to ensure that the impression is not removed until the material is fully set.

- Once set, remove the impression gently and assess the margins. If OK, then you can move on to the next step such as the opposing impression. If not, quickly dry the preparations and mouth again and make a new impression with the second pre-prepared tray.

## Tips

- Try in trays and paint adhesive for impressions only after packing your final cord – it will force you to wait for adequate retraction time.
- Wet retraction cord first before pulling it out before the impression – this will stop it sticking to the tissues and will therefore not cause trauma on withdrawal and start bleeding.
- With thicker tissues that are more difficult to retract, try using a heavier impression material in the sulcus, as it will maintain the displacement of the tissues.
- Use lip retraction to aid in establishing a dry field, visualisation and also seating the trays.
- Have a second tray of the same size painted with adhesive and be ready to make a second impression immediately after the first, in case there is a problem with the impression – this will avoid the retracted tissues collapsing and the need to place retraction cord again.

## References

1  Gargiulo AW, Wenz FM, Orban B. Dimensions and relations of the dentogingival junction in humans. *J Periodontol.* 1961;32:261–7.
2  Kois JC. Altering gingival levels: the restorative connection part I: biologic variables. *J Esthet Restor Dent.* 1994;6(1):3–7.
3  Cook R, Mealey B, Verrett R, et al. Relationship between periodontal biotype and labial plate thickness: an in vivo study. *Int J Periodont Restorative Dent.* 2011;31(4):345–54.
4  Donovan TE, Chee WW. Current concepts in gingival displacement. *Dent Clin North Am.* 2004 Apr;48(2):433–44.

## Further Reading

Baba NZ, Goodacre CJ, Jekki R, Won J. Gingival displacement for impression making in fixed prosthodontics: contemporary principles, materials, and techniques. *Dent Clin North Am.* 2014 Jan;58(1):45–68
Cook R. Relationship between periodontal biotype & labial plate thickness. 2012. http://www.ryancookdds.com/pdf/IT-Periodontal-Biotype.pdf
Nugala B, Kumar BBS, Sahitya S, Krishna PM. Biologic width and its importance in periodontal and restorative dentistry. *J Conserv Dent.* 2012 Jan–Mar;15(1):12–17.

# 6.5

# Aesthetic Posts and Cores

*Subir Banerji and Shamir B. Mehta*

## Principles

Restoration of the endodontically treated tooth can prove highly challenging, particularly where there has been a copious loss of coronal tooth tissue. Under such circumstances there is often a need to place a **post** (commonly referred to as a dowel) in the root canal chamber. The function of a post is primarily to retain a **core**, which will in turn provide support for the definitive restoration. A post will also provide protection to the remaining tooth structure by distributing occlusal stresses to the root along the post.

It is difficult to define the precise indications for a post. Historically, where there may have been less than half of the coronal volume remaining, the prescription of a post would have been given due consideration.[1] Where possible, however, the placement of a post should be avoided, as it may cause further weakening of the tooth, there may be risks of iatrogenic damage (including inadvertent perforations and disturbance of the apical seal), it may render access to the root canal system difficult (should root canal retreatment or post replacement be required) and further financial costs will be encountered when planning a post and core restoration.

There are a large variety of post and core systems in today's marketplace. They may be classified in accordance with their shape (tapered versus parallel), their composition (metallic versus non-metallic) and their method of fabrication (direct versus indirect).

Traditionally, the use of parallel-sided metal posts has commonly been advocated. However, the potential risks of root fracture (on account of a marked difference in the modulus of elasticity between root dentine and the post material, of up to and more than 13-fold) is a significant drawback.[2] The use of metallic posts is also associated with the risk of corrosion, the need for further tooth preparation to provide retention form, an alteration of the optical properties of the overlying restoration, concomitant darkening of the gingival margin (especially in patients with thin gingival biotypes in the aesthetic zone), as well as difficulties with removal.

In more recent times, the use of posts fabricated in **ceramic (zirconia)** or **composite** (based on epoxy resin) has become popular, providing an aesthetic alternative. While bio-compatible, zirconia posts have a similar modulus of elasticity to stainless steel.

*Practical Procedures in Aesthetic Dentistry*, First Edition. Edited by Subir Banerji, Shamir B. Mehta and Christopher C.K. Ho. © 2017 John Wiley & Sons, Ltd. Published 2017 by John Wiley & Sons, Ltd. Companion website: www.wiley.com/go/banerji/aestheticdentistry

Therefore, root fractures may be a more likely occurrence, as may endodontic failure, as a provisional post-retained restoration may be required (with an increased risk of bacterial ingress by the process of micro-leakage).

**Fibre-reinforced resin posts** have gained in popularity over the past few years. They have the potential to offer a number of advantages, which include:

- Aesthetics
- Reduced risk of root fracture (lower modulus of elasticity compared to metallic posts)
- Potential to chemically bond to resin-based luting agent, to form a 'monoblock'
- Ease of retrieval
- Direct technique (reduced costs and less need for laboratory-fabricated post and core), with lower risks of micro-leakage as a provisional restoration will not be required.

However, as fibre-resin posts are industrially light cured (with a high concomitant level of polymerisation conversation), there may be little remaining free resin to interact with the reactive chemical components present in resin lutes or resin composite cores. Consequently, the formation of a 'monoblock' may be far less effective than expected. The increased flexibility of these posts when compared with metallic posts also increases the risk of post-core fracture (particularly among teeth that receive higher occlusal loading in a lateral direction).[3]

This chapter provides a step-by-step approach to the planning and placement of a Fibre-White ParaPost (Coltene/Whaledent), an example of whicb is shown in Figure 6.5.1.

## Procedures

Where a post-retained restoration is planned, carefully assess the endodontic status of the tooth in question both clinically and radiographically. Of pertinent note is the quality of the root filling as well as the clinical absence of any periapical pathology, perforation or root fracture.

Evaluate the restorative prognosis of the tooth, noting the quality and quantity of residual tooth structure, the periodontal status and the patient's occlusal scheme (in both static and dynamic positions). The use of a calibrated periodontal probe to ascertain the presence of a circumferential collar of tooth tissue (of a minimum of 2 mm in the vertical dimension), commonly referred to as a **ferrule**, is advisable. This is critical in determining the prognostic outcome of all post-retained crown restorations.

Following rubber dam placement, plan the removal of gutta percha to permit the retention of a minimal seal of 5 mm in the apical portion of the tooth.[4] The removal of gutta percha for post preparation is best initiated with Gates Glidden burs, followed by refinement of the canal space using drill sets provided by the manufacturer.

There is no need to prepare the post space beyond what is necessary to fit the canal space; nor is it necessary to prepare any antirotational features. Naturally occurring undercuts should be preserved to aid core retention.

Using a pair of college tweezers, retrieve the post from the packaging and try-in the Fibre-White ParaPost (as seen in Figure 6.5.2). The retentive head of the post should extend through the resin composite core. Adjust the post if necessary to the desired length. It should be cut apically using a diamond bur in a high-speed handpiece with a water spray, keeping the bur perpendicular to the long axis of the post to avoid damage to the fibre structure and its mechanical characteristics. Ideally, the length of the post within the root should be at least equal to, or greater than, the height of the clinical crown.[3]

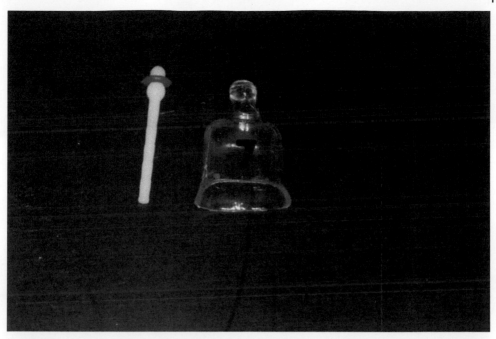

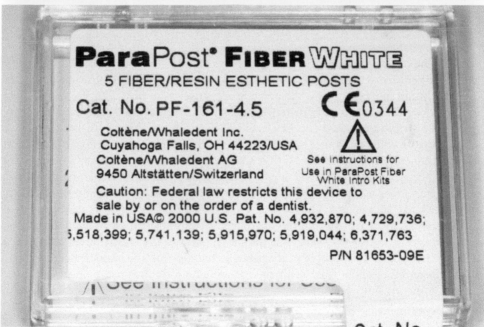

Figure 6.5.1 A Fibre-White ParaPost and core former (Para-Form, Coletene/Whaledent Inc., Cuyagoga Falls, OH, USA)

Prepare the canal space for adhesive luting. Treat the space using orthophosphoric acid for a period of 15 seconds; rinse with water for 10 seconds and gently dry with air. Absorbent points should be placed into the canal space to ensure the absence of any traces of etchant or moisture.

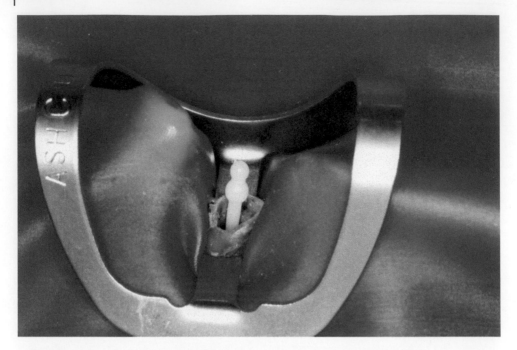

Figure 6.5.2  Try-in of a Fibre-White ParaPost

Using a proprietary micro-brush, apply your chosen self-cured (or dual-cured) activator to the canal space and the post as per the manufacturer's instructions. You may choose to remove excess agent using an absorbent point. Light cure if recommended.

Place the luting cement into the canal space. Insert the post into the canal space. Lightly move the post up and down the canal space in a vertical direction, to allow the effective distribution of cement. Once you are satisfied that the post is fully seated, using pressure with your finger to maintain the post in situ, apply an initial burst of light (to commence polymerisation). With a sharp probe, remove any excess cement and light cure in accordance with the manufacturer's recommendations, maintaining the tip of the light-curing unit over the head of the post, to permit optimal light transmission along the length of the post.

Prepare the root face and the retentive head of the post for adhesive bonding to a resin composite core. Make sure that you have removed the elastic identification ring from the head of the post. Apply your chosen etchant, prime and bond. Resin composite should be carefully applied, ensuring optimal contact with the post, pulp chamber and root face. Incremental layering may help reduce the incidence of voids within the resin core, and avoid the occurrence of a 'soggy bottom' (uncured basal layer) within the resin core. You may choose to use a 'core former', as shown in Figure 6.5.1.

Light cure as per the manufacturer's instructions. Following a period of time to allow for dark polymerisation (usually 7–20 minutes), prepare the core material to receive your prescribed indirect restoration. A ferrule of 2 mm is desirable. A completed tooth preparation with fibre-resin post-retained core is shown in Figure 6.5.3.

The definitive restoration should be contoured so as to conform to the existing occlusal scheme and provide an occlusal holding contact with the antagonistic tooth (in the intercuspal position, verified using articulating foil), with minimal contact during dynamic mandibular movements.

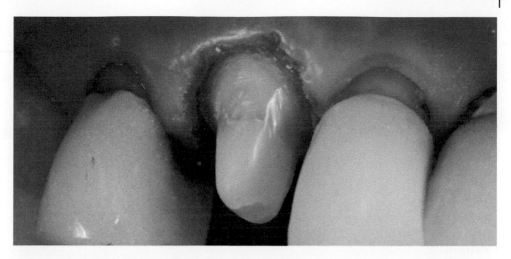

Figure 6.5.3  A completed resin fibre post and core restoration, with a 2 mm ferrule. *Source*: M Patel, Surrey, UK. Reproduced with permission from M Patel.

## Tips

- Your choice of luting agent and core material may influence the outcome of your definitive restoration.
- The prognostic outcome of teeth restored with such posts may be further guarded where the patient has a tendency for parafunctional tooth clenching/grinding, and/or among teeth that receive heavy occlusal loading in a lateral direction.[3]
- Always plan for failure!

## References

1 Christensen G. Posts: necessary or unnecessary? *J Am Dent Assoc.* 1996;127:1522–4.
2 Stewardson D. Non-metallic post systems. *Dent Update.* 2001;28:326–36.
3 Mehta SB, Millar BJ. A comparison of the survival of fibre posts cemented with two different composite resin systems. *Br Dent J.* 2008;205:E23.
4 Portell F, Bernier W, Lorton L, Peters D. The effect of immediate versus delayed dowel space preparation on the integrity of the apical seal. *J Endod.* 1982;8:154–60.

## 6.6

# Appraisal and Cementation

*Christopher C.K Ho*

## Principles

Cementation is the final stage in providing a successful restoration and requires as much care and diligence as the preceding stages. The final result may be suboptimal should a restoration not seat fully, leading to poor marginal integrity, recurrent caries and poor gingival health as well as occlusal interferences.

### Appraisal

Careful evaluation of the restoration is an important step to assess that the crown seats entirely, with excellent marginal integrity and fit. There are three stages to this appraisal.

#### Check the Crown on the Prepared Die

The crown should be checked on the prepared cast to ensure complete fit with no marginal deficiency or over-contouring. Check whether the die itself has been damaged at all, as it may be altered, and consequently may not allow your crown to seat in the mouth. It is good practice to have a second pour of the die or a 'verification die' to check the fit on an unaltered cast to ensure that the restoration seats on both dies (Figure 6.6.1).

#### Seat the Crown

The prepared tooth must be thoroughly cleaned of all temporary cement and plaque. The use of a pumice slurry or aluminium oxide air abrasion 27 micron at 40 psi is recommended (Figure 6.6.2). Once clean, the restoration is placed onto the preparation and should seat fully. There may be several reasons that the crown does not seat, including tight proximal contacts that cause binding of the restoration, trapped cement or soft tissues, inaccurate impression or poor fit of the restoration. The crown may be adjusted with the use of articulating film, disclosing material or aerosol disclosing sprays. Careful and judicious adjustment may allow the restoration to seat fully to the prepared depth; however, a new impression may be required should a crown not seat fully.

*Practical Procedures in Aesthetic Dentistry*, First Edition. Edited by Subir Banerji, Shamir B. Mehta and Christopher C.K. Ho. © 2017 John Wiley & Sons, Ltd. Published 2017 by John Wiley & Sons, Ltd.
Companion website: www.wiley.com/go/banerji/aestheticdentistry

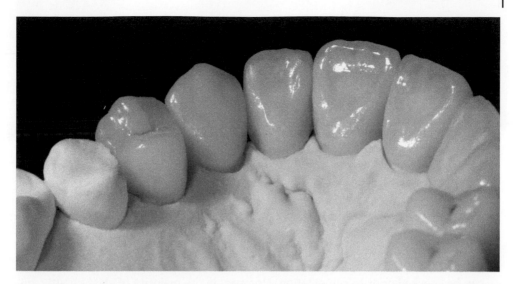

Figure 6.6.1 Assessment of crowns on the dies and unsectioned models to check fit, contact points and overall form and contour

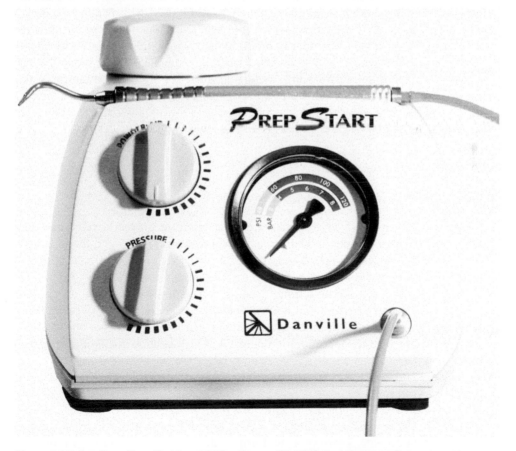

Figure 6.6.2 PrepStart (Danville Materials, San Ramon, CA, USA) air abrasion to clean preparation prior to seating of restorations. Alternatively a pumice slurry may be used to clean the preparations

### Seated Crown

Once the crown is fully seated the following should be assessed carefully:

- **Marginal fit**. This can be assessed by the use of a sharp explorer or by radiographic means. McClean and von Frauhofer in a five-year study on more than 1000 restorations concluded that 120 microns is the maximal tolerable marginal opening.[1] They also report that discrepancies less than 80 microns can be difficult to detect under clinical conditions. A good marginal fit could be considered to be from 40 to 100 microns.
- **Proximal contact**. Floss is used to assess tightness of contacts. Adjustment may be obtained by use of a small piece of articulating film between the proximal contacts or by a disclosing material.
- **Aesthetics**. Assess aesthetics with input from the patient to ensure that they are happy with the final shade, form and contours of the definitive restoration, as adjustments are relatively easy at the pre-cementation stage.
- **Occlusion**. With high-strength ceramics, all-metal and metal-ceramic crowns, this can be checked prior to cementation. However, in the majority of glass-ceramic restorations or thin all-ceramic restorations, occlusion should be checked once they are adhesively bonded, as their mechanical properties then improve. Articulating film and shimstock (approximately 8 microns) can be used with Millers forceps to assess occlusal contact. Posterior teeth should hold shimstock firmly in the maximal intercuspal position, while in anterior teeth shimstock may pull through when gently closed, although it would be held on firm clenching. Any adjustment should be carried out with fine diamond burs and careful polishing, as rough ceramic surfaces may cause opposing tooth wear. Sequential abrasives for polishing should be used in order to remove the micro-cracks that may be introduced during adjustment, or alternatively crowns may be re-glazed if heavy occlusal adjustment is required.

### Cementation

Cements can be classified as follows:

- **Conventional cements** – for example zinc phosphate, zinc polycarboxylate and glass ionomer (GI) cement. These rely on an acid base reaction resulting in the formation of an insoluble salt and water component. This category of cement has been used primarily in the cementation of metallic and porcelain-fused-to-metal (PFM) restorations. GI cement has a very thin film thickness, is moisture tolerant and, due to fluoride release, can have a remineralisation effect with demineralised tooth structure.
- **Hybrid** – for example resin-modified GI cement. These cements were created to be more insoluble, with the incorporation of resins as well as allowing light polymerisation.
- **Resin cements** – these can be separated into either self-etching/adhesive or conventional resin cements:
  - Conventional resin cements require pre-treatment of the tooth surface with an acidic primer and application of a dentin-bonding agent prior to application of the resin cement. These cements form a micro-mechanical bond to tooth and restorative material. Also, they are insoluble in oral fluids. There are two types of

traditional resin cements, dual-cured and light-cured versions. Most manufacturers and clinicians recommend using resin cements for all etchable glass-based all-ceramic restorations, porcelain veneers or minimal retention restorations such as onlays or partial coverage restorations.

○ Self-etching resin cements are the most recent addition to the resin cement family. They require no pre-treatment of the tooth surface and appear to have many of the clinical advantages of traditional resin cement systems, with the ease of use of more traditional types of cement. Many types of restorative material can be successfully cemented using self-etching resin cements, including metallic (gold), all-ceramic and PFM crowns. It must be understood that the bond strengths of self-etching resin cements are not as high as those for resin cements using the total etch technique. Consequently, if proper resistance and retention form of the preparation are lacking or the restoration has minimal thickness, the use of conventional resin cements is recommended.

In determining which type of cement material to use, the dentist should consider several factors such as the ability to attain isolation and control moisture, the type of restorative material, and whether the preparation is retentive or requires adhesive bonding. Cements made with zinc phosphate, polycarboxylate and glass ionomers work mainly with mechanical retention, so a retentive preparation is necessary. Adhesive cementation can help compensate for clinical scenarios where preparations have less than ideal taper and crown height. Adhesion can increase the bond strength to tooth structure, improving retention, and may give a better ability to distribute occlusal forces along the restoration.

## Procedures

Isolation is achieved to ensure good moisture control and to prevent fluid contamination of the preparation. The soft tissues should be healthy prior to cementation, and appropriate hygiene during the provisional phase is vital to prevent inflamed soft tissues and/or bleeding. Should there be bleeding, utilising a retraction cord along with a haemostatic agent is recommended.

The technique is as follows:

- Remove the temporary crown.
- Clean the preparation with pumice slurry or aluminum oxide 27 micron diameter delivery at 40 psi. Mark multiple restoration locations (Figure 6.6.3).
- Appraise and try-in the crown. Verify complete seating and marginal fit.
- Isolate with cotton rolls, rubber dam retraction cord(s) and achieve haemostasis.
- If using adhesive cementation, proceed with bonding procedures as instructed by manufacturer.
- Mix cement and coat the intaglio surface of the crown without overfilling it.
- Seat the crown slowly with firm finger pressure, allowing cement to extrude from the margins.
- Continue finger pressure on the crown or use cotton roll/wooden stick/implement for seating posterior restorations, helping to reduce film thickness.
- Follow manufacturer's instructions for mixing, setting times and removal. This also requires that restorations be kept from moisture contamination during the setting process.

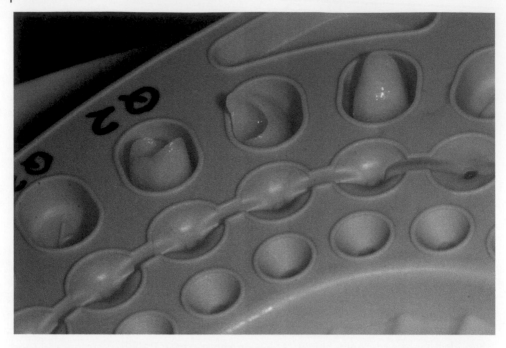

**Figure 6.6.3** Clearly marking multiple restoration locations after cleaning of crowns is important so as not to confuse placement of crowns. This may be with the use of place holders or can be as simple as writing tooth numbers on a paper towel

- Conventional cements should be allowed to set prior to removing their excess; conversely, in resin cements removal of excess cement prior to setting is recommended, as it can be very difficult to remove afterwards. The 'wave technique' is often used for resin cementation, where a light cure is applied by waving over the restoration margin for a couple of seconds allowing the cement to gel set, after which it can easily be removed and floss run between the interproximal surfaces (Figure 6.6.4). Once all excess is removed, complete polymerisation can be undertaken.

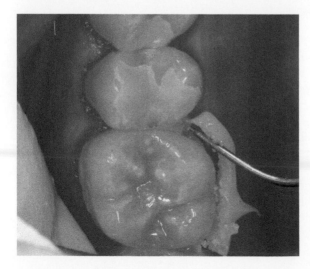

**Figure 6.6.4** Seating of the crown with a self-adhesive cement. As a dual-cure cement, after an initial gel set the excess can be removed. Alternatively the wave cure technique of waving a curing light over it for 1–2 seconds gel sets the cement, allowing simple removal

## Tips

- Obtaining a dry and uncontaminated field prior to cementation is critical and it is possible to use different haemostatic agents to obtain this. However, ferric-containing haemostatic agents such as ferric sulfate may interfere with polymerisation and lead to dark discoloration around the restoration margins. It is preferable to use aluminium chloride–containing haemostatic agents for this purpose.
- Try-in of ceramic restorations should be carried out dry initially so that margins can be evaluated with more precision. Try-in pastes can be used subsequently when assessing patient acceptance and approval prior to cementation, particularly in anterior restorations.
- Resin cements can be divided into light-cured, chemically cured and dual-cured. Chemically cured cements may be used for posts and Maryland bridges, while light-cured are useful for veneers. Dual-cured cements may be used for partial coverage restorations such as inlays, onlays and also full coverage restorations such as crown and bridgework. The dual-cured systems allow extended polymerisation times, yet are able to achieve adequate polymerisation in areas that the light cannot reach.
- Sharp scalers or a no. 12 scalpel blade can remove excess cement rather than using rotary instrumentation, which may remove the glaze layer and lead to a plaque-retentive, roughened surface.

## Reference

1 McLean JW, von Fraunhofer JA. The estimation of cement film thickness by an in vivo technique. *Br Dent J.* 1971;131:107–11.

## Further Reading

Wassell RW, Barker D, Steele JG. Crowns and other extra-coronal restorations: try-in and cementation of crowns. *Br Dent J.* 2002;193:17–28.

## 6.7

# Adhesive Bridges

*Subir Banerji and Shamir B. Mehta*

## Principles

The replacement of a missing tooth (or multiple teeth) should be based on the aim to gain an improvement in aesthetics and/or in oral function, as well as to prevent occlusal disharmony from developing. There are a number of options for tooth replacement. A **resin-bonded bridge (RBB)** is a form of fixed dental prosthesis that relies on resin composite to retain the appliance in situ. The terms 'minimally invasive bridge' and 'adhesive bridge' are often used synonymously with RBB. RBBs typically comprise a **pontic** that is anchored to the abutment tooth (or teeth) using a **metallic wing retainer**.

Evolution of resin-bonded bridges commenced in the 1970s with the introduction of the **Rochette bridge**. Such bridges are seldom in contemporary use (other than as fixed provisional restorations, for instance, prior to the placement of an implant-retained restoration) due to their lack of predictability. They typically comprise a perforated metal retainer, which is held in place by resin cement tags.

With the discovery of the ability to electrochemically etch metallic retainers coupled with the development of resin cements, predictable levels of adhesive bonding at the enamel–resin–metal interface can be attained, thus rendering it possible to prescribe RBBs with a higher level of clinical confidence. Indeed, current forms of resin-bonded bridges can offer equivalent levels of clinical success (over of a period of 5 years) to conventional (mechanically retained) bridges.[1]

Attaining high levels of success with RBBs is, however, very much dependent on:

- careful case selection
- attention to bridge design
- a meticulous clinical technique.[1,2]

The form of RBB that is most commonly prescribed in modern restorative practice is often referred to as the **Maryland bridge**. This stems from its inception at the University of Maryland, USA. This type of bridge has the merits of offering a minimally invasive, efficient, effective, economic and relatively simple way of replacing an edentulous space.

*Practical Procedures in Aesthetic Dentistry*, First Edition. Edited by Subir Banerji, Shamir B. Mehta and Christopher C.K. Ho. © 2017 John Wiley & Sons, Ltd. Published 2017 by John Wiley & Sons, Ltd.
Companion website: www.wiley.com/go/banerji/aestheticdentistry

## Procedures

Careful case selection is paramount for success with RBBs.[3] After having established the reasons for the replacement of a missing tooth (or teeth), try to determine your patient's expectations.

When carrying out an assessment and examination of a patient for whom prosthetic replacement is being considered, do not forget to undertake a full-mouth periodontal eval-uation (including clinical attachment levels, alveolar bone levels, standards and practice of oral hygiene, bleeding scores and mobility assessments). In addition, try to make sure that you carry out a caries risk assessment (including diet analysis and plaque scores), an assess-ment of the tooth morphology and anatomy, the quantity and location of the residual tooth tissue (the presence of copious, good-quality enamel is paramount for predictable resin bonding, which may be hampered in patients with developmental hard-tissue disorders), a detailed occlusal and aesthetic evaluation, an appraisal of the periapical and pulp tissue health, as well as examination of the edentulous space (noting any ridge anomalies).[4]

Your patient's oral health must be stable prior to embarking on any complex fixed prosthodontics.[4]

The use of colour photographs and articulated study casts (which may also include a diagnostic wax-up) may also be advisable.[4] The latter will permit evaluation of the inter-occlusal space for the retainer and pontic. It is important that the pontic is not involved in occlusal contact during dynamic mandibular movements (but a light occlusal stop should be maintained on the pontic in the intercuspal position).

In the event of there being inadequate interocclusal space for the metallic retainer (0.7 mm minimum thickness), tooth preparation may be required of either the abutment tooth or the antagonistic tooth. Space may, however, be gained through application of the principles of relative axial movement, which is discussed in Chapter 9.3. However, case selection and careful patient counselling are vital when placing restorations in supraocclusion.

Bridge design is an important determinant of success with RBBs. Higher levels of suc-cess have consistently been reported with cantilever designs rather than fixed designs. The latter appear prone to failure by decementation due to differential movement of abutment teeth (which are likely to present with differing pericemental surface areas) on occlusal loading. The mesio-distal length of the pontic should also be less than that of the abutment tooth, which may otherwise place great shear strain on the adhesive surface, leading to adhesive failure. In the event of a larger space (Figure 6.7.1), the use of two separate pontics cantilevered from either side or a splint pontic may be used.

Ideally the retaining wing should cover as much of the abutment tooth surface as pos-sible in order to optimise the surface area for adhesion. The term **wrap-around design** is often used in conjunction with RBB design, and here the retaining unit 'wraps' around the abutment tooth by 180°. However, the need to gain optimal adhesion may have to be counterbalanced against the aesthetic demands of your patient as well as the occlusal anatomy. For anterior teeth, it is sensible to evaluate the **dulling** effect that can arise when a metallic wing is luted in close proximity to a translucent incisal edge. This effect may be crudely demonstrated by taking a section of metallic foil and placing it on the palatal surface to assess the aesthetic impact. Management may require the retaining unit to be kept shorter than the ideal height (as shown in Figure 6.7.2) or the use of a masking restoration, placed over the incisal edge after cementation. For posterior teeth, full coverage of the palatal/lingual cusp may require further tooth reduction (unless the restoration is placed in supraocclusion). Where significant tooth reduction is less desir-able, an alternative design may be prescribed, as described in what follows.

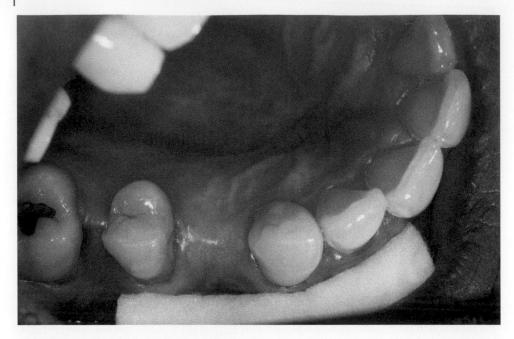

Figure 6.7.1 Upper right first premolar missing

The metallic retainer should ideally be formed of a base metal alloy (which can provide the required rigidity in thick sections); a minimum thickness of 0.7 mm is advocated. Nickel chromium is commonly used; the fit surface should be sandblasted with 50 μm aluminium oxide particles.

Existing restorations should be carefully evaluated and where necessary replaced with new adhesive resin composite restorations. Occasionally the defect may be utilised to enhance the retention and resistance form of the bridge. All preparations must be kept within enamel for predictable bonding; local anaesthesia is seldom required.

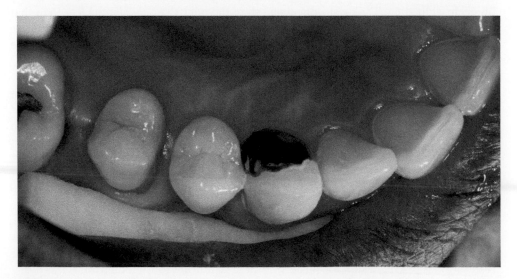

Figure 6.7.2 A adhesive bridge has been provided

Some practitioners do not undertake *any* tooth preparation. However, preparation can increase the surface area for bonding by the introduction of guide planes adjacent to the edentulous space, by the removal of any gross undercuts and the enhancement of adhesive bonding through the removal of the fluoride-rich aprismatic surface enamel.

The clinical technique is to prepare a chamfer margin on the abutment tooth in a supragingival position (finishing on enamel tissue), using your choice of metal crown preparation bur. The inclusion of a finishing line has a number of benefits: it will allow you to predictably seat your restoration in the desired position, it will help avoid over-contouring in the gingival area and it will provide a positive finishing line for the dental technician. For anterior teeth a cingulum rest may be prepared to direct occlusal forces down the long axis of the abutment; 0.7 mm of interocclusal clearance must also be given. This can be verified by the placement of an occlusal registrant medium, such as a polyvinyl siloxane (PVS) bite-registration paste, and measuring the thickness using an Iwansson crown gauge (UnoDent Ltd, Witham, Essex, UK). The preparation should end as close to the incisal edge as possible. A proximal guide plane can also be included to improve chemical retention form.

For posterior teeth, minimal preparation may also involve an axial preparation (of the retaining surface) to include the removal of any undercuts (to optimise retention form) and two 'D'-shaped occlusal rest seats (box preparations); one may be prepared adjacent to the pontic and the other at the opposing surface just prior to the contact area. An example is shown in Figure 6.7.1. This design will help to improve resistance form as well as aid in mechanical load distribution. The preparation of a guiding plane adjacent to the Pontic will also help improve retention form. Any sharp edges should be rounded off using a green stone.

Take good-quality full-arch impressions using an appropriate choice of rigid impression tray(s) and accurate materials. Sometimes, if the abutment tooth is involved with mandibular guidance, a facebow record may also be required.

Provide your dental technician with a carefully written prescription; ideally a modified ridge-lap pontic design is advocated, but in areas where aesthetics are crucial you may consider the use of an ovate pontic design. You may also decide to include a location lug for anterior teeth, which can be readily removed after cementation and the rough edge polished using a selection of abrasive discs.

On its return, the bridge should be tried in. Following verification of fit, the fit surface should be re-sandblasted (if it has become contaminated with saliva), or phosphoric acid etchant gel may be used instead. Ideally rubber dam isolation should be applied. You might also consider the use of the split dam technique.

The enamel surfaces of the abutment tooth should be cleaned using either an intraoral sandblaster or a slurry of oil-free pumice. Adjacent teeth may be isolated using polytetrafluoroethylene (PTFE) tape to avoid unwanted adhesion.

Phosphoric acid etchant gel is then applied to the enamel surfaces for 30 seconds and washed off (as described in Chapter 5.1). The cementation protocol will very much depend on the choice of cement applied. The cement should contain an agent that will promote adhesion between alloy and resin, such as in Panavia cements (Kuraray, Okayama, Japan), including 10MDP (10-methacryloxydecyl dihydrogen phosphate), which can form a chemical bond with nickel alloys, or 4-Meta (methylacryloxyethyl trimellitate anhydride), contained in C & B Metabond (Parkell, Inc., Edgewood, NY, USA), which also can form chemical active bonds with metallic alloys.

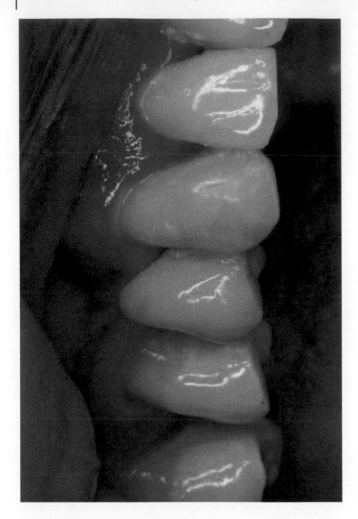

Figure 6.7.3 The adhesive bridge at the 9-year recall appointment

Carefully follow the manufacturer's instructions, making sure to remove any excess cement. The occlusal form should be verified, with light-holding contacts on the pontic in the intercuspal position and the absence of contact during dynamic movements. Oral hygiene instructions should also be given.

The results of the treatment described in Figures 6.7.1 and 6.7.2 are shown in Figures 6.7.3 and 6.7.4.

## Tips

- Make sure that you discuss all the possible options for tooth replacement in a clear, accurate, balanced, logical and comprehensive manner.
- Develop a good understanding of your chosen cement. For dual-cured materials with a short working time, you may opt to work in natural daylight only and turn off all other light sources, or use an orange light filter.
- For patients who display parafunctional habits, consider the provision of an appropriate post-operative occlusal splint.

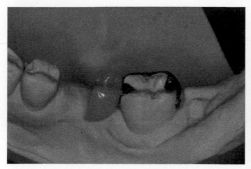
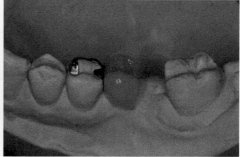
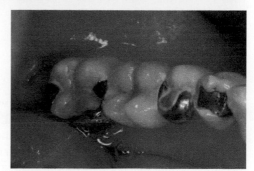

Figure 6.7.4  A missing lower left first molar tooth has been replaced with two cantilever adhesive bridges that have independent paths of insertion

## References

1 Pjetursson B, Tan W, Tan K, Brägger U, Zwahlen Z, Lang NP. A systemic review of the survival and complication rates of resin-bonded bridges after an observation period of 5 years. *Clin Oral Implant Res*. 2008;19:131–41.

2 Durey K, Nixon P, Robinson S, Chan MFW-Y. Resin bonded bridges: techniques for success. *Br Dent J*. 2011;211:113–18.

3 Morgan C, Djemal S, Gilmour G. Predictable resin-bonded bridges in general dental practice. *Dent Update*. 2001;28:501–8.

4 Maglad A, Wassell R, Barclay S, Walls A. Risk management in clinical practice 3. Crowns and bridges. *Br Dent J*. 2010;209:115–22.

## 6.8

# Fixed Partial Dentures

*Tom Giblin*

## Principles

Bridges, or fixed partial dentures (FPDs), were the main choice for fixed restoration of edentulous areas for decades, until dental implants were introduced, offering options in the replacement of teeth. Implant-retained crowns are regarded by many dentists as the treatment of choice, as they are seen to be less invasive to adjacent teeth and remain as single units, making them more easily cleanable. However, bridges still have many benefits where implant treatment is not possible.

Failures in FPDs include fracture of abutment teeth, due to the extra strain placed on them from taking the load of the pontics in occlusion; and recurrent decay under the abutment crowns, due to increased difficulty in cleaning under the bridge leading to cariogenic plaque accumulation, but also the breakdown of the luting cement. In addition, insufficient periodontal support may also lead to failure.

Poor retentive properties, especially in the posterior, can cause crown dislodgement over time. Abutment tooth fracture can also occur if the teeth are over-prepared, especially in the anterior where the loads are largely lateral to provide for thicker, more aesthetic porcelain. It should be remembered that adequate ferrule and retention need to be established, even with the use of boxes and grooves to help improve retention.

Chipping and fracture are other complications that can occur in porcelain FPD restorations. This is usually due to poor restoration design, the materials used or inadequate fabrication techniques. It is important when fabricating a FPD that the framework is of sufficient thickness to resist flexure and fracture, and that it is designed to minimise the amount of unsupported veneering porcelain.

### Occlusion

Knowledge of occlusion is essential when planning an FPD, as the occlusal loads imparted on the teeth need to be shared over a reduced root surface area. Destructive lateral and non-axial forces and excessive flexure of the bridge have to be avoided to prevent complications in the long term.

Posterior bridges should be designed with the primary contacts axially directed over the abutment teeth, ensuring that the loads are directly down the axis of the teeth. Off-

*Practical Procedures in Aesthetic Dentistry*, First Edition. Edited by Subir Banerji, Shamir B. Mehta and Christopher C.K. Ho. © 2017 John Wiley & Sons, Ltd. Published 2017 by John Wiley & Sons, Ltd.
Companion website: www.wiley.com/go/banerji/aestheticdentistry

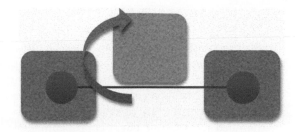

Figure 6.8.1 Off-axis pontics may induce a torque moment

axis contacts can impart a torque moment around the abutment, leading to premature failure (Figure 6.8.1).

On pontic teeth, contact should be light or slightly out of occlusion to minimise the bending moment of the bridge span. The contacts should also be as close as possible to a line drawn between the centre of the two abutment teeth.

This usually excludes bridges that are curved, as the pontics are often outside this line. In this case, the contacts should be placed on the abutment teeth and avoided on the pontic. A case like this can cause what is known as the 'bucket handle' effect, where the whole pontic acts like a lever around the abutment teeth (Figure 6.8.2). This effect is the reason for long-span anterior bridges being especially risky.

In the upper anterior, due to the tooth contacts being on an incline plane on the palatal, the forces are primarily directed laterally towards the labial. These forces can cause significant displacement of the tooth in the socket. To avoid this, when designing the restoration the bridge should be left slightly out of occlusion, so that at full clench the loads are taken axially on the posterior teeth. This minimises the flexure of the teeth in the socket and the stress placed on luting cement.

This works well in static occlusion; however, that may change in function.

### Design: Span Lengths and Thickness

In any bridge, the span length is a critical factor in long-term success. The longer the span, the greater the flexure on the framework, and this rises exponentially as the length of the span increases.

The framework should be as thick as possible to increase rigidity without compromising the aesthetics of function. A properly designed framework should also be thick enough to keep the veneering porcelain to a thickness of 1–2 mm to reduce chipping.

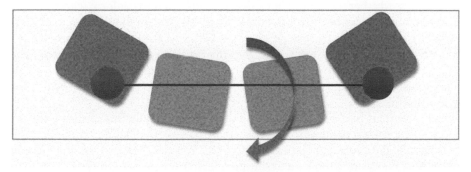

Figure 6.8.2 The 'bucket handle' effect of curved bridges

### Abutment Design

Tooth preparation for FPDs can often be difficult, as the abutment teeth need to be prepared in parallel, even if the axes of the teeth are not. This can often lead to over-prepared teeth or a greater taper, thus reducing the retentive value of the tooth and increasing the likelihood of crown dislodgement. It can also increase the chance of endodontic issues or fracture of abutment teeth.

The need for a ferrule effect is probably more important on bridges than on single teeth, as the forces imparted on the abutment teeth are higher and of a different nature to a single crown. While splinting teeth together will effectively eliminate the mesial-distal torque of a crown, it may increase the bucco-lingual torque due to the increased occlusal surface area and potential off-axis loading of the bridge. Boxes and grooves should be used as additional retentive features to aid in mechanical retention where practical.

### Pontic Design

When designing a bridge, it is important to decide the type of pontic that is best suited for the situation. Knowing that many RPDs fail due to decay from food trapping and bacterial build-up, a hygienic design of pontic may be chosen to reduce future complications. In the case of good hard and soft tissue, and where aesthetics are desired, an ovate pontic may be the best option. This acts most like a natural tooth and is optimal · for the creation and maintenance of papillae. The modified shape of an ovate pontic with a slight buccal concavity at the gingival margin can actually increase the thickness and volume of the surrounding soft tissue. If there is insufficient bone or soft tissue, a ridge lap design may be the best decision.

### Resin-Bonded Bridges

Resin-bonded bridges (RBBs) comprise pontics that are retained only by bonding to the adjacent teeth without traditional mechanical retention, such as the Rochette bridge or Maryland bridge. Adhesive bridges are covered in more detail in Chapter 6.7.

## Procedures

When preparing FPDs, time should be taken first to assess the abutment teeth, the hard and soft tissue levels, the restorative space and the occlusion. The preparations should also be planned to determine the path of insertion of the bridge in relation to any adjacent teeth, and then to assess whether the abutment teeth can be prepared to conform with this.

Prior to commencement of the tooth preparation, the dentist should anticipate how they are going to temporise the bridge (Figure 6.8.3). If there is currently an edentulous space, a wax-up should be requested from the laboratory and a matrix made. The laboratory may also be able to prepare the teeth on the cast and make a prefabricated temporary to use to save clinical time. The laboratory-prepared cast can also be used as a guide for the clinician.

The most important part of a bridge preparation is the parallelism of the abutment teeth. The easiest way to achieve this is to start by placing parallel depth cuts on the buccal surfaces of the abutment teeth as a reference. You can then prepare the teeth in relation to these indicating grooves and stay parallel to the other abutments.

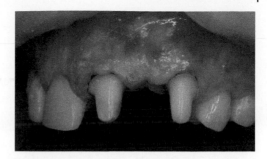

Figure 6.8.3 An upper left central incisor and canine repaired for a three-unit bridge

Throughout tooth preparations, the clinician should regularly check preparation alignments from all planes (buccal, lingual occlusal, medial and distal) to ensure a common path of insertion and avoid undercuts. If perspective is difficult to achieve, a periodontal probe held adjacent to the axial wall of the abutment teeth should give a visual aid to compare the preparations.

When making the temporary, ensure that the thickness of the pontic and connectors is adequate – acrylic material is weaker and may fracture more easily than the final bridge.

## Tips

- Good retraction helps when doing complex preparations. Use an Optragate (Ivoclar Vivadent AG, Schaan, Liechtenstein) or similar retraction, which will also give you better visual access to determine parallelism.
- When making the temporaries, after injecting the matrix with bisacryl, dry the teeth and flow the temporary material around the margins of the preparations, just like when making an impression. This will ensure a much better fit from the temporaries, improve retention and, due to the better marginal fit, also provide better soft-tissue health, which makes it much easier to cement the final restorations.
- If you are unsure about your preparations, especially in multiunit cases, stop, take a quick quadrant impression with alginate and pour it up with a fast-set stone or plaster. It should take under 10 minutes, but you will pick up more about your preparations on a cast than you will in the mouth.

## Further Reading

Misch CE. *Contemporary implant dentistry*. 3rd ed. Amsterdam: Elsevier, 2014.

Salama H, Salama MA, Garber DA, Adar P. The interproximal height of bone: a guidepost to esthetic strategies and soft tissue contours in anterior tooth replacement. *Pract Periodontics Aesthet Dent*. 1998 Nov—Dec;10(9):1131–41.

Tarnow DP, Magner AW, Fletcher P. The effect of the distance from the contact point to the crest of bone on the presence or absence of the interproximal dental papilla. *J Periodontol*. 1992;63:995–6.

Torabinejad M, Anderson P, Bader J, et al. Outcomes of root canal treatment and restoration, implant-supported single crowns, fixed partial dentures, and extraction without replacement: a systematic review. *J Prosthet Dent*. 2007 Oct;98(4):285–311.

Walton TR. An up-to-15-year comparison of the survival and complication burden of three-unit tooth-supported fixed dental prostheses and implant-supported single crowns. *Int J Oral Maxillofac Implants*. 2015 Jul-Aug;30(4):851–61.

## 6.9

# The Role of CAD/CAM in Modern Dentistry

*Charles A.E. Slade*

*Video: The Role of CAD/CAM in Modern Dentistry*
*Presented by Charles A.E. Slade*

## Principles

The processes of modern CAD/CAM dentistry can be broken down into several distinct phases, with the possibility of moving between digital and analogue workflows at several stages. Indeed, many dentists could be unaware that considerable aspects of their indirect restorations may be digitally produced already (Figure 6.9.1).

Data acquisition can be achieved directly from the patient or indirectly by scanning models or impressions. The goals for a successful scan are identical to those for an impression. It is essential to acquire an accurate copy of the teeth, tooth or implant being treated in addition to the surrounding tissue and adjacent teeth. Similarly, a representation of the remaining teeth in the arch, opposing surfaces and the dynamic interocclusal relationship between the opposing arches must also be recorded.

All scanners use a light source and a still or video camera or cameras to produce a digital image, in which the inherent accuracy of the image is a function of the accuracy of the camera, the speed of data acquisition and, significantly, the algorithm employed to model the data. In some systems a light powder, usually titanium oxide in a carrier medium, is applied to all the surfaces to be recorded to provide contrast or accurate reference points for the software to link the multiple images. Maintaining homogeneity and even thickness of this layer was a source of possible variation.[1] The advent of powderless scanners has removed this source of inaccuracy with no limitation of scan accuracy,[2] eliminating one of the main barriers to the technique. However, multiple reflective surfaces can still slow scan speeds significantly.

The three-dimensional (3D) image of any object is constructed of triangles, whose density of distribution is related to the density of the data present at any point on the object. You will notice in Figure 6.9.2 that the areas of low contour change are populated with sparse large triangles, while marginal areas show small, densely populated regions.

*Practical Procedures in Aesthetic Dentistry*, First Edition. Edited by Subir Banerji, Shamir B. Mehta and Christopher C.K. Ho. © 2017 John Wiley & Sons, Ltd. Published 2017 by John Wiley & Sons, Ltd.
Companion website: www.wiley.com/go/banerji/aestheticdentistry

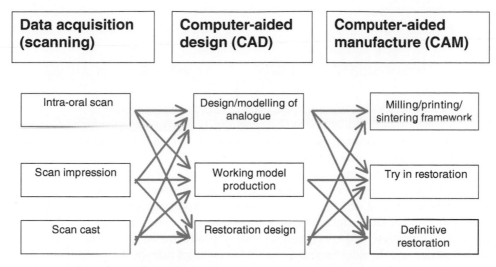

| Data acquisition (scanning) | Computer-aided design (CAD) | Computer-aided manufacture (CAM) |

Intra-oral scan → Design/modelling of analogue → Milling/printing/sintering framework

Scan impression → Working model production → Try in restoration

Scan cast → Restoration design → Definitive restoration

Figure 6.9.1 Phases of CAD/CAM dentistry

These data sets create the 3D image, but also constitute a source of error, as there is a trade-off between accuracy and size of data file: doubling the data points and hence the accuracy quadruples the processing time. Files are stored and manipulated using Standard Tessellation Language, usually referred to as 'STL' files, which ideally are open source and directly available for manipulation without the need for third-party rendering.

These data files can be used to design and produce limited restorations 'in house' with chairside/bench-top milling machines and small furnaces, or sent to a remote laboratory where the restorations of a vast array can be designed and produced.

The software uses intelligent algorithms to create the scan and to some extent is capable of determining and correcting errors based on assumptions of the probable shapes of the missing data, as can be seen in Figure 6.9.3.

This and the inability of a digital scan to reproduce sharp angles absolutely (Figure 6.9.4) are limiting factors in scanning, and demand preparations to minimise

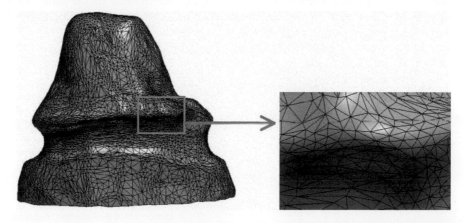

Figure 6.9.2 Triangulation and density distribution of data points across the varying surface of the preparation

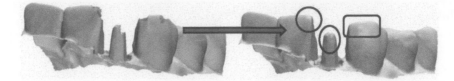

Figure 6.9.3 Actual scan data image (left) and image corrected with algorithm (right)

these effects. The shape of the image being scanned is an approximation of the possible angular features of a dental preparation.

More advanced programs remove unwanted soft-tissue incursion and highlight areas where greater data is required. Unlike an impression, this simply demands that the missing area be re-scanned, and the new data is overlaid and interlaced to the existing scan.

Despite this, the latest digital scanners are at least as accurate as a gold standard conventional impression[3] and are equally capable of producing acceptable fit accuracy on both chamfer and shoulder finishing lines at the external margin.[4]

Digital production of the restoration also demands an understanding of production techniques and suitable alteration of preparation morphology. Milling sharp internal angles is not possible and thus rounded internal angles are mandatory. When the correct preparations are employed, the fit accuracy of restorations is significantly improved with the digital platform even over a two-stage silicone impression.[5]

## Procedures

Scanning practice varies slightly according to the case being treated and the manufacturer's software. A full arch scan of both arches and acquisition of the retruded contact position and/or position of maximum intercuspation along with data for articulation is optimal.

Not all cases will require this level of data, in the same way that, in a conventional workflow, articulation of an indirect restoration is specific to the tooth treated and the restorative aims of the case. It is possible to take a sectional scan of a treated tooth and opposing and adjacent surfaces. However, while there is a saving in scan time and size of data file, this approach, even if digitally articulated, carries exactly the same occlusal limitations as a sectional impression would in an analogue workflow, albeit with less inaccuracy in impression and articulation.

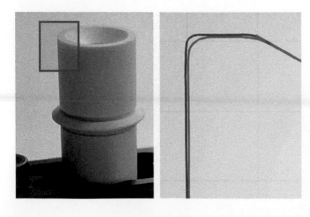

Figure 6.9.4 The two lines in the box on the right show the two-dimensional digital representation, by two scanners, of the surface marked by the box on the image on the left

There are several possible workflows. This example will consider a simple single restoration and the author's preferred software and pattern of working.

A data file is created for the patient, which may contain full-face photographs, intraoral shade tab photos taken with a digital camera along with scanned images, for instance a patient's own photographs, enhancing the information for the technician. Similarly, tooth-specific information can be annotated and drawn onto the prescription via the trackpad.

The proposed restoration, including construction detail, is selected from the pre-populated menu. This pre-sets appropriate reduction values for the specific restoration and prescribed restorative material within the system, as well as creating a laboratory prescription. Restorative clearance is measured against the antagonist surfaces, with the goal of minimal reduction rather than simply reducing existing tooth tissue to a specific formula. The parameters of reduction are customisable by the user, although deviation from manufacturer's tolerances will affect the outcome, both aesthetically and mechanically, of the final restoration.

The patient's teeth may be scanned prior to any intervention, allowing the shades of all teeth to be measured and automatically recorded by the system before any dehydration that will result from the preparation. To minimise time and cost, depending on prevailing legislation, this scan may be carried out by another member of the dental team at a prior appointment. It is not critical to record in high detail areas that will not in any way influence the outcome, although there is nothing to stop the clinician recording a complete 3D image of both arches and immediate soft tissues if desired.

The intercuspal position record is rapidly acquired and can be verified bilaterally. An retruded contact position record is possible, requiring the inclusion of a bite, Lucia Jig or gothic arch trace to verify and hold the mandibular position while the scan records the respective bilateral positions of the arches.

When you perform the tooth preparation, remain cognisant of the differences between a CAD/CAM and a conventional restoration.

With the preparation complete and suitable isolation in place, the prepared tooth is then scanned. You will need to start this aspect of the scan from a pre-existing data point, which sounds daunting but simply means the adjacent unprepared tooth surface or other recognisable, previously scanned area. The software will indicate once it has matched enough data points to stitch the new image accurately into the existing scan. The clinician can then review the preparation in 3D, rotating the image to check that all areas of the preparation are completely represented and that other significant structures, such as adjacent contact points and regions below the survey point of adjacent teeth, are fully recorded. Any area that is lacking data is clearly highlighted in the viewing software and simply re-scanned into the existing picture. An HD photo can be superimposed over any area to improve visualisation of the preparation and stump shade by the laboratory.

Similarly, a critical appraisal of the physical preparation parameters is simple for the clinician. If improvements are identified, these can be effected and the altered areas added into the scan. It is likely that the simplicity of improving the scan or preparation is the underlying reason that studies comparing CAD/CAM scans and conventional impressions show a significant increase in the number of re-scans in comparison to re-taken impressions. Re-scanning allows alterations of preparations with a significant reduction in time and cost,[6,7] as well as an improvement in preparation quality over the analogue pathway.

At this point there is a clear choice in the digital pathway. It is possible to mill a limited range of restorations in surgery. These mills are slightly limited in application by milling axis, size and the need to replace cutting tools easily. The restoration is designed by the clinician and sent to the milling station, where the restoration can be milled in a multitude of shades, even using graduated colour blocks to mimic the absence of monochromatic structures in the natural dentition. The restorations can be further customised by staining and glazing, again in surgery. There is a trade-off that this pathway entails: the immediacy of the restoration is undeniably attractive, as is the absence of a laboratory bill at the end of the month. The calculation of chairside time on design and finishing the restoration should not be under-estimated; consideration also needs to be given to the loss of scope of restorative solutions available and the ultimate accuracy of the fit of the final restoration. The inability to articulate digital models anatomically in the chairside milling system is a significant limitation, in the author's opinion.

The advantages that dedicated laboratory software, with semi-adjustable articulation, can bring to the definitive restoration are significant. My preferred route is to send the digital file direct to the technicians, who can immediately commence 3D printing models or design of the restoration. The downside is that a provisional restoration is required, which can be either pre-made digitally or conventionally done chairside, and the patient requires a second appointment. The removal of the clinician from the design/manufacture stages, improved fit quality and vast range of restorative solutions will be a significant factor for some clinicians. Even with a two-stage procedure, the reduction in laboratory stages and disposables (impressions, models etc.) along with reduced manufacturing costs leads to a significant reduction in cost per unit.[6] Patient-orientated advantages are a general expectation of technology, improved patient acceptance of treatment and the comfort of eliminating impressions. For patients with a severe gag reflex or those for whom remaining static is impossible, digital scanning is especially elegant, as the image can be built in small sections at a time.

Following either of the digital restoration construction pathways, the restoration is fitted in the same a manner as a 'conventional' indirect restoration. Studies show that there are significantly fewer adjustments required at the fit appointment within the digital pathway. There is an undeniable simplicity in the data acquisition and refinement, if required, along with the absence of many complex critical stages with numerous set times and technique-sensitive chemical reactions both in surgery and the laboratory, even excluding the possible physical deformation of both of the impressions.[8]

The progression of dentistry along a digital pathway is unquestionable from a cost, predictability and accuracy point of view. We have tools available to us that were unimaginable previously and to ignore them could be costly. We are at a critical point in the evolution of dental restoration provision. The evolution is as fundamental and inevitable as the progression from a typewriter to a laptop.

## Tips

- Scan the dental arches prior to preparation of the tooth or teeth.
- If you can't see it you can't scan it – make sure that all margins are visible!
- Use the skills of the whole team to improve clinical efficiency.
- Be critical of the level and amount of data actually required.

- Use the simplicity of 3D viewing to critique your preparation and the simplicity of re-scanning an altered preparation to achieve optimal quality.
- Make sure that there are no sharp line angles in your preparation.

## References

1 Dehurtevent M, Robberecht L, Béhin P. Influence of dentist experience with scan spray systems used in direct CAD/CAM impressions. *J Prosthet Dent.* 2015;113(1):17–21.
2 Ender A, Mehl A. Influence of scanning strategies on the accuracy of digital intraoral scanning systems. *Int J Comp Dent.* 2013;16(1):11–21.
3 Lee SJ, Betensky RA, Gianneschi GE, Gallucci GO. Accuracy of digital versus conventional implant impressions. *Clin Oral Implants Res.* 2015 Jun;26(6):715–9.
4 Re D, Cerutti F, Augusti G, Cerutti A, Augusti D. Comparison of marginal fit of Lava CAD/CAM crown-copings with two finish lines. *Int J Esthet Dent.* 2014;9(3):426–35.
5 Pradíes G, Zarauz C, Valverde A, Ferreiroa A, Martínez-Rus F. Clinical evaluation comparing the fit of all-ceramic crowns obtained from silicone and digital intraoral impressions based on wavefront sampling technology. *J Dent.* 2015 Feb;43(2):201–8.
6 Joda T, Brägger U. Digital vs conventional implant prosthetic workflows: a cost/time analysis. *Clin Oral Implants Res.* 2015 Dec;26(12):1430–5.
7 Lee SJ, Gallucci GO. Digital vs. conventional implant impressions: efficiency outcomes. *Clin Oral Implants Res.* 2013;24(1):111–15.
8 Story D, Coward T. The quality of impressions for crown and bridges: an assessment of the work received at three commercial dental laboratories. Assessing qualities of impressions that may lead to occlusal discrepancies with indirect restorations. *Eur J Prosthodont Restorative Dent.* 2014;22(1):11–18.

## 6.10

# Ceramic Repair

*Christopher C.K. Ho*

## Principles

Ceramics are widely used in dentistry due to their ability to re-create natural optical characteristics. They have been developed to enhance bio-compatibility and durability; however, fractures have become an increasing complication due to the advent in popularity of tooth-coloured materials and subsequently less use of metal. The mode of fracture can occur with the veneering porcelain or a framework fracture. In glass ceramics, inceram and alumina restorations, framework fracture has often been the mode of failure, while in zirconia restorations, veneering porcelain chipping or even delaminating has been identified.

The majority of ceramics consist of crystalline fillers that vary in proportion, from relatively low concentrations in glass-based ceramics to higher concentrations in polycrystalline high-strength materials, resulting in superior mechanical properties.

The failure of ceramic can occur due to several factors, including the following:

- **Trauma** – from micro-trauma (i.e. parafunctional forces) and macro-trauma (i.e. physical trauma).
- **Preparation design** – sharp line angles, grooves and knife-edge margins may predispose a restoration to more stress with subsequent fracture.
- **Ageing** – low-temperature degradation due to liquid penetration leading to phase transformation of zirconia materials has been shown to reduce mechanical properties.
- **Thermal conductivity** – zirconia has a low thermal conductivity with a different coefficient of thermal expansion to many of the veneering porcelains. Developments have been made to more closely match the thermal coefficients as well as understanding the heating and cooling times required.
- **Framework design** – appropriate design of the framework to properly support veneering porcelain while also understanding the ratio of framework thickness to veneering porcelain thickness. Moreover, anatomically designed copings are better able to reduce chipping.
- **Inappropriate adjustment of ceramics chairside** – with induced micro-cracks leading to failure.

### Options for Repair

There may be several options for repairing the restoration, depending on the size, position and type of fracture that has occurred:

*Practical Procedures in Aesthetic Dentistry*, First Edition. Edited by Subir Banerji, Shamir B. Mehta and Christopher C.K. Ho. © 2017 John Wiley & Sons, Ltd. Published 2017 by John Wiley & Sons, Ltd.
Companion website: www.wiley.com/go/banerji/aestheticdentistry

- **Small chips** – these may be satisfactorily contoured and polished, especially in non-aesthetic areas and where food or plaque will not accumulate and predispose patients to caries or periodontal disease. Furthermore, polishing should be performed to minimise any surface flaws that may lead to subsequent failures.
- **Direct repair:**
  - Bonding the fractured portion of ceramic back onto the restoration with resin cement
  - Directly repairing with composite resin
  - Preparing the fractured ceramic restoration for a veneer or an over-crown, and bonding a new restoration to the existing restoration
- **Indirect repair** – removal of restoration and re-firing or replacing veneering porcelain by a dental ceramist. This may be possible with a screw-retained implant restoration, but in cemented conventional crown and bridgework it may be difficult to carry out without damaging or distorting the cemented restoration during its removal.

The repair of ceramic requires an understanding of how retention can be attained by providing micro-mechanical retention and enhancing the bond with silane primers or phosphate monomers.

### Micro-mechanical Retention

- **Air abrasion/intra-oral sandblaster**. Roughening of ceramic surfaces can be achieved by air abrading with 50 micron aluminium oxide at 2 bar air pressure, which can clean, roughen and activate the ceramic surfaces. There has been concern that the use of air abrasion can lead to surface flaws due to the high energy with which these particles are blasted onto the surface, which in turn may be of concern with weaker porcelains. In glass (silica) ceramics it may therefore be best to use acid etching, as this is capable of roughening the ceramic sufficiently for bonding. Air abrasion is necessary for oxide ceramics and metals because acid etching produces insufficient roughening of those surfaces.
- **Acid etching with hydrofluoric acid** (2.5–10%). Glass-based ceramics can be etched with acid to increase roughness. The intra-oral use of hydrofluoric acid should be approached with extreme caution due to its highly corrosive nature, and clinicians are encouraged to use rubber dam for appropriate isolation. Zirconia and metals cannot be sufficiently etched with the use of acid.

### Chemical Bonding

- Silane primers enhance the covalent bonds between ceramic and resin as well as promoting the wettability of the surface for the penetration of resin. Metal oxides such as zirconia and metal restoration do not contain silanol groups and may be silicoated by a process called tribochemical coating. This has been made possible through the development of a chairside system (CoJet, 3M, St Paul, MN, USA), which consists of 30 micron aluminium oxide particles that are doped in silica. The particles are air abraded onto the surface of the ceramic or metal, which roughens the surface as well as embedding silica into the surface layer. This silica-enriched surface can then be bonded to predictably.
- Phosphate monomers are molecules that can facilitate chemical bonding of resin to metal or ceramics. They are available as primers (e.g. Alloy primer or Clearfil ceramic primer, Kuraray Noritake, Okayama, Japan; Monobond Plus, Ivoclar Vivadent, Schaan, Liechtenstein) as well as in modified phosphate monomer-containing resin cements (Panavia, Kuraray Noritake; SuperBond C&B, Sun Medical, Shiga, Japan).

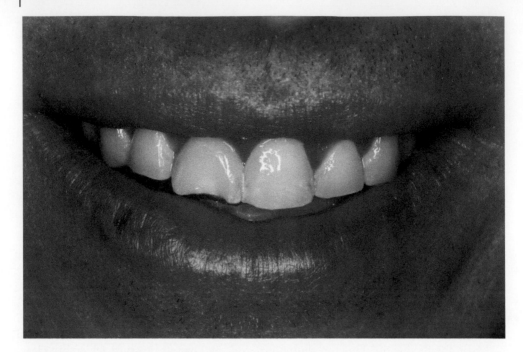

Figure 6.10.1  Fractured all-ceramic crown

The repair of an all-ceramic crown is illustrated in Figures 6.10.1, 6.10.2 and 6.10.3.

## Procedures

The repair of ceramics intra-orally is with air abrasion, etching or a combination of both followed by the application of a silane primer (Table 6.10.1). More recently the use of phosphate monomers in both primers and resin cements has been developed, as well as silicatising surfaces with CoJet.

### Glass (Silica-Based) Ceramics

- Attain adequate isolation with rubber dam or liquid rubber dam.
- Lightly roughen the porcelain with a fine diamond and bevel the margin.
- Option of either:
  - Air abrasion only or with CoJet; or
  - Acid etching with hydrofluoric acid, for feldspathic porcelains for 60 seconds compared to lithium siliciate materials for 20 seconds only. Wash and dry thoroughly.
  - Apply fresh silane primer and air dry to evaporate the solvent.
  - Apply an unfilled resin that does not contain HEMA (2-hydroxyethyl methacrylate) or another hydrophilic monomer, as porcelain is a very hydrophobic material. Air dry.
  - Apply composite and sculpt to correct tooth contours.
  - If possible, delay finishing of the margins as the bond will mature and improve. This may not be realistic, and careful finishing may be carried out with fine diamond burs and polishing rubbers.

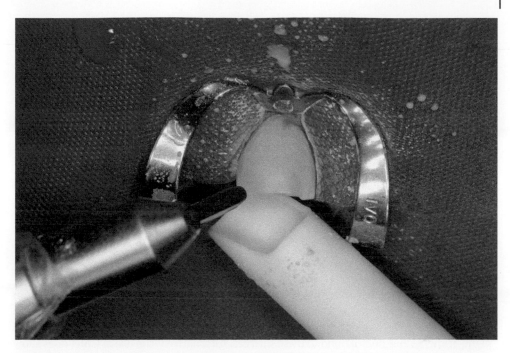

Figure 6.10.2 CoJet air abrasion to roughen and silicoat the surface of the crown to allow adhesive bonding

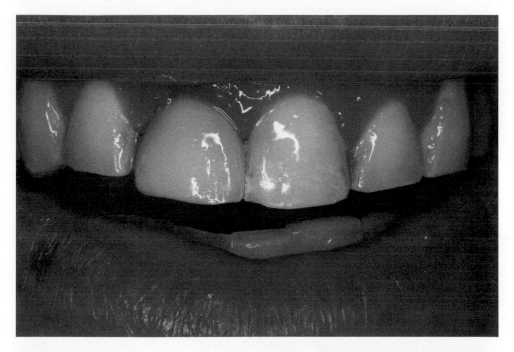

Figure 6.10.3 Repaired all-ceramic crown with direct resin composite displaying satisfactory aesthetics

Table 6.10.1 Preparation of substrate materials for ceramic repair

| Material | Micromechanical retention | Chemical treatment |
|---|---|---|
| **All-ceramic (glass ceramic)** e.g. feldspathic porcelain, leucite containing, Empress Esthetic (Ivoclar Vivadent); lithium disilicate, eMax (Ivoclar Vivadent) | Hydrofluoric acid, or air abrasion, or air abrasion and hydrofluoric acid | Silane |
| **All-ceramic (polycrystalline)** Alumina/zirconia based | CoJet | Silane or Silane and phosphate monomer primer (e.g. Alloy primer, Clearfil Ceramic Primer or Monobond Plus |
| **Porcelain-fused-to-metal (PFM)** | CoJet | Silane and phosphate monomer primer (e.g. Alloy primer) |

## Metals and Oxide Ceramics (Zirconia)

The use of acids on these materials is ineffective in creating an etch pattern for retention and thus mechanical treatment with the use of air abrasion is indicated. This then requires chemical treatment with phosphate monomer–containing primers or resin cement, as silane primers alone do not bond to these surfaces. Alternatively, the use of CoJet does allow the application of silane primers or a phosphate monomer–containing primer or cement.

In some cases it may not be practical to repair directly with resin, and it may be possible to prepare the surface of the restoration for a veneer or an over-crown that can be impressed and an indirect restoration fabricated and bonded to the existing restoration.

## Tips

- It may be difficult to determine what type of glass-based ceramic has been used, especially if a fracture has occurred to a restoration that you did not complete. If this is the case, then the use of an acid etching time of 60 seconds is recommended to etch the ceramic surface sufficiently.
- Ensure that your silane primer is kept fresh, as these materials may have a short shelf life and may thereafter be ineffective.
- If metal has been exposed, after the surface treatment it may be advisable to use an opaque tint or resin to block out the metallic appearance.

## Further Reading

Kern M, Barloi A, Yang B. Surface conditioning influences zirconia ceramic bonding. *J Dent Res.* 2009;88(9):817–22.

Kimmich M, Stappert CF. Intraoral treatment of veneering porcelain chipping of fixed dental restorations: a review and clinical application. *J Am Dent Assoc.* 2013;144(1):31–44.

Magne P, Paranhos MP, Burnett LH Jr. New zirconia primer improves bond strength of resin-based cements. *Dent Mater.* 2010;26(4):345–52.

Wolfart M, Lehmann F, Wolfart S, Kern M. Durability of the resin bond strength to zirconia ceramic after using different surface conditioning methods. *Dent Mater.* 2007;23:45–50.

# Part VII

# Indirect Ceramic Veneer Restorations

## 7.1

## Planning for Porcelain Laminate Veneers

*Christopher C.K. Ho*

## Principles

### Treatment Planning

A comprehensive examination with a complete history and clinical assessment is a critical step in this treatment modality. The prevention of disease and control should be considered a first priority, with planning for aesthetic improvement such as veneers considered after this has been completed.

The treatment planning begins with the following:

- Discussion of a patient's objectives and the ability of the dentist to achieve the desired outcomes.
- Initial examination. A systematic approach documenting clinical findings, including periodontal conditions, existing restorations, occlusion and so on. A radiographic examination and study models should complete this initial examination. A photographic series of the patient including extra-oral photos of the full smile and lateral smiles as well as intra-oral photos should be part of the documentation process.
- Informed consent. With the information gathered, discussions should be held to inform the patient fully about the treatment. This should be done in a simple manner, detailing the treatment steps and limitations of treatment. Care must be exercised not to over-promise the final outcomes, and also to determine whether the patient is expecting unachievable results.

It must be remembered that as health professionals we abide by *Primum non nocere*, a Latin phrase that means 'First, do no harm'. If a patient can be treated with conservative options, then this must be discussed and recommended to patients as part of the treatment planning process.

Here are some examples:

- Crooked teeth and diastemas may be treated with orthodontic treatment, which would be advantageous, as there would be no preparation of teeth or long-term replacement required. Orthodontics may also be a phase of treatment to position the teeth prior to veneers, allowing for less invasive preparation. The introduction of new orthodontic techniques like Invisalign™ may help to remove some of the objections to conventional orthodontics.

*Practical Procedures in Aesthetic Dentistry*, First Edition. Edited by Subir Banerji, Shamir B. Mehta and Christopher C.K. Ho. © 2017 John Wiley & Sons, Ltd. Published 2017 by John Wiley & Sons, Ltd.
Companion website: www.wiley.com/go/banerji/aestheticdentistry

- Discoloured teeth might be bleached with vital bleaching or, in the case of a discoloured non-vital tooth, a non-vital 'walking' bleach may be carried out.
- Small chips on teeth might be restored with direct resin.

### Indications for Porcelain Veneers [1]

1) Type I – Teeth resistant to bleaching:
   a) Tetracycline discoloration.
   b) No response to external or internal bleaching.
2) Type II – Major morphologic modifications:
   a) Conoid teeth.
   b) Diastema and interdental triangles to be closed.
   c) Augmentation of incisal length and prominence.
3) Type III – Extensive restoration:
   a) Extensive coronal fracture.
   b) Extensive loss of enamel by erosion and wear.
   c) Generalised congenital and acquired malformations.

### Contraindications for Veneers

- Minimal enamel for bonding.
- Major changes in tooth colour.
- Major changes in tooth positions, such as severe crowding.
- Large restorations within tooth, minimal enamel and reduced tooth rigidity.
- Bruxism (unprotected) or other parafunctional habits, for instance pen chewing, ice crushing.
- Psychological.

### Diagnostic Wax-Up or Mock-Up

Utilisation of a diagnostic wax-up (Figure 7.1.1) can help plan the desired aesthetic appearance. This should incorporate the patient's wants that were expressed in the initial treatment planning discussions.

The diagnostic wax-up provides visualisation of the desired treatment and a blueprint of the final restorations. Additionally, a wax-up allows the fabrication of putty keys for provisionalisation and reduction guides for the preparation process. The contours and form of the final teeth can be transferred from the desired wax-up to the provisionals, allowing the patient to have a preview of their desired appearance and to re-confirm that they are happy with the planned changes. It is certainly advantageous for a patient to view the changes prior to constructing the veneers, due to the cost of re-making restorations if patients are not happy.

### Material Choices

There are different types of ceramics available to fabricate veneers, but there are two basic types of materials used: low-fusing feldspathic porcelain and lithium disiliate or leucite-reinforced ceramics.

#### Feldspathic Porcelain
This is also referred to as powder liquid or stacked veneers. It is used in the layering or build-up technique of most modern porcelains. This material contains mainly silica

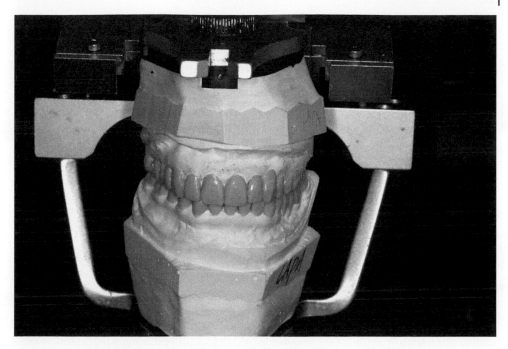

Figure 7.1.1 Diagnostic wax-up on articulated models

and feldspar. Additional components include pigments and opacifying agents. There is no outstanding inherent strength (up to 100 MPa flexural strength), but feldspathic porcelain is twice as strong as human enamel (50 MPa). In the form of a bonded veneer, it gains much of its strength from the underlying tooth structure, the so-called lamination effect. One of the advantages of feldspathic porcelain is the ability to build within each veneer different colours, characteristics and even opacity. Another advantage is the ability to use a minimal thickness veneer with a depth reduction of 0.3 mm. This preparation is more conservative, and more likely to remain in enamel, especially if a reductive approach is required in the preparation.

### Lithium Disilicate and Leucite-Reinforced Ceramics

These ceramics were introduced in the 1990s and are made of pre-sintered ingots, which consist of silicate glasses containing a crystal phase. They can be fabricated using a pressed approach, where the restoration is created in wax and the lost-wax technique is used to create the final restoration. The pressing procedure consists of a homogeneous ceramic ingot being heated and then forced under pressure into a wax-formed void (investment). The process eliminates porcelain shrinkage, porosity and inconsistencies that may be present with brush build-up techniques. The alternative technique is the use of CAD/CAM technology and milling the glass ceramics. Two of the most popular materials include Empress, leucite containing (Ivoclar Vivadent, Schaan, Liechtenstein), and e.max, lithium disilicate containing (Ivoclar Vivadent). These materials have several advantages, including more flexural strength. Due to this higher strength capability, it is possible even to increase incisal length. It has been reported that up to 4 mm of missing tooth structure can be restored with leucite-reinforced ceramic. [2] These materials have good marginal integrity and wear compatibility. They are also available in different translucencies and opacities, allowing the ceramist better colour masking.

## Periodontal Considerations

The patient's periodontal status must be optimal prior to treatment. This ensures long-term stability of the periodontal apparatus and minimises any chance of marginal gingival recession. Periodontal therapy should be completed as well as proper plaque control methods practised with the patient for long-term maintenance. This also enables the clinician to work with healthy periodontal tissues and not to have excessive bleeding due to inflammation while working on the patient. The concept of 'biologic width' should be respected, with preparation margins not invading the minimum space of 3 mm between the most coronal level of the alveolar bone and the gingival level. The surgical correction of gingival asymmetries, gingival recession, excessive gingival display (gummy smile) and altered passive eruption should be completed and time allowed for the maturation of the tissues prior to veneers being constructed (Figure 7.1.2). This may range from 3–6 months depending on the case.

## Informed Consent

Porcelain veneers are often an aesthetic and elective procedure and as such require a full discussion on the benefits and risks, with the functional and aesthetic objectives defined within this process. Alternative means of achieving the patient's goals must be mentioned and a discussion held on the procedures involved, including the steps from start to completion. The patient must be educated on the care and maintenance of the veneers, and mention made of the longevity of the veneers and their eventual replacement.

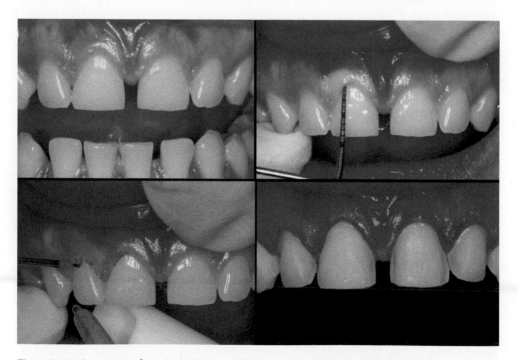

**Figure 7.1.2** Correction of gingival contours with measuring of biologic width and gingivectomy with diode laser

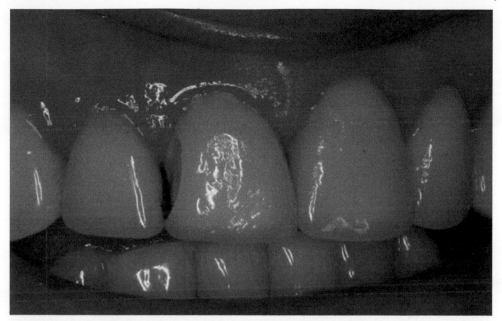

Figure 7.1.3 Complications with porcelain laminate veneer with fracture

Maintenance and Complications

The survival rate of porcelain veneers has been shown in the literature to be very high. Friedman, in a review of 3500 veneers over 15 years, found a 7% occurrence of complications in clinical service, or a success rate of 93% (Figure 7.1.3). Of the 7% failures, fractures accounted for 67% of total failures, leakage 22% and debonding 11%. [3]

Fradeani et al., in a review of 182 veneers, found a probability of veneer survival of 94.4% at 12 years, with a low clinical failure rate (approximately 5.6%). [4]

## Procedures

- **Treatment planning** – comprehensive history taking with an understanding of the patient's needs, and a complete medical and dental history identifying any possible risk factor(s) that may influence the long-term success of treatment.
- **Comprehensive examination** – hard and soft tissue examination, including occlusal assessment and periodontal examination. It is important to evaluate the patient's dento-labial features and to understand features of smile design, addressing any that may be improved. It may be that the patient does not understand what makes a smile beautiful; an example may include gingival asymmetry. In many a case with uneven gingival contours, carrying out veneers would not give the patient an aesthetic result without addressing the gingival contours.
- **Records** – photography (see Chapter 2.2) and radiography should be undertaken to assess the case prior to initiation of treatment. Assessing the teeth to ensure that there is no pathology or attachment loss with periapical radiographs is an important step in treatment planning.
- **Other diagnostic tests** – such as transillumination to assess teeth for fractures, pulpal sensibility testing and so on.

- **Study models** – these are articulated and assessed for occlusion, as well as planning.
- **Diagnostic wax-up or mock-up** – used to plan the required changes as well as being transferred onto the patient's teeth to allow a 'test run' or 'trial smile', giving them the ability to gauge whether they are happy with the prescribed changes. Often a patient is unsure of the final aesthetics until given some time to accustom themselves to the changes.
- **Informed consent** – the patient should be given all the available options, the advantages and disadvantages of each procedure, along with risks, complications and success rates. It may also be at this stage that it is prudent to address where it may not be possible to meet the patient's needs.

## Tips

- To communicate clearly the correct final orientation of the incisal plane of the planned veneers, it is important that the ceramist receives a 'stick bite' or 'symmetry bite' (Figure 7.1.4). This can be as simple as two sticks within the bite registration to register the midline

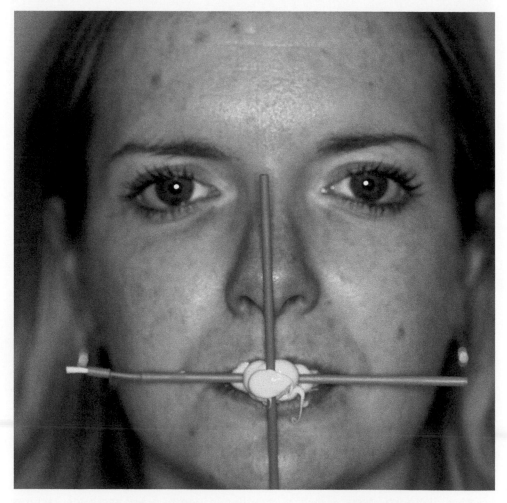

Figure 7.1.4 Symmetry bite or stick bite – This allows the orientation of the facial vertical plane and the interpupillary line to be transferred to the dental ceramist, enabling the correct alignment of incisal edges relative to these planes in the final restorations

and the interpupillary line to the teeth. There are also commercial tools available to carry out this procedure, including the Kois Dento-Facial Analyser (Panadent, Orpington, UK), and Symmetry Facial Plane Relator (Clinician's Choice, New Milford, CT, USA).

- It is important to explain to patients that veneers can fracture; they are just like natural teeth in that they can chip and break. Although veneer failures are rare, they are possible, although it should be explained that the veneers can easily be repaired or replaced.
- It is important to explain to patients the aftercare needed with veneers. An instruction sheet is seen in Table 7.1.1.

Table 7.1.1  Post-operative instructions on the care of veneers

**Temporary changes in speech**

Your teeth will feel different to your lips and tongue when you first close your mouth. This is normal and to be expected when changes have been made to the shape and size of the teeth. Sometimes your speech may change or be affected in the beginning until your tongue adapts to the changes. Even though the changes are slight (measurable only in millimetres), your mouth is extremely sensitive and will exaggerate those feelings at first. Usually after a couple of days the feelings lessen and your mouth will feel normal again.

**Daily hygiene**

We recommend that you brush with an ultra-soft toothbrush twice a day and floss nightly to extend the life of your veneer. As with your natural teeth, the veneer may pick up stains from tobacco, coffee, tea, red wine, colas etc. Having regular dental cleans will usually remove these stains. Do not use baking soda or any abrasive toothpaste. Avoid routinely rinsing with mouthwashes containing alcohol. Alcohol softens bonding and weakens the bond of porcelain. Select non-alcoholic mouthwashes or a solution made of hydrogen peroxide and water.

**Diet and habits to avoid**

As with natural teeth, avoid chewing excessively hard foods on the veneered teeth, such as:

- Hard sweets
- Nuts
- Spare ribs
- Hard bread and rolls
- Ice
- Raw carrots.

This puts stress on the veneer and could result in a fracture or a chip.

Do not bite extremely hard objects with one tooth. Avoid habits such as:

- Opening packages with your teeth
- Biting thread
- Chewing ice
- Nail biting
- Pipe smoking.

**Playing sports**

Extreme force or trauma can break porcelain veneers, just as the same force can break natural teeth. Use care when playing sports or other potentially traumatic situations. We recommend wearing a sports mouthguard in these instances.

**Continuing care**

Visit us for examinations and continuing care at regular six-month examination periods. Often, problems that are developing with the veneers can be found at an early stage and repaired easily, while waiting for a longer time may require re-doing the entire restorations. We will arrange your continuing care appointment with you at the end of your treatment.

## References

1  Magne P, Belser U. *Bonded porcelain restorations in the anterior dentition: a biomimetic approach*. Berlin: Quintessence; 2003.
2  Castelnuovo J, Tjan AH, Phillips K, Nicholls JI, Kois JC. Fracture load and mode of failure of ceramic veneers with different preparation. *J Prosthet Dent*. 2000;83:171–80.
3  Friedman MJ. A 15-year review of porcelain veneer failure: a clinician's observations. *Compend Cont Educ Dent*. 1998;19;625–32.
4  Fradeani M, Redemagni M, Corrado M. Porcelain laminate veneers: 6- to 12-year clinical evaluation – a retrospective study. *Int J Periodontics Restorative Dent*. 2005;25(1):9–17.

## 7.2

# Tooth Preparation for Porcelain Laminate Veneers

*Christopher C.K. Ho*

Video: Tooth Preparation for Porcelain Laminate Veneers
Presented by Christopher C.K. Ho

## Principles

Relative to crowns, porcelain laminate veneers (PLVs) are a conservative treatment option to improve anterior aesthetics and have a long history of documented success. The preparation for PLVs should be based on the final smile design, with the shade and position of the margin of the restorations being taken into consideration. It is important that whatever tooth reduction is required, it is based on the definitive wax-up/planned outcome and not the original tooth. Failure to do this may result in excessive and unnecessary removal of tooth enamel.

All efforts should be made to contain the preparation within enamel, as this provides opportunity for a reliable and durable bond between restoration and remaining tooth tissue. Preparation into dentine should be avoided because of the less reliable bond to dentine and the difference in elastic modulus and flexibility between dentine and porcelain. This puts the porcelain at risk of fracture when placed under tensile loading. In a 12-year study by Gurel of 583 veneers, 7.2% or 42 veneers failed.[1] Those veneers bonded to dentin and teeth with preparation margins in dentin were approximately 10 times more likely to fail than those bonded to enamel.

Meticulous tooth preparation is required with porcelain laminate veneers. The aims of tooth preparation are to:

- Provide sufficient thickness for the porcelain for adequate fracture resistance and not to over-contour the final restoration.
- Provide a definite margin, so that the ceramist has a finishing line, allowing correct emergence of the veneer from the gingival margin.
- Maintain the preparation within enamel wherever possible.
- Provide a finished preparation that is smooth and free of any sharp internal line angles.
- Provide definite seating landmarks, allowing proper seating of the veneer.

*Practical Procedures in Aesthetic Dentistry*, First Edition. Edited by Subir Banerji, Shamir B. Mehta and Christopher C.K. Ho. © 2017 John Wiley & Sons, Ltd. Published 2017 by John Wiley & Sons, Ltd.
Companion website: www.wiley.com/go/banerji/aestheticdentistry

## Procedures

### Labial Preparation

The preparation of the labial contour of anterior teeth needs to be addressed in three planes: incisal, middle third and cervical (Figure 7.2.1). The labial contour has a convex surface.

- Careful depth reduction of tooth structures is carried out to provide a minimum of 0.3 mm (feldspathic porcelain) or 0.6 mm (Empress, e.max) preparation. The enamel thickness at the gingival third is 0.3–0.5 mm, up to 0.6–1 mm at the middle third and 1.0–2.1 mm at the incisal third.[2] All efforts should be made to keep preparation within the enamel for long-term adhesion and also to avoid any unnecessary tooth structure removal.
- Veneers may be used to mask discoloration. A porcelain veneer needs a minimum thickness of 0.2–0.3 mm for each shade improvement if discoloured, or alternatively a more opaque porcelain can be chosen.
- In short, the thickness of porcelain veneers is determined by the amount of desired shade change and the final tooth position, which is dictated by functional and aesthetic parameters.
- The use of depth cutters or grooves and dimples has been recommended to control tooth preparation, as standardised objects allow accurate judgement of depth. Burs that are specially constructed to provide graded depth cuts are then reduced together with a chamfer bur (Figures 7.2.2 and 7.2.3). An alternative is to use depth grooves or dimples. Dimples are depth pits prepared on the surface of the tooth using a 1 mm diameter round bur sunk to half its diameter to attain 0.5 mm depth. Note that the orientation of the teeth with regard to the arch form will also influence the depth of tooth tissue to be removed (see Figure 7.2.4).

### Incisal Edge Reduction

There are four different preparation designs possible (Figure 7.2.5), with two (feather and window preparation) that involve no reduction of the incisal edge or preparation of the lingual surfaces and other preparations that involve a reduction of the incisal edges.

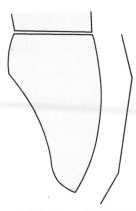

Figure 7.2.1 Three-plane contour of labial surface of maxillary anterior tooth *Source*: Wilson 2015.[3] Reproduced with permission from Elsevier.

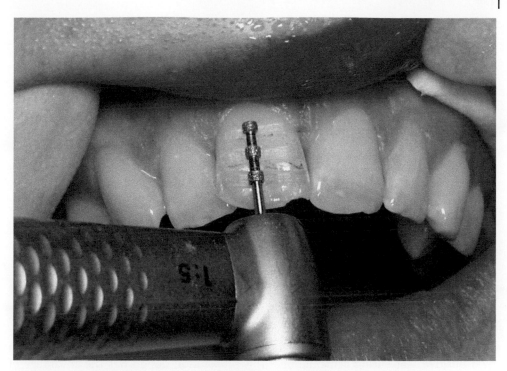

Figure 7.2.2 Use of depth cutting bur to initiate depth of reduction required

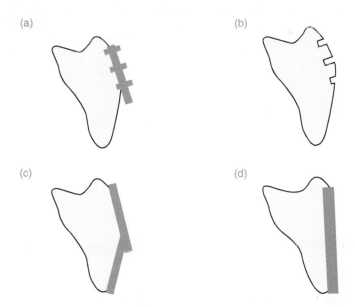

Figure 7.2.3 (a) Cross-sectional view of depth cuts with depth cutting bur. (b) Cross-sectional view of depth cuts. (c) Connection of depth cuts with burs; note the convex contour required. (d) Poor preparation with one plane reduction may encroach into close proximity to the pulp, with irreversible damage. *Source*: Wilson 2015.[3] Reproduced with permission from Elsevier.

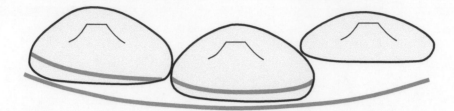

Figure 7.2.4 Occlusal view of the amount of reduction required to develop the arch form outlined by the orange line. It is important that you visualise prior to preparation whether the reduction of tooth structure is actually necessary to attain the final tooth position and contour. Note that one tooth would not even require preparation, as to attain the desired arch form would be purely additive

- **Feather preparation**. The preparation is taken or feathered to the incisal edge, without reducing the incisal edge. The disadvantage of this preparation is that the margins can be subjected to shear forces in protrusion.
- **Window preparation**. This involves preparing the veneer short of the incisal edge, retaining the enamel over the incisal edge. The disadvantage here is the difficulty of hiding the margin.
- **Bevel preparation**. A bevel is carried over the incisal edge from buccal to palatal, with 1–2 mm of incisal reduction. According to Calamia, a tooth preparation that incorporates incisal overlap is preferable, because the veneer is stronger and provides a positive seat during cementation. [4] This preparation design has the advantage of simple tooth preparation, and the aesthetic characteristics are easier to fabricate with the ceramist, as it is possible to develop incisal translucency. The proper seating of the veneer is also enabled with the positive seat that is provided. The margin should not be in a position where it will be subjected to protrusive forces during excursive movements, therefore reducing the stress within the veneer while distributing the occlusal load over a wider surface area.

(a)          (b)

(c)          (d)

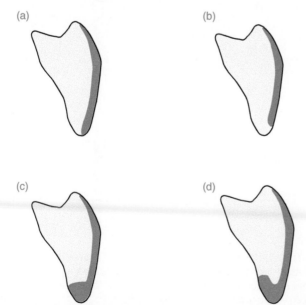

Figure 7.2.5 (a) Feather preparation. (b) Window preparation. (c) Bevel preparation. (d) Incisal overlap preparation

- **Incisal overlap**. The incisal edge is reduced with the preparation, then extended onto the palatal aspect. A positive seat is provided with this preparation, although there is a need to evaluate carefully the path of insertion to ensure that no undercuts are present.

The ideal choice of incisal preparation has not been determined. An overlap or bevel design is often used due to the advantages created by a positive seat during cementation. The aesthetic potential with this method allows ceramists to build more characteristics within the restoration. It is also the design of choice when increasing the length of the tooth.

### Proximal Preparation

This preparation can be made proximally by stopping short of breaking the contact, or by preparing through the contact point.

- If contact points are left intact, it is preferable to leave the contact point with the margin ending approximately 0.25 mm or more labial to the contact region.
- The visibility of the tooth:porcelain interproximal interface may be viewed from different angles and might be hidden by the use of an L-shaped preparation or elbow preparation to hide the margins interproximally (Figure 7.2.6).
- Breaking the contact is often used in changing the shape or position of teeth. With the additional space interproximally, this allows the ceramist freedom to adjust the contours and position of the teeth and address any width discrepancies between them.
- Preparations may extend futher proximally with the presence of caries and existing restorations.

### Cervical Margin

- Recommended chamfer design with a maximum depth of 0.4 mm. This allows the veneer to reproduce natural tooth contours and not be over-contoured. Additionally, it allows simple seating of the veneer, and minimises stresses, enhancing the future fracture resistance of the veneer.
- Use of thin, translucent porcelain often allows a 'contact lens' effect, where the margins are blended with no discernible demarcation. This enables margins to be either equigingival or supragingival.
- A supragingival margin has many advantages, with less risk of exposing dentine and less chance of injury to the soft tissues during preparation. Due to the likelihood of the margin being in enamel, there is less chance of micro-leakage associated with enamel bonding.

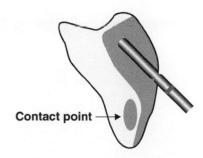

Figure 7.2.6 L-shaped proximal preparation to hide proximal margins. *Source*: Wilson 2015.[3] Reproduced with permission from Elsevier.

**Contact point**

- Subgingival margins may be required when there are caries or previous restorations extending subgingivally. Due to the deeper placement of the margin, often onto dentine, there is a greater possibility of micro-leakage and staining. It is also more difficult for the patient to clean and for dentists to finish the restoration after cementation.

### Existing Restorations

Bonding veneers onto a composite restoration increases the risk of failure, especially when the preparation margin is on an existing filling. [5,6] It is preferable to incorporate the restoration within the veneer so that it is removed completely if possible.

### Finishing the Preparation

A thorough final assessment of the preparation should be made, preferably with magnification. Ensure that there is adequate reduction and internal line angles are rounded, for example the junction between the lingual, labial and proximal planes of reduction of the preparation should be rounded with no sharp angles. These areas may intitiate stress concentration within the ceramic, predisposing it to fracture. The margins should be defined and smooth, with none located at wear facets or in occlusion.

## Tips

- Using a silicone index prepared from the diagnostic wax-up may assist in assessing the amount of reduction. When seen from the occlusal view, this can be cut in horizontal slices that can be peeled back to assess different vertical positions of the reduced teeth. Utilisation of a silicone index derived from the wax-up allows visualisation of the reduction required to achieve the form and contours of the pre-planned shape and length of the final veneers (Figures 7.2.7 and 7.2.8).

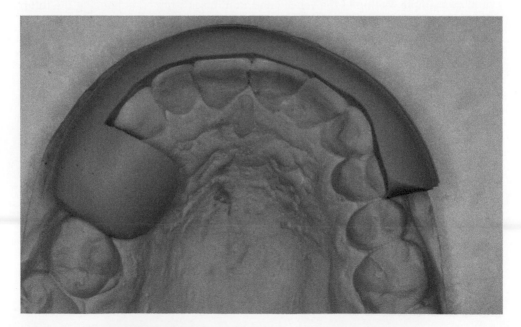

Figure 7.2.7 Silicone index seen from the occlusal view

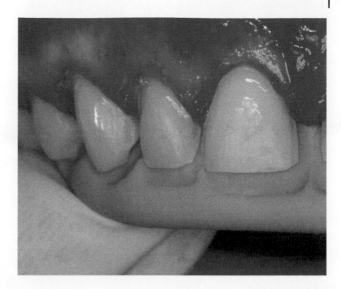

**Figure 7.2.8** Silicone index assessing the vertical reduction.

- During the final stages of preparation the use of discs and polishing rubbers can assist in smoothing the line angles of the teeth.
- When an existing restoration is very large, the tooth possesses less structural rigidity, allowing flexure and possible failure of a veneer. In these cases a decision should be made to use a full coverage restoration. This also applies to situations where there has been extensive loss of enamel, with the tooth being less rigid, and furthermore the lack of enamel means that adhesive bonding is less predictable over the long term.

## References

1  Gurel G, Sesma N, Calamita MA, Coachman C, Morimoto S. Influence of enamel preservation on failure rates of porcelain laminate veneers. *Int J Periodontics Restorative Dent.* 2013;33(1):31–9.
2  Ferrari M, Patroni S, Balleri P. Measurement of enamel thickness in relation to reduction for etched laminate veneers. *Int J Periodont Rest Dent.* 1992;23:407–13.
3  Wilson N. *Essentials of esthetic dentistry: principles and practice of esthetic dentistry.* Amsterdam: Elsevier; 2015.
4  Calamia JR. The etched porcelain veneer technique. *NY State Dent J.* 1988;54:48–50.
5  Christensen GJ, Christensen RP. Clinical observations of porcelain veneers. A three year report. *J Esthet Dent.* 1991;3:174–9.
6  Dunne SM, Millar BJ. A longitudinal study of the clinical performance of porcelain veneers. *Br Dent J.* 1993;175:317–21.

## 7.3

# Provisionalisation for Porcelain Laminate Veneers

*Christopher C.K. Ho*

*Video: Provisionalisation for Porcelain Laminate Veneers*
*Presented by Christopher C.K. Ho*

## Principles

Provisionalisation is an integral stage of treatment procedures, and allows the ability to communicate with the patient and laboratory about the planned aesthetic changes. Often patients are planning veneers for an enhanced cosmetic appearance, and as such it is a subjective process, with many patients not able to determine their desires or visualise the final result just by discussing the changes verbally. Using provisionals allows an opportunity for a 'trial smile' so that patients can preview the final planned result. There are some clinicians who feel that provisionalisation is not necessary with veneers, due to the minimal tooth reduction required. However, this step is strongly recommended and essential in the planning process. It is much easier to modify provisional restorations to please a patient than to send finished veneers back and forth to your dental ceramist or, worse still, to have to remove permanently cemented veneers due to patient dissatisfaction.

The provisional restorations are duplicated from the diagnostic wax-up incorporating the proposed changes that the patient, clinician and ceramist have planned. This may include increases in incisal length, shade changes, form and contour changes.

The main aims in provisionalisation are the following:

- **Health.** Pulpal protection and periodontal health and gingival stability are the focus here.
- **Function.** The provisional restorations can be used to assess and alert to any functional and phonetic problems with the proposed changes. The patient can be asked to perform excursive movements in both laterotrusion and protrusion. Pronouncing 'V' and 'F' sounds should create a light contact between the central incisor and the 'wet-dry' line of the lower lip.
- **Aesthetics.** The provisional restorations can be used to assess the basic shade to be chosen, incisal edge position, form and shape of teeth, dental midline location, lip support, parallelism of incisal plane to interpupillary line as well as the curvature of the lower lip. Evaluation of aesthetics provided by the provisionals at this stage is crucial in guiding the patient to the amount of display necessary for an aesthetic smile.

*Practical Procedures in Aesthetic Dentistry*, First Edition. Edited by Subir Banerji, Shamir B. Mehta and Christopher C.K. Ho. © 2017 John Wiley & Sons, Ltd. Published 2017 by John Wiley & Sons, Ltd.
Companion website: www.wiley.com/go/banerji/aestheticdentistry

## Procedures

There are various techniques for fabricating provisionals.

### Freehand Sculpting

Composite resin can be anatomically sculpted from a single veneer to multiple veneers. The prepared tooth can be spot etched (normally in the mid-labial region), with bonding agent applied and light cured, prior to building up the composite. This procedure requires more creative skills to build the correct tooth shape and form, and dentists have complete control over the build-up rather than relying on the ceramist. Note that prior to cementation of the veneers, the surface of the tooth that has been spot etched must be carefully smoothed to remove the resin in order to have a fresh surface to which to bond, and also to ensure that there is no remnant of composite that would prevent complete seating of a veneer.

### Silicone Template

A silicone template developed from the wax-up (Figure 7.3.1) can be used intra-orally.

- **Shrinkwrap technique.** Bisacryl resin composite – temporary materials such as Luxatemp (DMG America, Englewood, NJ, USA) or Protemp (3M, St Paul, MN, USA) – can be used and then allowed to set. After this has polymerised the template is removed, which often leaves the temporary veneers shrinkwrapped onto the prepared teeth due to polymerisation shrinkage. Alternatively, if the temporary veneers are removed they can be trimmed, polished and then re-cemented to the teeth by re-bonding with flowable resin (spot etching). Or the temporary veneers can be cemented with non-eugenol cement, such as Tempbond Clear (Kerr, Orange, CA, USA), a clear cement that when cemented temporarily allows a natural translucent appearance in comparison to opaque temporary cements. If the temporary veneers stay on the teeth once the silicone template is removed, then any excess flash is removed with carbide burs or the use of a no. 12 scalpel blade.

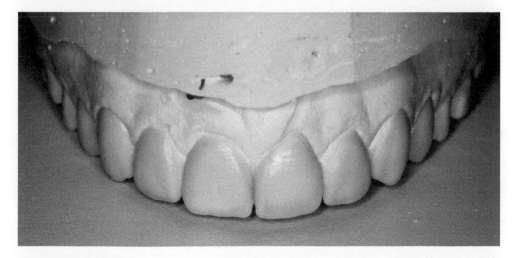

Figure 7.3.1 Diagnostic wax-up

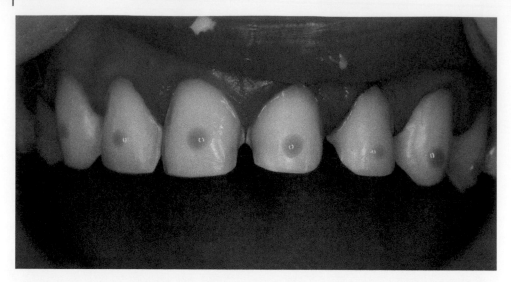

Figure 7.3.2 Spot etch of phosphoric acid applied on mid-labial of tooth. After washing off the etch, the whole prepared surface has bond applied

- **Spot etch technique** (Figure 7.3.2). The prepared tooth can be spot etched (normally in the mid-labial region), with bonding agent applied, and light cured. Following that, bisacryl resin is loaded into the silicone putty and then placed over the prepared teeth (Figure 7.3.3). As the tooth has been spot etched, the provisional material will adhere at that region and not be displaced. Any excess flash is then removed with carbide burs or a no. 12 scalpel blade (Figure 7.3.4).

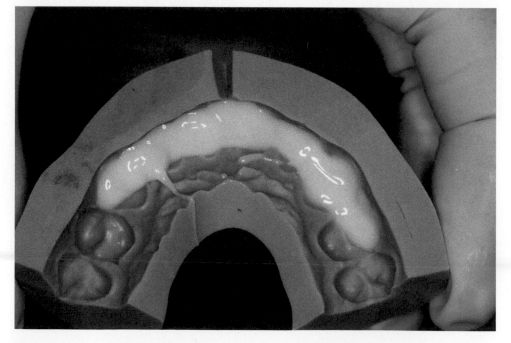

Figure 7.3.3 Loading of bisacryl resin into silicone template of diagnostic wax-up. Note that the template has been notched between 11/21 teeth to allow easier insertion intra-orally

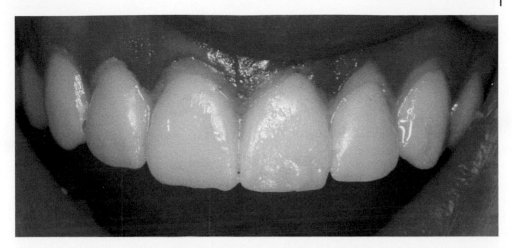

Figure 7.3.4 Provisional material after removal from silicone key. Note that voids and areas of deficiency can be added with flowable composite resin to repair or modify. Any excess is removed with a no. 12 scalpel blade or multifluted carbide finishing burs. Ensure adequate contouring of the interdental spaces to allow sufficient space for access for cleaning

A delayed approach of assessing the provisional restorations is recommended, so that the patient is not pressured into deciding whether they do or do not like the provisionals on the day of preparation. The patient is often anaesthetised with associated facial palsy and cannot adequately assess aesthetics at this time. Furthermore, the patient will often ask friends and family about the proposed changes and can accustom themselves to their new look given the extra time. If there are major changes to the lengths of teeth or occlusion, then time is also required to allow the patient to adapt to the new changes.

If the patient is happy with the provisional restorations, then the ceramist may construct the final restorations using the original wax-up as a blueprint. If the provisional restoration requires modifications, the temporaries can be adjusted or composite resin can be added and an impression of the temporaries can be made. This can then be used as a template and communication tool to the ceramist about additional changes.

## Tips

- Any voids or deficient margins present are easily repaired with flowable composite resin. There is no need to apply adhesive for this purpose.
- The use of clear temporary cement (e.g. Tempbond Clear; Tempspan Clear, Pentron, Orange, CA, USA) is recommended for veneers, as opaque cement will make the veneer opaque and distinct, not allowing the patient a correct preview of anticipated changes.
- There should be minimal to no sensitivity, as there is minimal reduction for veneers, with many cases being limited to enamel only. Should there be exposed dentine, the use of bond (non-etched) that has been placed over the prepared tooth normally blocks out any sensitivity. If there is continuing sensitivity the use of commercial desensitisers is normally sufficient to block any discomfort.
- Ensure that oral hygiene is optimal in the temporary phase so that there is minimal inflammation and bleeding during the adhesive cementation.
- Warn patients of the temporary nature of the veneers and the possibility that they may dislodge, so that patients are not concerned if this does happen inadvertently.

## 7.4

# Appraisal and Cementation of Porcelain Laminate Veneers

*Christopher C.K. Ho*

*Video: Appraisal and Cementation of Porcelain Laminate Veneers*
*Presented by Christopher C.K. Ho*

## Principles

### Appraisal and Try-In of Veneers

It is important to assess veneers on models to check marginal fit as well as to evaluate the integrity of the porcelain to ensure that there are no defects or fractures prior to cemenation. It is vital to have confirmation from the patient that they are happy prior to proceeding with the cementation procedures.

It is preferable not to use local anaesthetic for the patient to approve the final aesthetics prior to cementation. However, if local anaesthesia is required, an alternative is to use the AMSA local anaesthetic block technique, so that the injection achieves pulpal anaesthesia of the central incisors through the second premolar without collateral numbness of the face and facial muscles of expression. This is best achieved with the computer-controlled injection system – the Wand (Milestone Scientific, Livingston, NJ, USA) – which delivers a virtually painless palatal injection.

### Cementation

Correct preparation of the fitting surface of the veneer involves micro-mechanically roughening the surface by etching with hydrofluoric acid. This removes a layer of glass, leaving a roughened surface. There is a salt residue on the surface, which should be removed to enhance the final bond strength. The surface is then silanated and ready for cementation. Isolate carefully to enhance access and restrict moisture contamination.

The veneers are adhesively bonded with light-cure resin cement, which allows sufficient working time to seat the veneer and possesses better colour stability. There are various shades of cement that can be utilised, which have minimal influence on the final shade due to the low film thickness of the cements once luted. Using opaque cements may help to block out discoloration as well as increase the value of the final shade of the veneer. If opaque cement is used it should be applied sparingly, as too much will make the veneer distinct and not lifelike in appearance.

*Practical Procedures in Aesthetic Dentistry*, First Edition. Edited by Subir Banerji, Shamir B. Mehta and Christopher C.K. Ho. © 2017 John Wiley & Sons, Ltd. Published 2017 by John Wiley & Sons, Ltd.
Companion website: www.wiley.com/go/banerji/aestheticdentistry

# Procedures

## Appraisal

The provisional veneers can be carefully removed using a spoon excavator to lever them from the proximal walls. If this is unsuccessful, the provisional material can be sectioned with a vertical cut and a torquing movement applied with an instrument to remove separate fragments.

The tooth surface should be cleaned of any residual resin cement or provisional material, to ensure perfect adaptation of the veneers. If a spot etched temporary veneer was placed, then the etched area will need be prepared with a fine diamond to allow a clean surface to which to bond. This will also ensure that there is no resin present that would interfere with the seating of the veneer.

The tooth is then cleaned with fine pumice slurry or air abraded with 27 micron aluminium oxide, carefully avoiding the soft tissues to minimise any chance of gingival bleeding. Small finishing strips can be used interproximally to clean the contact areas.

Each veneer should be assessed to ensure that the marginal fit around the die is accurate. It is good practice to assess each veneer with transillumination to ensure there are no fractures within the porcelain. The veneers should then be appraised on the preparation individually to assess fit. This is best done dry (without water or try-in gels), as marginal adaptation is then better visualised. Do not apply excessive pressure while trialling the veneers, as they are brittle prior to bonding.

Incomplete seating is normally due to resin cement that has not been removed, remaining provisional material or tight contact points. Once each individual veneer has been assessed, then all the veneers should be assessed in place, evaluating the proximal contacts. It may be necessary to use the try-in gels at this stage to allow temporary seating of the veneers.

The veneers should be checked with the patient in relation to colour, form and length, as well as whether they are pleasing to the patient or may require modification. There are different water-soluble try-in gels that a clinician can use to alter the colour of the veneer, from lowering or raising the value to opaquing the restoration to mask discoloration.

At this stage the patient should not be asked to check occlusion, as this may cause fracture of an unbonded veneer.

## Treating the Fitting Surface of the Veneer

Once the final aesthetics of the veneers are approved, the restorations are prepared for cementation.

The veneers (being silica-based restorations) must be etched with hydrofluoric acid, which allows a micro-mechanical bond when adhesively bonded. The fitting surface is etched with 9.5% hydrofluoric acid for 20 seconds with lithium disilicate (e.max) or 60 seconds for other silica-based ceramics. The use of hydrofluoric acid dissolves the glassy matrix surrounding the crystalline phase within the porcelain, leaving retentive areas between the acid-resistant crystals.

The treatment of the veneer with hydrofluoric acid etching is often carried out by the ceramist, and if this is the case it should not be repeated. Instead, the fitting surface can be treated with >30% phosphoric acid for more than 15 seconds. This helps to remove the calcium fluoride salt precipitates and to make the surface more active for the silane primer prior to bonding.

Although many laboratories etch porcelain for dentists, it is best to treat the veneer with hydrofluoric acid etching after try-in, as this minimises the contamination of the etched surface. It has been reported that die stone contamination with the etched veneers being placed onto the die stone can reduce bond strength, and thus it is preferred to etch veneers after clinical try-in. [1]

The acid should be thoroughly cleansed with air–water spray and the porcelain should then be placed into a container of distilled water (or 95% alcohol or acetone) and put into an ultrasonic bath for 4 minutes to remove any residues remaining on the surface. Restorations are removed, dried and silane primer is applied to the fitting surface, which helps provide a chemical covalent bond to the ceramic. This is allowed to remain on the veneer for 1 minute and after that the veneer should be gently blown with air to evaporate any remaining solvent.

Heat treatment of the silane may enhance the effect of silane coupling and this may be achieved by placing the restoration in a dry furnace at 100 °C for 1 minute, or using 2 minutes of hot air from a hair dryer. [2]

### Isolation and Haemostasis

The application of rubber dam is recommended to achieve adequate isolation, which helps to provide a clean, dry environment and minimises contamination from saliva and blood. It also plays a crucial role in preventing ingestion or aspiration of instruments, tooth debris, dental materials or other foreign bodies.

As well as the provision of isolation and moisture control, there is the added benefit of retraction of lips, cheeks and tongue. This allows improved access, visualisation and protection of soft tissues from rotary instrumentation.

Due to the requirement for adhesive bonding, it is best not to utilise a ferric-containing haemostatic agent, as this may inhibit polymerisation and cause marginal staining. In these cases the use of aluminium chloride is recommended.

### Cementation

The prepared surfaces are etched with phosphoric acid and adhesive is applied. The use of different coloured or opaque cements should have been chosen at the try-in phase, with the ability to modify slightly the final colour or opacity of the veneer.

### Bonding Veneers

Light-cure composite resin cement is preferred for cementation of the veneers, as it has a longer working time than dual-cure or chemically cured composites. This allows sufficient time to remove excess composite prior to curing and thus reduces the finishing procedures.

The colour stability of light-cure resin cements is much better compared to dual-cure or chemically cured composites. Dual-cure resin cements contain tertiary amines that may undergo long-term colour change ('amine discoloration') with overall darkening and thus are normally contraindicated with veneers due to their thin nature and translucency.

For porcelain with a thickness of more than 0.7 mm, light-cure composites do not reach maximum hardness. It may be necessary to increase the exposure time or utilise a dual-cure resin cement in these cases. [3]

There are different techniques for bonding the veneers, but they can be basically categorised into two different techniques: wave or tacking. Both techniques involve first gently placing the veneer over the tooth, starting from the incisal edge and progressively placing the veneers towards the apical region, with slight pressure towards the palatal. It is also important for the resin cement to be squeezed out from all margins, to avoid voids within the cement margins.

- **Wave technique.** This involves seating the veneer, followed by waving the curing light over the margins for only a few seconds. It partially polymerises the resin cement into a gel state that can then be easily removed. Any excess cement around the margins can be further removed with a brush or a gum stimulator (Figure 7.4.1). This allows a smooth margin with minimal tendency for the resin to be dragged out of the margin. Floss should also be used gently to clean out interdental areas. Eventual removal should always be by pulling the floss towards the palatal to avoid dislodging the partially set cement (Figure 7.4.2).
- **Tacking technique.** This involves using a tacking tip from the curing light, typically 2–4 mm in diameter, which spot tacks the veneer, stabilising it in the correct position (Figure 7.4.3). While the veneer is being tacked, the clinician provides a seating pressure that is also directed slightly mesially to ensure complete seating (Figure 7.4.4). This slight mesial pressure is not intended to change the proximal contact points inadvertently, which can be an issue when you go on to seat the final veneers and find that there is no room to seat them due to the contact points being too tight. Once the veneer is tacked into place, there is a similar clean-up phase with the use of a brush or a gum stimulator to remove the excess.

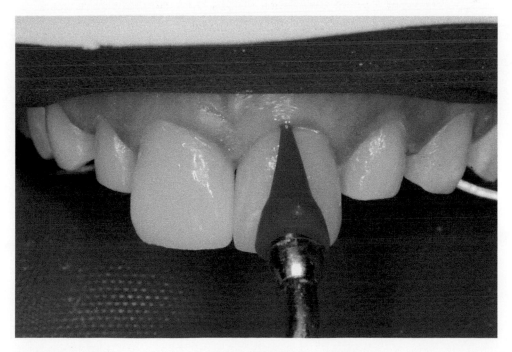

Figure 7.4.1 Use of a gum stimulator to remove unset excess resin cement

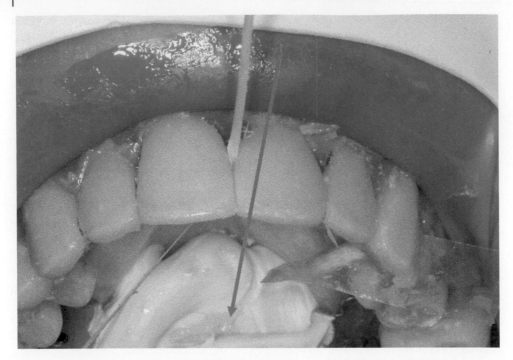

Figure 7.4.2 Floss should be pulled towards the palatal so as not to dislodge the veneer

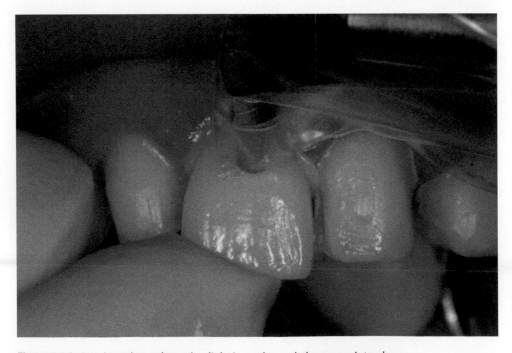

Figure 7.4.3 A tacking tip on the curing light is used to tack the veneer into place

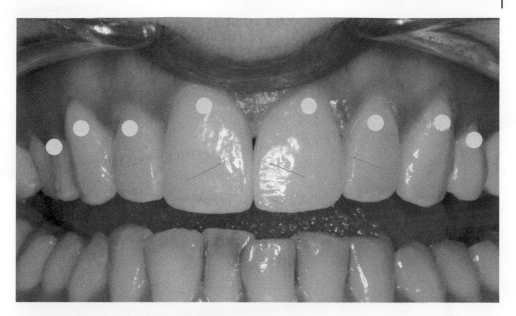

Figure 7.4.4  Veneers are tacked into place while pressure is placed towards the mesial and palatal (orange circle denotes the tacking tip position)

### Use of Opaque Cements

When there is a need to block out discoloration, there may be a need to use opaque resin cements containing composites with metal oxide particles, for instance titanium oxide. The opacity can be unpredictable due to slight variations in film thickness, which may alter the value of the veneer, resulting in bright spots. The resin cement also has opacity, which will negate the lifelike qualities of the veneer. Furthermore, the veneer becomes optically distinct and does not blend in at the margins, which results in a visible margin. If using opaque cement, it is best not to use 100% opaque cement, but a mix of a normal translucent cement and opaque cement. Using translucent resin cement is recommended to maximise the 'contact lens effect', allowing margins to blend in. This improves the aesthetic longevity of the veneers, as the soft-tissue recession that occurs with age will not reveal the distinct line seen with crowns and opaque veneers.

### Finishing and Polishing

If the bonding procedure was completed smoothly with a well-fitting veneer, there should be minimal cement to clean up from around the margins. It is preferable not to use a rotary instrument to finish the margins, as this may remove the glaze layer, increasing the roughness of the porcelain and causing increased plaque retention. It can also cause wear of antagonists, unless polished to a smooth surface. Instead, the use of a no. 12 blade to remove excess cement carefully is the preferred technique (Figure 7.4.5).

Polishing instruments are well suited to flat surfaces, but may not perform so well in interdental and gingival areas. If it proves necessary to polish the margins with rotary instrumentation, the careful use of very fine diamond is suggested, followed by polishing rubbers and diamond polishing paste. Any interproximal excess cement

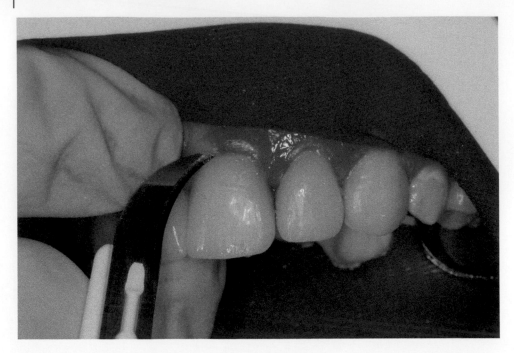

Figure 7.4.5 Use of no. 12 scalpel blade to remove excess cement

may be removed by interproximal saws and polishing strips. There are a variety of commercial kits available to polish the surface finish of the porcelain.

The occlusion is carefully checked initially with centric occlusion, followed by other excursive movements. Egg-shaped diamonds with water spray can be used to adjust the porcelain. Any adjustments must be further polished.

The patient is recalled within two weeks to evaluate the porcelain veneers. At this appointment the clinician should check and adjust occlusion if necessary, remove any excess resin that was not detected at cementation stage, and carry out any further adjustments of the veneers that you or the patient deem necessary.

## Tips

- When flossing excess cement from around partially set veneers, proceed with flossing and pulling out lingually so as not to dislodge the veneer.
- The use of a no. 12 scalpel or sharp scaler may assist in removing excess cement around the margins without resorting to rotary instrumentation.

## References

1 Magne P, Cascione D. Influence of post-etching cleaning and connecting porcelain on the microtensile bond strength of composite resin to feldspathic porcelain. *J Prosthet Dent.* 2006;96:354–61.
2 Roulet JF, Soderholm KJ, Longmate J. Effects of treatment and storage conditions on ceramic/composite bond strength. *J Dent Res.* 1995;74:381–7.
3 Linden JJ, Swift EJ, Boyer DB, Davis BK. Photoactivation of resin cements through porcelain veneers. *J Dent Res.* 1991;70:154–7.

# Part VIII

# Partial Removable Prosthodontics

## 8.1

# Aesthetic Removable Dental Prosthetics

*Subir Banerji and Shamir B. Mehta*

*Video: Aesthetic Removable Dental Prosthetics*
*Presented by Subir Banerji and Shamir B. Mehta*

## Principles

Removable partial dentures (**RPDs**) are commonly prescribed as definitive appliances for the restoration of aesthetics and function (masticatory and phonetic), which may become compromised following the loss of teeth and the investing tissues, as well as for the preservation of occlusal stability. RPDs may sometimes be used in a **transitional** manner while carrying out stabilisation of oral disease or to enable the verification of planned occlusal changes, where there may be an occlusal anomaly such as the loss of occlusal vertical dimension.

RPDs can provide a minimally invasive and economic option for the replacement of multiple missing teeth (and supporting tissues), especially where there may be more than one edentulous space, while also concomitantly offering the benefit of lip and cheek support. They also give the potential for contingency planning when the residual dentition presents with a guarded prognosis.

However, by virtue of not being 'fixed' prostheses, they may not offer the same level of masticatory function or feeling of self-confidence as is optimally desired. Furthermore, there is the potential for the exacerbation of oral disease (in the presence of a removable appliance) in an unfavourable environment. The latter can, however, be further controlled by paying careful attention to appliance design and the implementation of an effective preventative regime.[1,2]

It is important that the planning and design of RPDs are primarily viewed as the role and responsibility of the dental practitioner, and are undertaken as part of whole patient care and overall restorative planning. This chapter will outline the stages in RPD design. The appropriate use of a design sheet is advisable.

## Procedures

Following a comprehensive patient assessment (including a detailed evaluation of the edentulous spaces, any existing appliances, potential abutment teeth and the prognostic

*Practical Procedures in Aesthetic Dentistry*, First Edition. Edited by Subir Banerji, Shamir B. Mehta and Christopher C.K. Ho. © 2017 John Wiley & Sons, Ltd. Published 2017 by John Wiley & Sons, Ltd.
Companion website: www.wiley.com/go/banerji/aestheticdentistry

outcome of the residual dentition), it is worth fabricating a set of accurate study casts, which may require mounting on a suitable form of dental articulator.

It is important also to identify the presence of any features that may reduce the intra- or interocclusal spaces, such as tilted, rotated, drifted and over-erupted teeth as well as any hard or soft tissue factors that may compromise the insertion of an RPD. A detailed static and dynamic occlusal assessment should be carried out, additionally noting the freeway space (FWS), the presence of any occlusal interferences and/or any slides between the intercuspal position (ICP) and the first point of tooth contact in centric relation (CRCP). Aspects that may compromise the provision of an RPD or its ability to restore aesthetics and function should be identified and managed at this stage.

Having determined the edentulous spaces that are to be replaced by the RPD, commence with the selection of an appropriate **path of insertion** (and withdrawal) or POI using a **dental surveyor** (as seen in Figure 8.1.1). The selection of a POI will be influenced by a number of factors:

- Provision of retention to displacement in a vertical direction
- Enabling the utilization of guide planes
- Use of hard and soft tissue undercuts
- Elimination of unsightly 'black' spaces that will also serve as food traps.

Sometimes the choice of a given POI may require tooth preparation, which may be achieved by either additive (bonding) or subtractive means. The selected POI should be scribed on the cast as a source of reference. The use of undercut gauges (Figure 8.1.2) is helpful when attempting to measure undercuts for the placement of dental clasps.

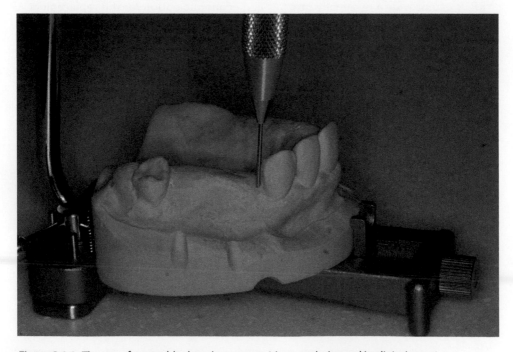

Figure 8.1.1 The use of a portable dental surveyor with an analysing rod in clinical practice

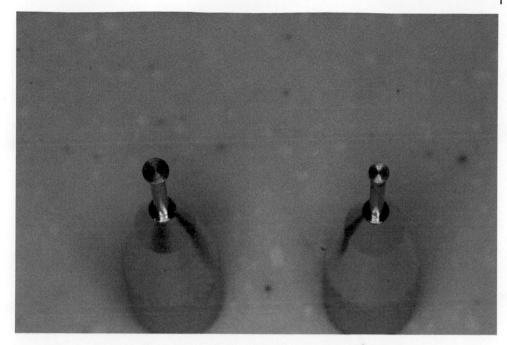

**Figure 8.1.2** Undercut depth gauges for flexible clasp (left) and non-flexible clasp (right) designs

The means by which **support** is to be provided should be determined. This may be derived from the mucosa, teeth or a combination. When using **rest seats** (occlusal, cingulum or incisal) to provide tooth support, it is imperative that space is provided to incorporate the rest seat as well for the attachment of the seat to the major connector (via a minor connector). This may require preparation of the abutment tooth. Where an indirect restoration is to be provided on an abutment tooth, features such as the presence of an undercut for direct retention and a ledge for a bracing component (together with the rest seat) should be included. The preparation form should account for the incorporation of these features.

For bounded saddles, rest seats should be sited as close to the saddle as possible to optimise load distribution. For free-end saddled dentures (where support will be provided anteriorly by the teeth and posteriorly by the mucosa), owing to the differences in relative displaceability when an occlusal load is applied, in order to minimise torqueing forces on the abutment tooth the use of a mesially placed rest seat on the distal abutment, a distal guide plane, the use of a ginigival-approaching 'I-bar clasp', the use of narrower teeth and maximisation of the covering of the ridge by the saddle may all be advisable.

Determine the means by which **retention** to vertical displacement will be provided. This may be by adhesive and cohesive forces, muscular control, the inclusion of guide planes to limit the direction of the POI as well as to provide frictional resistance, and the use of direct retainers. Direct retention is typically provided by the means of dental clasps (Figure 8.1.3). There are a plethora of clasp designs and materials for their fabrication. In general, the choice of a clasp will depend on the position and size of the undercut, the depth of the undercut, the relationship of the survey line to the gingival margin and occlusal surface, the aesthetic demands of the patient (taking into account

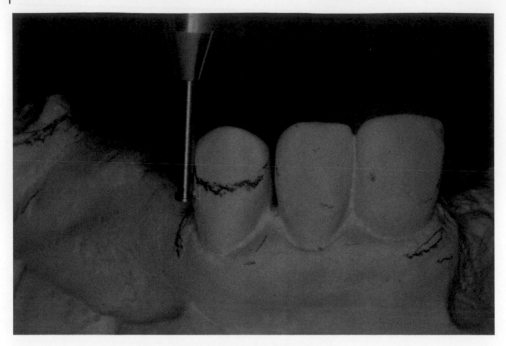

Figure 8.1.3 Use of an undercut depth gauge for a rigid clasp design

the smile line) and the presence of anatomical factors that may prove unfavourable. In some cases, modification of the survey line or POI may be required to optimise retention and/or to negate the use of anterior clasps. Resin-based tooth-coloured clasps are being used more commonly, although they are prone to fracture.

Direct retention can also be provided by the means of **precision attachments** or **telescopic crowns**, which will avoid the display of clasps in the aesthetic zone.

**Reciprocation** will be required to oppose the action of the clasp, which will not only avoid unwanted tooth movement, but improve the efficacy of the clasp. This will require the provision of a bracing arm on the abutment tooth or a plate connector.

The choice of **major connector** design should be subsequently determined. For mucosally supported dentures, ideally as much surface area should be covered as possible; however, gingival margin coverage should be avoided. For mandibular tooth-supported dentures the choice of a lingual bar, sublingual bar, labial bar or plate will be determined by the depth of the lingual sulcus. There is an array of materials that can be used to form the major connector, broadly encompassing metals and acrylic. In recent years, there has been a trend towards the use of thermoplastic flexible base (and clasp materials). However, adjustments, repairs and additions may prove difficult. De-bonding of acrylic teeth can also be a concern.

The ability of the appliance to provide resistance to rotational displacement (**stability**) should also be assessed. For a tooth-supported appliance this may require the inclusion of indirect retention, which may be provided by prescribing rest seats or components placed perpendicular to an axis that passes through an imaginary line formed between the tips of the most distal opposing clasp units.

Finally, review the design. For predictable outcomes, designs should be kept as simple as possible.

## Tips

- Denture design should take place early when planning for care. Patients need to be provided with a clear overview of the merits and disadvantages of these appliances and the choices they have concerning design and aesthetics, as well as the need for good preventative care.
- You may wish to apply concepts such as the shortened dental arch when assessing the need for tooth replacement.[3]
- To further enhance the aesthetic outcome, pay close attention to the selection of artificial teeth (often applying the concepts of smile design). Teeth may be further characterised by the addition of stains, craze lines, wear facets or the inclusion of dental restorations. Minor imbrications and tilting may also enhance the aesthetic outcome. Characterisation of the flanges will help to improve the aesthetic result by the inclusion of stains to mimic pigmentation (where natural pigmentation may be present) or by introducing stippling.

## References

1 Bergman B, Hugoson A, Olsson C. A 25-year longitudinal study of patients treated with removable partial dentures. *J Oral Rehab.* 1995;8:595–9.
2 Carlson G, Hedegard B, Koivumma K et al. Studies on partial denture prosthesis. IV. Final results of a four-year longitudinal investigation of dentogingivally supported partial dentures. *Acta Odontol Sand.* 1965;23:433.
3 Kayser A. How much reduction of the dental arch is functionally acceptable for the aging patient. *Int Dent J.* 1990;40:183–8.

## Further Reading

Davenport J, Basker R, Heath J, Ralph J, Glantz P. *The clinical guide series, a clinical guide to removable partial denture design.* London: BDJ Books, 2000.

Part IX

Aesthetic Management of Tooth Wear

## 9.1

# Aesthetic Management of Tooth Wear: Current Concepts

*Subir Banerji and Shamir B. Mehta*

## Principles

The irreversible wearing away of the dental hard tissues is a consequence of the natural ageing process. The condition of **tooth wear (TW)** is used to describe the surface loss of the dental hard tissues from conditions other than caries, trauma or developmental disorders.

Where the observed level of TW for any given patient is considered to be extensive so as to be associated with concerns relating to the presence of symptoms of pain or discomfort, aesthetic or functional compromise, or indeed the rate of wear exceeds what may be considered normal for the age of the patient (perhaps better termed physiological), the suffix **pathological** may be added.

With an ageing population, lifestyle and habit changes, it is not uncommon in the developed world to encounter patients presenting with pathological wear on a regular basis across the entire age spectrum, ranging from younger children to the geriatric patient.

TW often has a multifactorial aetiology. Individual factors include **erosion**, **abrasion**, **abfraction** and **attrition**. It would appear that erosion is a factor in the majority of patients with TW. Acidic substrates, which lead to erosive wear, may be derived intrinsically or extrinsically. A sevenfold increase in the rate of consumption of soft beverages in the UK between the 1950s and 1990s has been reported as taking place, with adolescents accounting for 65% of all purchases.[1] In more recent times, with more individuals pursuing a healthier lifestyle and consuming copious quantities of fresh fruits and vegetables, it is also likely that this will have an aetiological impact. Table 9.1.1 provides a list of the typical pH values of commonly consumed beverages.

Table 9.1.1 Typical pH values of commonly consumed beverages.[2]

| Manufacturer | Brand | PH value |
| --- | --- | --- |
| Pepsi-Cola | Diet | 2.95 |
| Coca-Cola | Regular | 3.25 |
| Lucozade | Sport Orange | 3.78 |
| Tango | Diet Orange | 2.80 |
| Orange juice | | 3.50 |

*Practical Procedures in Aesthetic Dentistry*, First Edition. Edited by Subir Banerji, Shamir B. Mehta and Christopher C.K. Ho.  © 2017 John Wiley & Sons, Ltd. Published 2017 by John Wiley & Sons, Ltd.
Companion website: www.wiley.com/go/banerji/aestheticdentistry

The successful management of a patient presenting with TW requires the clinician not only to derive an accurate diagnosis based on a recording of a contemporaneous dental history and to undertake a meticulous patient assessment (as described in Part 2), but also to understand the processes involved in **passive management** (prevention and monitoring) and to possess a suitable level of knowledge of how to successfully restore cases where **active intervention** is indicated.

This chapter will focus on the passive management phase.

## Procedures

Having established that your patient has pathological TW, it is advisable to record the **severity** and **location** of the pattern of wear. Wear may be broadly classed as **localised** or **generalised**. The former may be further described as anterior, posterior, maxillary or mandibular. A detailed subclassifcation system will be discussed in subsequent chapters, which will aid in the process of systematic treatment planning and provision.

The severity of TW may be described purely by observation or recorded with the aid of dental indices. The Tooth Wear Index by Smith and Knight is commonly used.[3] A plethora of other indices have also been introduced.

The primary objective should be to manage any **acute conditions** (if present). This may range from easing a sharp cusp or incisal edge to the prescription or application of a de-sensitising agent or appropriate dental material to seal patent dentinal tubules, the placement of a resin composite veneer where there may be an aesthetic compromise, the extirpation of the dental pulp, the management of the acute symptoms of temporomandibular joint dysfunction or the extraction of a tooth with a hopeless prognosis.

The long-term, successful management of the patient will largely depend on the ability of both patient and clinician to identify and prevent the causative factor(s) from inflicting further harm.

A **dietary analysis** is invaluable. Ask the patient to keep a diet diary of their food and beverage intake for three consecutive days. A reduction in the quantity and frequency of the consumption of fruits, fruit juices, carbonated drinks or any other acidic substances should be encouraged, perhaps limited to meal times only. The consumption of hard cheese or dairy products after the ingestion of acidic beverages can reduce their erosive effect.

Sugar-free chewing gum, which may contain fluoride or carbamide, may be helpful in simulating salivary flow, which may help to buffer the pH levels and further protect the dental hard tissues from erosive wear. Patients with xerstomia should be managed appropriately and this may involve referral to a specialist colleague.

Further **habit changes** may be helpful, such as drinking acidic beverages through a wide-bore straw to minimise contact with the teeth. Oral hygiene instructions may be advisable, such as the avoidance of over-zealous brushing (especially after acid exposure) or of using abrasive toothpastes or mouthwashes with low PH, coupled with other habit changes such as refraining from pen/pencil biting.

**Topical fluoride application**, either in the form of toothpaste containing 1.1% neutral sodium fluoride or an appropriate rinse, may be particularly helpful in reducing the impact of erosive substrate exposure. Neutral sodium fluoride gels, alkaline preparations such as milk of magnesia or sodium bicarbonate solution or de-sensitising gels containing potassium nitrate or amorphous calcium phosphate (Recaldent or Tooth Mousse, GC Corp, Tokyo, Japan), placed within modified bleaching trays with reservoirs, may also be beneficial to help with **neutralisation**, **desensitisation** and **remineralisation**, respectively. Caution is advocated for patients with gastric reflux, as the splint may unintentionally act as a reservoir for the acid produced.

If there are symptoms of jaw joint dysfunction, or a confirmed diagnosis of parafunctional tooth clenching and/or grinding habits, then a hard **occlusal stabilisation splint** should be considered. As a short-term emergency measure a soft, vacuum-formed PVC (polyvinyl chloride) splint can be fabricated. Soft splints have the risk of unwanted tooth movements as well as the potential to cause an increase in the level of muscle activity, which in turn may culminate in poor tolerance and compliance. Ideally, a hard, full coverage indirect heat-processed acrylic splint (as described in Chapter 3.6) should be prescribed.

For areas with **exposed dentine**, the application of a dentine-bonding agent, fissure sealant resin or glass ionomer cement can be considered. This helps to reduce dentinal hypersensitivity as well as protect the affected surfaces from further wear and tear.

If an underlying medical condition such as gastric reflux or bulimia is suspected, then **referral to a medical colleague** is required.

For the majority of patients, passive management is all that may be needed. To assess the efficacy of the preventative strategy, it is important to be able to monitor the condition of the worn surfaces. This may involve the use of an index to record the level of wear, taking and recording high-quality clinical photographs, periodic study casts (at 6–12-month intervals), with the use of a sectional PVS (polyvinyl siloxane) index as a guide formed on the initial cast. These monitoring techniques are not highly sensitive. The use of digital technology such as software to map surface changes may have a beneficial role for the future.

Finally, where active treatment has been decided at the outset, a process of prevention and monitoring for a minimum 6-month period should be undertaken (other than with cases with excessively high wear rates, such as among bulimic patients), not only to ensure successful containment of the causative factor, but also to provide an opportunity to establish effective rapport with the patient and to provide details relating to definitive care provision, which may be complex, as discussed in subsequent chapters.

## Tips

- Take time to identify possible aetiological factors for tooth wear.
- Where possible avoid advanced restorative care without effectively preventing the causative factors from inflicting further harm.
- Failure to do this will culminate in premature restorative failure.
- Intra-oral photographs showing the pattern and extent of wear are useful to inform the patient about the problem.
- The diagnostic build-up of one or two teeth with some composite can make the patient more aware of the problem.
- The presence of sensitivity is often an indication that the tooth wear process is active.

## References

1 Shaw L, Smith A. Erosion in children. An increasing clinical problem? *Dent Update.* 1994;21:103–6.
2 Kelleher M, Bishop K. Article 1, Tooth surface loss. In: *Tooth surface loss: an overview.* London: BDJ Books; 2000. p. 3–7.
3 Smith B, Knight J. An index for measuring the wear of teeth. *Br Dent J.* 1984;156:435–8.

## Further Reading

Mehta SB, Banerji S, Millar BJ, Suarez-Feito J-M. Current concepts on the management of tooth wear part Assessment, treatment planning and the strategies for the prevention and passive management of tooth wear. *Br Dent J.* 2012;212:17–27.

## 9.2

# The Direct Canine Rise Restoration

*Subir Banerji and Shamir B. Mehta*

*Video: The Direct Canine Rise Restoration*
*Presented by Subit Banerji and Shamir B. Mehta*

## Principles

In Chapter 3.1, the requirements for a mechanically stable occlusal scheme were outlined, hence the concept of the **mutually protective occlusal scheme**. In summary, this includes the presence of even, stable occlusal stops on all of the teeth (being of a slightly higher intensity on the posterior teeth) in the intercuspal position, with the absence of contact between the posterior teeth (**disclusion**) during excursive movements. Guidance to the mandible should be provided by the anterior dentition, with occlusal loads being equally shared. With a **canine-guided occlusal scheme**, guidance during lateral excursive movements is provided by the canine teeth only.

In the absence of posterior disclusion during excursive and protrusive mandibular movements, the posterior teeth will make antagonistic contact, which may ultimately manifest as:

- Pathological wear
- Partial or indeed complete tooth fracture
- Premature restorative failure (additionally affecting the anterior dentition)
- Increased loading of teeth and occlusal trauma (and its sequelae)
- Contributing to temporomandibular joint disorders or dysfunction.

Figure 9.2.1 depicts an example of a patient with mild posterior tooth wear due to wear of the canine tooth.

The absence of posterior disclusion in a patient who may have previously presented with a canine-guided occlusal scheme may occur following the process of tooth wear affecting the canine teeth, iatrogenic intervention (adjustment of the canine teeth or following the placement of a dental restoration with an altered occlusal morphology), orthodontic tooth movement, dental caries, periodontal disease, trauma or indeed after a dental extraction.

The anatomy and location of the canine teeth, commonly with a lengthy, bulbous root, render them suitable for the process of providing posterior disclusion, as earlier described.

The practical section in this chapter will describe the process of **restoring canine guidance**, where it may have been altered by the process of wear, which may be

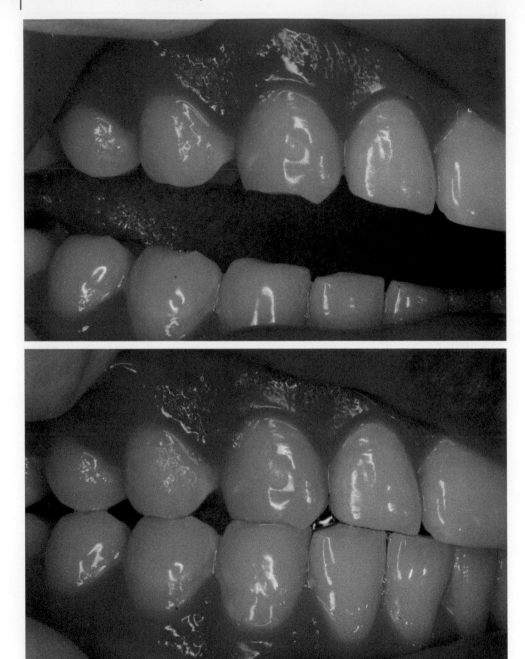

Figure 9.2.1 An example of a patient with mild posterior tooth wear, due to wear of the canine tooth

considered as a means of preventing many of the conditions listed earlier, including the protection of newly placed posterior supracoronal restorations from destructive lateral loading during dynamic mandibular movements.[1] This form of restoration may be referred to as a **canine riser or Stuart lift**, which, by altering the cuspal incline of the canine teeth, aims to provide a canine-guided occlusion.[2]

## Procedures

A complete occlusal assessment should be carried out as described in Chapter 3.1. A long-cone periapical radiograph of the canine teeth should be taken to provide you with further insight into the morphology and size of the root, the level of alveolar support, the presence of any apical pathology (including root resorption), evidence of ankylosis, carious lesions, status of any existing restorations and the morphology of the pulp chamber. Endodontically treated canine teeth or brittle canine teeth (as may be encountered in the geriatric patient) may be unsuitable for this form of restoration due to heightened risks of tooth fracture.

A detailed periodontal analysis and aesthetic evaluation are also advisable.

Mock up a riser restoration simply by drying the tooth and placing resin composite (without any bonding) on the canine as a means of attaining consent and allowing the patient to visualise the aesthetic outcome.

The technique described here relates to the placement of resin composite in a **direct manner** to restore a worn maxillary canine. However, it can equally be applied to restore a worn mandibular canine tooth, or perhaps both, dependent on the level of wear observed and the aesthetic demands of the patient.

Clearly, the placement of direct resin composite requires the presence of a good quantity and quality of enamel tissue for predictable adhesive bonding, as well as the need to attain effective moisture control. Resin composite has the merits of being aesthetic, as well as allowing for contingency planning, should the patient be unable to tolerate the restoration. Adjustments can be made readily, or the restoration removed with no harm being incurred. Resin composite is also a relatively inexpensive material. If the patient can tolerate the restoration, a more robust restorative material can be considered in the longer term.

The appropriate shade of resin composite is then chosen. The centric stop on the canine tooth should be identified and marked using articulating paper. This mark should ideally remain in situ during the course of the procedure. Following isolation, the enamel is cleaned using air abrasion or a slurry of oil-free pumice. Cleaning should be confined to the hard tissues superior to the centric stop and should be extended over the incisal edge towards the facial surface.

Isolation of the adjacent teeth is recommended to avoid inadvertent resin adhesion. This can be achieved by either the placement of a suitable matrix, such as cellulose acetate strip(s), a metal matrix or PTFE (polytetrafluoroethylene) tape, as shown in Figure 9.2.1. Then 37% orthophosphoric acid is applied to the cleaned enamel surfaces for a period of 30 seconds. This is washed off and the surface gently air dried. Adhesive resin is applied to the etched hard tissues, as per the manufacturer's recommendations, gently air dried to permit solvent evaporation and then light cured.

For a severely worn canine tooth a dentine shade of resin composite may be required along with the enamel shade, taking great care only to add material superior (incisal) to the marked centric stop. The inadvertent placement of composite resin on or inferior (gingival) to the centric stop will culminate in an increase in the patient's occlusal vertical dimension.

The dentine shade is added in a manner that restores the dentine tissue that has been lost, and then light cured. Resin should be placed in increments no greater than 2 mm to permit adequate curing. The selected enamel shade is placed to restore the enamel layer. The enamel layer should be extended onto the facial surface to cover as much of the labial enamel as possible, without compromising the aesthetic or oral hygiene requirements of your patient. After light curing the enamel layer, a final translucent layer of resin composite may be applied.

The efficacy of the restoration placed should be evaluated; ideally it should provide canine guidance, which can be verified by asking your patient to demonstrate a lateral excursive movement. This should result in disclusion on both the working and non-working sides. Articulating paper can be used to aid the verification process. Further increment of resin can be applied if required. The ramp provided should harmonise with the residual occlusion, otherwise displacement and/or mobility of the canine teeth will result.

A delay of approximately 20 minutes prior to finishing and polishing, to permit dark polymerisation, reduces the risk of micro-fracture initiation.

Using a fine needle-shaped diamond bur, remove any gross excess resin. Interproximal contacts should be flossed and any unwanted adhesive removed accordingly. Caution must be taken with the finishing and polishing protocol, to make sure that the ability of the restoration to provide posterior disclusion is maintained.

Finishing can then be completed using a set of Dura-Green and Dura-White Stones (Shofu Inc., Kyoto, Japan), so as to provide a harmonious marginal finish as well as to impart micro-characterisation, as described in Chapter 5.5. The restoration should be polished using your chosen polishing protocol. Finally, a layer of glycerine is applied to the restoration and light cured, to ensure polymerisation of the surface layer, which may otherwise remain unpolymerised due to the air-inhibition phenomenon.

Your patient should be instructed to maintain a soft diet for 24 hours, to permit complete polymerisation of the resin composite. Figure 9.2.2 provides a post-operative view where a canine riser restoration has been placed.

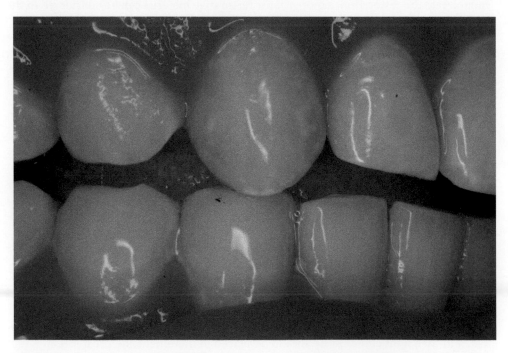

Figure 9.2.2 Post-operative view, following the placement of a direct resin composite–based canine riser restoration

A silicone key may be constructed and kept with the patient's records to guide future additions or repairs and for monitoring the wear pattern of the restoration.

## Tips

- The canine rise restoration has a plethora of applications in restorative dentistry, from the prevention of wear to fractures as well as improving the life span of restorations that you place on a daily basis.
- Should aesthetic compromise be a potential concern, try applying resin without any adhesive bonding – 'dry and try'.
- Caution may be needed where the canine tooth is suboptimal, or where the tooth is brittle, such as following endodontic therapy or in an elderly patient, due to sclerosis.
- During each recall visit, reassess the efficacy of your riser restoration.

## References

1 Murray MC, Brunton PA, Osborne-Smith K, Wilson NH. Canine risers: indications and techniques for their use. *Eur J Prosthodont Restor Dent.* 2001 Sep-Dec;9(3–4):137–40.
2 Thayer KE, Doukoudakis A. Acid etch canine rise occlusal treatment. *J Prosthet Dent.* 1981 Aug;46(2):149–52.

## 9.3

# Anterior Freehand Direct Restoration

*Subir Banerji and Shamir B. Mehta*

*Video: Anterior Freehand Direct Restoration*
*Presented by Subir Banerji and Shamir B. Mehta*

## Principles

Tooth wear (TW) may be subclassified in a variety of different ways: **localised**, **generalised**, **anterior**, **posterior mandibular** or **maxillary**. Although a significant proportion of pathological TW cases may be effectively managed using a passive-preventative approach, as described in Chapter 9.1, for certain patients active restorative intervention will be indicated, for instance where there may be:

- Aesthetic concerns
- Symptoms of pain and discomfort
- Functional difficulties
- The presence of an unstable occlusion
- A rate of tooth surface loss that is of extreme concern to either the dental operator or the patient, which furthermore if neglected may culminate in exposure of the dental pulp.[1]

The protocol for **active restorative intervention** may vary considerably, depending on various aesthetic and functional-mechanical considerations, as well as the quantity and quality of residual tooth tissue.

Maxillary anterior teeth are more likely to be affected by pathological TW, especially where erosive agents are causative (perhaps due to the lack of direct buffering from saliva, which mandibular anterior teeth may benefit from, coupled with the action of the tongue to hold acidic substrates in close proximity to these teeth). This chapter will largely focus on the management of maxillary anterior TW using simple restorative techniques. However, the principles for restoration apply equally to the lower anterior dentition.

*Practical Procedures in Aesthetic Dentistry*, First Edition. Edited by Subir Banerji, Shamir B. Mehta and Christopher C.K. Ho. © 2017 John Wiley & Sons, Ltd. Published 2017 by John Wiley & Sons, Ltd.
Companion website: www.wiley.com/go/banerji/aestheticdentistry

In deciding how to optimally restore maxillary anterior teeth affected by the process of wear, there are six key aspects to consider:

1) Pattern of anterior, maxillary tooth surface loss
2) Interocclusal space availability
3) Space requirements for the dental restorations being proposed
4) Quantity and quality of available dental hard tissue and enamel respectively
5) Aesthetic demands of the patient
6) Speech.[1]

For cases of anterior maxillary wear involving visible facial surfaces, restorative techniques will invariably require the prescription of tooth-coloured aesthetic materials, hence **dental ceramics** and/or **resin composite**.

Where possible, restorative techniques should be minimally invasive (as the affected dentition will have sustained injury and volumetric loss already) but also offer the potential for adjustment should the planned changes be poorly accepted or tolerated. Contingency planning should be given due consideration. For these purposes, the use of **resin composite applied directly** offers a suitable option.

Direct composite resin when used in the management of cases of TW offers the **advantages** of providing:

- Acceptable aesthetic outcome
- Non-invasive procedure
- Diagnostic tool
- Acceptable level of tolerance by pulpal tissues
- Minimal abrasion to antagonistic surfaces
- Ease of repair and adjustment
- Cost-effective material
- Restorations may be applied within a single visit.[2]

The disadvantages of direct resin composite restorations for this purpose include:

- Polymerisation shrinkage, which may culminate in marginal leakage and staining
- Accelerated wear rate (when compared to metals/ceramics) and possible inadequate wear resistance for posterior use
- Bulk fracture(s)
- Discoloration
- Need for optimal moisture control
- Need for good quality/quantity of dental enamel
- Complexity of application, particularly for palatal veneers, and limited control over occlusal and interproximal contours.[2]

It is generally accepted that resin composite restorations when applied to areas of high loading should be placed in the thickness range of 1.5–2.0 mm. Thus, in order to place this quantity of material, there is a need to provide the desired level of **interocclusal clearance**.[1] This may occasionally be present in the intercuspal position, where an open bite may exist, or the patient presents with a rate of wear that exceeds the rate of dento-alveolar compensation (which serves to maintain the function of the masticatory system). In some cases, the required interocclusal clearance may also be present where there is a discrepancy between intercuspal position and retruded contact position (see Chapter 3.1).

Where interocclusal clearance is not present, the operator may choose to follow traditional prosthodontic protocols and create space to accommodate restorations/restorative materials through the process of tooth reduction and to conform to the existing occlusion. Alternatively, an overall increase in the occlusal vertical dimension may be considered, although this may result in highly complex restorative care, as discussed further in Chapter 9.7.

A further approach is to place the material in **supra-occlusion**, hence the idea of **relative axial movement**, perhaps more commonly referred to as the **Dahl concept**.[3-5] This refers to the axial tooth movements that occur when a localised appliance or localised restoration(s) are placed in supra-occlusion and the occlusion re-establishes full arch contacts over a period of time. The re-establishment of occlusal contacts is thought to occur through a process of controlled intrusion and extrusion of dento-alveolar segments, with an element of mandibular repositioning involving the mandibular condyles and neuro-muscular adaptation. This will be discussed in more detail in Chapter 9.4.

There are a variety of techniques available to predictably place resin composite in a direct manner, which are also discussed further in Chapter 9.4. For relatively simple cases of isolated anterior wear, such as the palatal surfaces of the upper incisor teeth, a **freehand technique** may be used. This may involve a conformative approach when the intercuspal position would not be changed, or there is space available in this position, or a localised relative axial movement is being anticipated. The practical section that follows provides a description of how relatively simple palatal wear affecting the anterior maxillary dentition may be restored in a freehand manner.

The freehand application of resin composite requires the operator to have a very good working knowledge of the concepts of dental anatomy, aesthetics and occlusion, as well the skills to apply resin composite in such a manner to attain a desirable and predictable aesthetic outcome. However, this technique is cost and time effective, as further laboratory stages are not required.

## Procedures

Having carried out a comprehensive examination, including an occlusal and aesthetic assessment, begin by selecting an appropriate shade(s) of resin composite. This is perhaps best done while the teeth are hydrated. The use of a trial shade may help the process.

Mark the centric stops using articulating paper. Apply an appropriate form of isolation. It is best to remove any pre-existing composite restorations. Thoroughly clean the teeth using oil-free pumice slurry or air abrasion. The process should be extended on all surfaces where resin bonding will take place.

Condition the appropriate surfaces for adhesive bonding, as described in Chapter 5.1.

Place the selected enamel shade of composite resin onto the palatal surface of the affected tooth. With an appropriate plastic instrument, adapt the resin material to form the palatal contour. A paddle-shaped instrument, burnisher or interproximal carver is useful for this purpose. Resin placement should be carried over the incisal

Box 9.3.1 Relevant features to note when restoring maxillary incisor teeth

Height to width ratio, which should be approximately 1.2:1 for a maxillary central incisor

The relationship of the incisal edge to the lip line and the naso-labial angle at rest

The morphology of the restored teeth in frontal and lateral planes

The presence of symmetry across the midline

The overall shape of the teeth, which may reflect the personality and/or facial profile of your patient

edge onto the facial surface. It is important to maintain a minimal thickness of resin composite of 1.5–2.0 mm in all areas of loading to ensure the required mechanical integrity.

Once the desired contour is achieved, the composite resin is light cured. You may choose to place a final layer of translucent resin shade to enhance the aesthetics. The analogous process is continued for subsequent anterior maxillary teeth.

After a period of 30 minutes to permit dark polymerisation, using articulating paper, initially verify the desired occlusal scheme and adjust using a diamond bur. The aim should be to provide shared contacts between the anterior teeth during protrusive mandibular movements, as well as posterior disclusion.

Assess the proportion, size and symmetry of the restorations across the midline. Features to note are listed in Box 9.3.1.

Gross finishing may be undertaken using a set of tungsten carbide composite finishing burs, followed by Durastone (Shofu Inc., Kyoto, Japan), as described in Chapter 5.6. Prior to discharging your patient, re-assess the occlusion to ensure the desired occlusal scheme has been achieved. It is good practice to complete the polishing stage at a subsequent visit, after the patient has had a chance to adapt to these restorations. The use of polishing discs may help with the refinement of embrasure spaces. However, caution needs to be exercised to avoid 'flattening' of the facial surface, with a subsequent loss of anatomical form. Interproximal areas can be polished using appropriate polishing strips, taking care to not open patent contact areas. Re-check the occlusion.

High-gloss polishing may be attained using silicone carbide–impregnated brushes, followed by a diamond polishing paste applied using a suitable polishing wheel. Restorations may then be coated in glycerine and light cured, to permit polymerisation of the surface layer, which may be affected by the air-inhibition phenomenon.

Finally, you may wish to record the shape of the restored teeth using a PVS (polyvinyl siloxane) material, which may be stored and used in a contingency if restorative failure is encountered.

Where restorations may culminate with being placed in a supra-occlusal position, a more controlled approach as described in Chapter 9.4 may be more suitable.

Figures 9.3.1, 9.3.2, 9.3.3, 9.3.4 and 9.3.5 show an example of a patient where localised anterior maxillary tooth wear has been managed by the freehand, direct addition of resin composite in supra-occlusion to restore the worn palatal and incisal surfaces. This has resulted in the separation of posterior tooth contacts (Figure 9.3.4), which has subsequently re-established contact over a period of time (Figure 9.3.5).

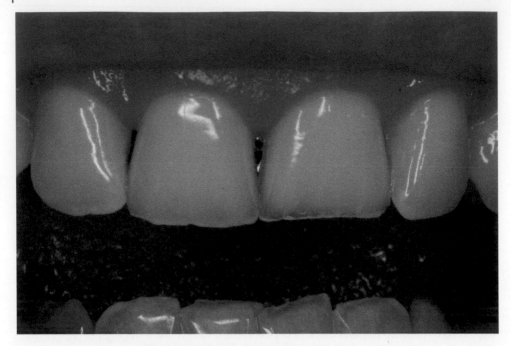

Figure 9.3.1 Pre-operative view: localised anterior maxillary wear

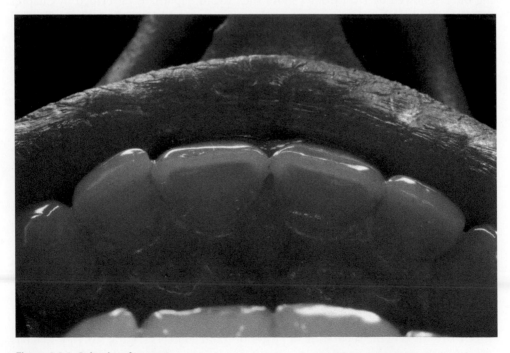

Figure 9.3.2 Palatal surface wear

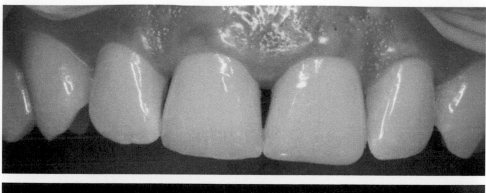

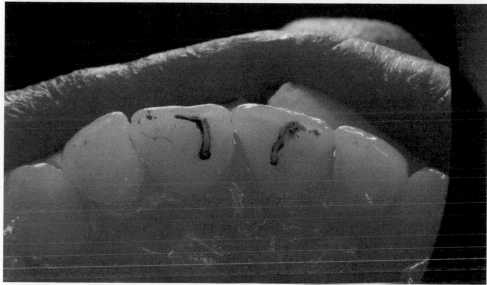

Figure 9.3.3 Freehand addition of resin composite to the maxillary central incisor teeth placed in supra-occlusion. Upon protrusion of the mandible the protrusive guidance is equally shared between the upper central incisors.

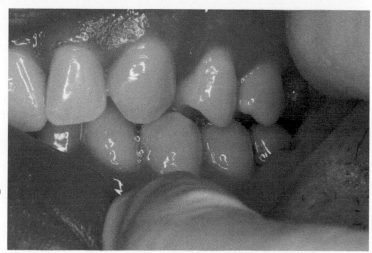

Figure 9.3.4 Separation of posterior units, by virtue of anterior supra-occlusal restorations

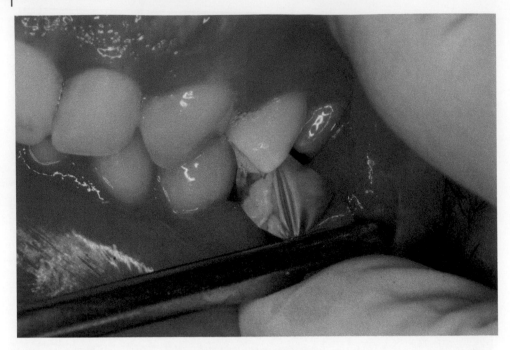

Figure 9.3.5  The re-establishment of posterior tooth contacts

## Tips

- Carefully advise your patients of the risks versus benefits of this approach, including the need for regular monitoring and maintenance. Resin composite restorations are prone to chipping, fracture, de-bonding, leakage, discoloration and secondary caries.
- In cases where the phenomenon of relative axial movement is being utilised, the patient must be informed before commencement of treatment about the anticipated change in the feel of the 'bite'.
- Simply placing a restoration at the early stages prevents the need for complicated management in the future.

## References

1 Mehta SB, Banerji S, Millar BJ, Saures-Fieto JM. Current concepts in tooth wear managements. Part 1: assessment, treatment planning and strategies for the prevention and passive monitoring of tooth wear. *Br Dent J.* 2012;212(1):17–27.
2 Kilpatrick N, Mahoney E. Dental erosion: part 2. The management of dental erosion. *N Z D J.* 2004;2:42–7.
3 Dahl B, Krungstad O, Karlsen K. An alternative treatment of cases with advanced localised attrition. *J Oral Rehab.* 1975;2:209–14.
4 Dahl B, Krungstad O. Long term observations of an increased occlusal face height obtained by a combined orthodontic/prosthetic approach. *J Oral Rehab.* 1985;12:173–80.
5 Poyser N, Porter R, Briggs P, Chana H, Kelleher M. The Dahl concept: past, present and future. *Br Dent J.* 2005;198:669–76.

## 9.4

# Maxillary Anterior Direct Build-up with Indices

*Subir Banerji and Shamir B. Mehta*

*Video: Maxillary Anterior Direct Build-up with Indices*
*Presented by Subir Banerji and Shamir B. Mehta*

## Principles

For more challenging anterior tooth wear (TW) cases, there is a need for a protocol that provides the operator with a greater level of control, predictability and contingency planning. This can be accomplished by the use of a **diagnostic wax-up**, which should be carefully formulated on the basis of an accurate occlusal and aesthetic prescription. The latter may be directly **indexed** using either a **polyvinyl siloxane (PVS)** material or a fabricated stone duplicate, which can then be used to form a thermoplastic template to assist with resin composite placement. This chapter will focus on the use of the former.

Cases of anterior TW that may benefit from the use of a more controlled approach include:

- Where there may be extensive TW extending to include a significant portion of the proximal walls
- Occlusal changes that may involve an overall increase in the occlusal vertical dimension, especially where multiple posterior restorations are being planned
- Where attainment of the functional or aesthetic end point may be challenging
- Where is a need to apply resin composite in a 'layered' manner.

The five principles for the restoration of worn teeth, as discussed in Chapter 9.3, apply in an analogous manner for all levels of TW, and should be given consideration when planning restorative rehabilitation.

For cases where resin composite is to be used as the dental material of choice, it is important to make sure that a minimum thickness of 1.5–2.0 mm of material is placed in all areas of functional loading. Accordingly, wax patterns should be made to conform to this dimension. The occlusal end point should aim to provide even contacts in the intercuspal position, shared occlusal contacts on mandibular protrusion and a canine-guided occlusal scheme. It should be noted that in cases where there is also TW on the

*Practical Procedures in Aesthetic Dentistry*, First Edition. Edited by Subir Banerji, Shamir B. Mehta and Christopher C.K. Ho. © 2017 John Wiley & Sons, Ltd. Published 2017 by John Wiley & Sons, Ltd.
Companion website: www.wiley.com/go/banerji/aestheticdentistry

posterior teeth, then this would also need to be addressed. Where it is just localised in the maxillary anterior dentition, the passive axial re-establishment of the posterior teeth following the anterior build-up would allow the desired occlusal contacts to be established and this should be confirmed. There may, however, be a need to include alterations to this generic approach given the individual circumstances, such as the presence of a large direct restoration or endodontically treated tooth (particularly in the presence of a post-retained core).

The aesthetic prescription is perhaps most appropriately established by undertaking an intra-oral mock-up, as described in Chapter 2.5. The use of biometric guides such as those listed in Chapter 9.3 may be helpful.

A number of studies have evaluated the efficacy of resin composite to treat wear of the anterior dentition. A success rate of approximately 90% has been described for labial direct composite veneers reported over a short to medium evaluation period.[1-4]

## Procedures

Carefully inspect the diagnostic wax-up when it is returned from the dental laboratory. Figure 9.4.1 shows the use of a Golden Mean gauge to ascertain the desired proportions. It is worth carrying out an intra-oral mock-up using the information from the wax-up, as described in Chapter 2.5.

Prepare a **palatal silicone index**, commonly referred to as a **silicone key**. An example is shown in Figure 9.4.2. This index will assist you with resin placement in an incremental, layered manner. It will allow the worn-down tooth to be re-constructed in an anatomical way and also optimise resin polymerisation, by applying suitable increment sizes that will permit complete polymerisation. The silicone key will in essence provide

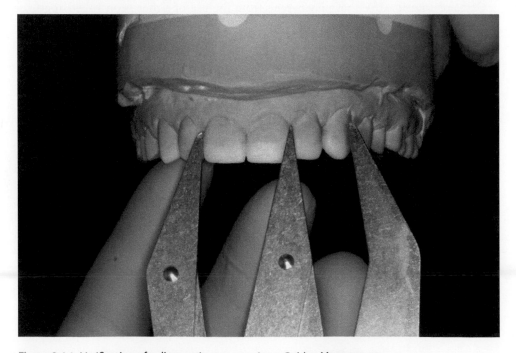

Figure 9.4.1  Verification of a diagnostic wax-up using a Golden Mean gauge

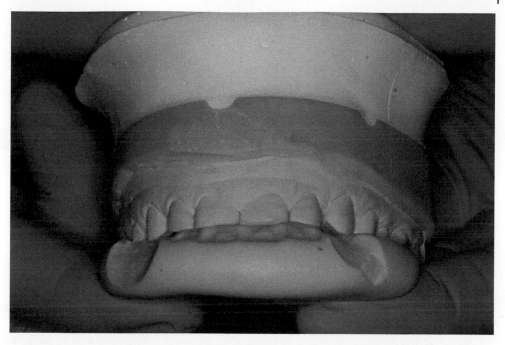

Figure 9.4.2  Silicone key made from the wax-up, which can be used to assist with the layering of resin composite, to augment the worn-down dentition

a 'negative' of the occlusal prescription as established by the wax-up, allowing the occlusal prescription to be 'copied'.

To prepare the index, on a suitably damp dental cast of the wax-up apply your chosen PVS material. Duplication of the wax-up in stone can lead to the loss of fine detail. The use of a transparent PVS material (such as Memosil 2, Heraus Kulzer GmbH, Hanau, Germany) can be helpful in permitting light curing from a palatal direction; this is particularly relevant for cases of TW where there has been a significant loss of palatal enamel, with a minimal loss of incisal edge tissue. Otherwise a putty consistency can be used. The PVS material should be extended to the premolar areas, and wrapped around the latter teeth to provide support and stability. The index material should be sufficiently bulky to provide rigidity, such that it does not readily exhibit flexion on intra-oral insertion and seating. On the facial aspect, the index should only extend up to the incisal edge. Any excess material should be carefully cut away using a putty knife or a scalpel.

Select the appropriate shade(s) of resin composite; for further details refer to Chapter 5.4. It is also worth producing a hand-drawn sketch of the desired postoperative outcome, including the topography of the incisal edge.

With an appropriate form of isolation in situ, having managed any defective pre-existing restorations, you may choose initially to bevel the facial enamel and prepare the palatal enamel to receive a butt finish. The latter may help to improve micro-mechanical retention as well as the aesthetic outcome. The differing forms of marginal finish (between the facial and palatal surfaces) reflect the differing enamel prism orientations encountered on the two surfaces. For further details, refer to Chapter 5.3.

Thoroughly clean the teeth using oil-free pumice slurry or air abrasion. Adjacent teeth should be protected using an appropriate form of matrix, as described in Chapter 9.2.

Commence the build-up procedure on a maxillary canine tooth. Condition the surface for adhesive bonding initially by applying a suitable etchant (using a total etch technique), which is then thoroughly washed off and dried (avoiding desiccation). This is followed by the careful application of the chosen bonding agent.

Prior to index placement, place an appropriate quantity of enamel shade on the surface of the tooth to be restored; the use of pre-warmed resin composite may prove helpful. The amount of resin dispensed will depend on the level and pattern of TW present. Position your index, making sure that it is correctly seated. Using your chosen instrument (a paddle-shaped instrument or an interproximal carver is useful for this purpose), form the **palatal enamel wall**. This is commonly also referred to as the 'palatal shelf'. The shelf should be extended to the incisal edge and finished just short of the interproximal areas. Light cure according to the manufacturer's recommendations. The use of flowable resin composites is not recommended, as they do not offer the required mechanical strength.

Place a suitable matrix to encompass both of the interproximal areas, commonly referred to as the **interproximal pillars**. The use of a Teflon-coated 'dead-soft matrix' may be particularly helpful, as it can be shaped with a burnisher in a customised manner and will retain its form. The presence of a Teflon coating will help to prevent adhesion of the resin-based materials to the matrix. The matrix may be held in situ using a suitable form of interproximal wedge.

Place the selected enamel shade onto the affected tooth against the matrix strip, on either the mesial or distal surface. Using the index finger of your left hand (for a right-handed operator), carefully support the matrix. Using a suitable instrument, carefully adapt the material between the matrix and the palatal shelf; the pillar should form a substitute for the enamel tissue lost in this area of the tooth. A goat's-hair brush can be useful in adapting the material, particularly when using warmed resin composite. You may also choose to gently 'tug' the matrix in a palatal direction to improve adaptation. The pillar should be built to the profile of the facial enamel layer. Carefully roll the matrix strip over the facial surface and light cure. Repeat the process for the opposing wall.

You will now have formed an **envelope**, into which you can apply your dentine shade (if required) to replace lost dentine tissue. The material should be placed to the level of the inner surface of the first bevel.

Using a fine-bladed instrument, finish the dentine layer in accordance with the desired incisal edge anatomy. For a younger patient, in order to develop translucency, finish the dentine layer short enough against the palatal shelf to develop the desired level of incisal edge translucency. Mamelons may be sculpted too if required using either a fine-bladed instrument or a pointed cone-shaped burnisher. Light cure. For further refinement, subsurface resin tints may be carefully applied to the dentine layer and light cured.

Finally, apply the enamel shade over the dentine layer to the second bevel and light cure. The enamel layer should be sculpted to form the desired emergence profile. You may choose to place a final layer of translucent resin shade to further enhance the aesthetics. The analogous process is continued for subsequent anterior maxillary teeth.

After a period of 30 minutes to permit dark polymerisation, using articulating paper initially verify the desired occlusal scheme and adjust using a diamond bur. Assess the proportion, size and symmetry of the restorations across the midline, as discussed in Chapter 9.3.

Gross finishing may be undertaken using a set of tungsten carbide composite finishing burs, followed by Durastones (Shofu Inc., Kyoto, Japan). Prior to discharging your patient, re-assess the occlusion to ensure that the desired occlusal scheme has been obtained.

It is good practice to complete the polishing stage at a subsequent visit, as resin augmentations can be very demanding. During this visit, together with a review, micro-characterisation of the restorations may be performed to further enhance the aesthetic outcome.

Figure 9.4.3 provides an example of anterior maxillary wear treated by the addition of resin composite in a 'supra-occlusal' position. Occlusal contacts were re-established 9 months after restoration.

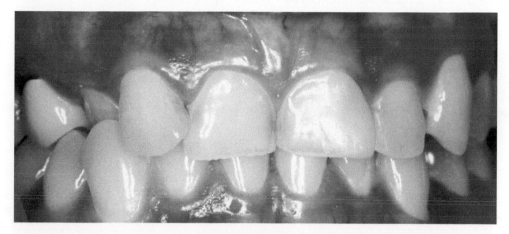

Figure 9.4.3a Pre-operative view of a patient with localised anterior maxillary tooth wear – facial view

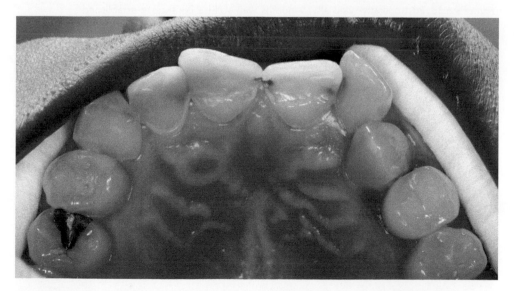

Figure 9.4.3b Pre-operative occlusal view – dental caries was stabilised prior to active wear management

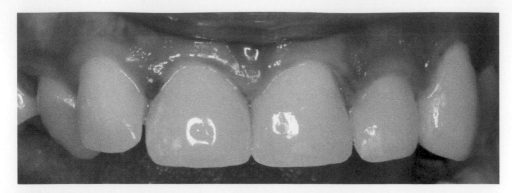

Figure 9.4.3c  Post-operative view – resin was added to restore wear without any tooth reduction using a PVS index guide and restorations were placed in supra-occlusion

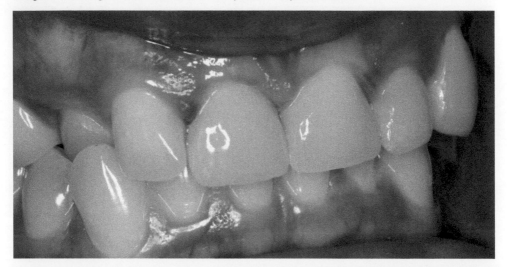

Figure 9.4.3d  Post-operative view after 9 months, with occlusal contacts re-established

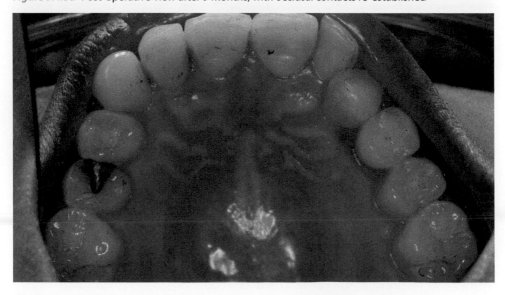

Figure 9.4.3e  Post-operative occlusal-palatal view, centric stops marked

## Tips

- When constructing an index, try using a non-perforated impression tray to enable the index to be separated without damaging the diagnostic wax-up.
- Make sure that your patient fully understands the limitations of resin composite and the maintenance requirements of these restorations, including risks of bulk fracture, wear, chipping, de-bonding, discoloration, secondary caries and marginal leakage.
- Keep a stone-cast duplicate of the diagnostic wax-up as part of your records of the treatment.

## References

1 Welbury R. A clinical study of microfilled composite resin for labial veneers. *Int Jour Paediat Dent.* 1991;1:9–15.
2 Hemmings K, Drabar U, Vaughn S. Toothwear treated with direct composite at an increased vertical dimension, results at 30 months. *J Prosthet Dent.* 2000;83:287–93.
3 Redman C, Hemmings K, Good J. The survival and clinical performance of resin based restorations used to treat localised anterior tooth wear. *Br Dent J.* 2003;194:566–72.
4 Poyser N, Porter R, Briggs P, Kelleher M. Demolition experts: management of the parafunctional patient: 2. Restorative management strategies. *Dent Update.* 2007;34:262–8.

## 9.5

# Mandibular Anterior Direct Build-up: Injection Moulding Technique

*Subir Banerji and Shamir B. Mehta*

*Video: Mandibular Anterior Direct Build-up: Injection Moulding Technique*
*Presented by Subir Banerji and Shamir B. Mehta*

## Principles

The principles for the restoration of the worn anterior mandibular dentition are no different to those for the management of the worn antagonistic teeth, as discussed in Chapters 9.3 and 9.4. However, pragmatically, worn lower anterior teeth can pose the treating clinician a few additional challenges.

Often, as a consequence of pathological tooth wear, patients may present with rather diminutive lower front teeth with little remaining hard tissue. The lack of a sufficient quantity and quality of tooth enamel renders adhesive bonding somewhat unpredictable. Under such circumstances, there may be a need to undertake surgical crown lengthening procedures, and to consider the prescription of conventionally (mechanically) retained indirect restorations, such as crowns or overlays.

The freehand application of direct resin composite to restore worn lower teeth may prove to be technically challenging, especially in cases of severe tooth surface loss. The use of a silicone index may also prove difficult where teeth are severely retroclined or in a patient with a shallow lingual sulcus and a raised tongue position. Effective moisture control can sometimes prove difficult.

The use of a thermoplastic template formed on a refractory cast of a diagnostic wax-up was briefly alluded to in Chapter 9.4. This involves the placement of resin composite into such a template, which is then seated over the worn teeth and the resin composite subsequently light cured. There are, however, an array of disadvantages associated with this protocol:

- Difficulty with the augmentation of the interproximal areas, with gross interproximal excess being encountered
- Difficulty with resin layering, resulting in monochromatic restorations, with risks of inadequate polymerisation due to incomplete light transmission to the basal layers of the material placed
- Air entrapment

*Practical Procedures in Aesthetic Dentistry*, First Edition. Edited by Subir Banerji, Shamir B. Mehta and Christopher C.K. Ho. © 2017 John Wiley & Sons, Ltd. Published 2017 by John Wiley & Sons, Ltd.
Companion website: www.wiley.com/go/banerji/aestheticdentistry

- A large polymerisation exotherm
- Difficulty estimating the amount of material required, often resulting in under-filling and the subsequent development of voids or gross excess, necessitating lengthy and cumbersome refinement.

Nevertheless, the use of a **modified template** may overcome many of these drawbacks. A technique is described in this chapter involving the use of a guided **resin injection moulding technique**, which can be applied to restore the worn lower anterior dentition rapidly, predictably and effectively.

The use of indirect resin composites also offers an option, and is discussed further in Chapter 9.6.

## Procedures

Once you have verified your diagnostic wax-up (Figure 9.5.1), form an accurate stone duplicate onto which the PVC (polyvinyl chloride) template will be fabricated. The thermoplastic stent most suitable for this purpose is of a 0.5 mm thickness. Templates may be developed by either **vacuum forming** or **pressure forming**. The former is advocated, as the use of pressure to form the template can result in a relatively inflexible matrix, which may be difficult to prepare, place and remove and may be vulnerable to breakage of the stone cast.

Once the stent has been adapted to the cast, trim the template using a pair of scissors. The template should extend past the second premolar teeth. Trim away excess material around the template margins. Gingivally, it is essential that there is at least 3–4 mm of material apical to the gingival margin to provide resilience. The template should be cut to follow a neat straight line, as opposed to a scalloped finish.

With the template positioned on the cast, with a heated scalpel blade make slits in the template in the interproximal areas, extending at least 3 mm apical to the contact area. It is imperative to use an adequately heated blade to ensure that neat incisions are produced without dragging warmed template material when cutting. Check the cuts made, and remove any carbonised residue and debris with a pair of college tweezers.

Place the sectioned matrix onto the pre-operative cast. You may choose to use a duplicate cast of the study model to avoid any unwanted damage to the reference record. Using a rugby ball–shaped diamond bur, make access vents in the template for each tooth that requires restoration. The vents should be placed approximately 3 mm coronal to the occlusal plane, on the facial aspect of the matrix. The access vent should be wide

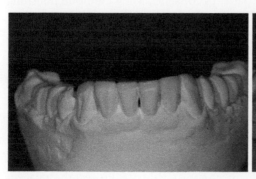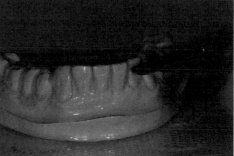

Figure 9.5.1 A 0.5 mm PVC stent formed on a duplicate model of a diagnostic wax-up

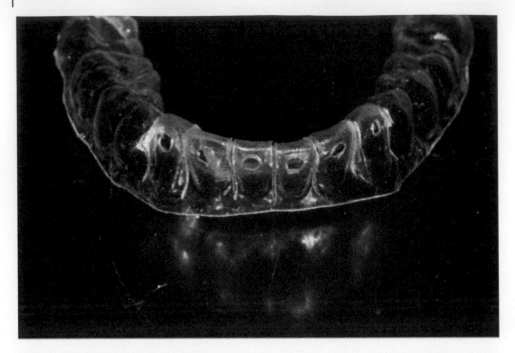

Figure 9.5.2 Template modified for use

enough to permit the passive insertion of the tip of your chosen resin composite material. Figure 9.5.2 depicts a template ready for use.

Prior to stent placement, floss your patient's interproximal contacts and make a note of interproximal areas that may offer resistance to flossing. Try-in your modified template. Check it for retention and stability. A poorly fitting template should be abandoned.

Using a pair of scissors, cut 1.5 cm sections of a wide, straight steel matrix band. Ideally, a thin matrix should be used and four sections produced. With the template in situ, for each tooth to be treated attempt placing the sectioned matrices in each of the mesial and distal surfaces. Where this may prove challenging, review your stent to make sure that the slits have been correctly cut. If so, you may need to undertake very minor interproximal reduction (with your patient's consent), using diamond polishing strips.

Once you are satisfied that the matrices can be readily inserted and are retentive, remove the template. You may choose to bevel the facial enamel in the manner described in Chapter 5.3 and prepare a lingual butt margin. You may also elect to roughen the interproximal surfaces using a medium-textured interproximal polishing strip. Any existing restorations should be assessed, and replaced if deemed to be undesirable.

For patients with moderate to advanced wear, there may be the need to replace dentine, accomplished by the formation of a **dentine 'cone'**. Prior to tooth conditioning, prepare the teeth to improve the potential for micro-mechanical retention using either a slurry of oil-free pumice on a rubber cup or an air-abrasion device. Protect the adjacent surfaces using an appropriate form of isolation. You may choose to apply a split dam for tooth isolation. Apply your chosen adhesive protocol. Floss the interproximal contacts and cure according to the manufacturer's instructions.

Using your chosen shade of dentine material, apply resin composite to form the dentine cones. A fine-bladed interproximal carver is helpful for this exercise. The material should be finished to the inner surface of the labial bevel, allowing adequate space for an enamel layer. Light cure.

Floss each of the interproximal areas. Remove any excess adhesive material with a sharp probe. Re-position the template, and make sure that the matrix strips prepared earlier can be re-positioned in the desired manner.

Select a tooth to restore. Re-condition this tooth for adhesive bonding, using isolation to protect the neighbouring teeth. Teeth should ideally be restored on an individual basis (one at a time), but given experience with this technique multiple teeth can be restored. Place the matrices into the mesial and distal interproximal areas. The matrices should pass 3 mm apical to the contact area. For a right-handed operator, place the thumb of your left hand between the matrices; this will avoid excess material flowing lingually, help to stabilise the template and permit an improved adaptation of the matrices. Ideally, using pre-warmed resin, insert the resin compule into the access vent and carefully backflow resin composite into the matrix. Flowable resins are not advocated for this technique. Using a flat plastic instrument, apply gentle pressure to the template (in a labio-lingual direction) to improve adaptation. Remove excess material around the access vent, otherwise you will risk locking the template in situ. Light cure according to the manufacturer's instructions.

Carefully remove the matrices and prize away the template. Inspect the resin augmentation. At this stage, any voids may be repaired by further resin additions. Refrain from adding bulk increments, otherwise the template will not re-seat.

Using a fine needle-shaped diamond bur, remove any flash excess. Caution must be applied not to remove excess material. Using an interproximal polishing strip in an 'S'-shaped motion, so as to avoid flattening and subsequent loss of patent of the interdental contacts, carefully remove excess material interproximally and round off any sharp corners at the line angles of the restored tooth.

Repeat this procedure for the next tooth and continue until the injection moulding technique is completed. After a period of 30 minutes, to permit dark polymerisation, with a set of composite finishing tungsten carbide burs complete any gross finishing. A pointed cone-shaped bur can be very helpful for completing the lingual surface, as well as the establishment of the required embrasure spaces. A flame-shaped bur can assist with the refinement of the labial profile. You may choose to use an interdental bur to refine areas around the contact point.

Verify the occlusal form using articulating foil and paper. Resin addition or subtraction may be undertaken until the desired aesthetic and functional parameters are derived. Fine polishing may be delayed for a subsequent session. Check the embrasure spaces, connectors and contact areas and emergence profile to make sure that you are satisfied. Apply a thin layer of glycerine and light cure to permit polymerisation of the surface layer.

Figures 9.5.3, 9.5.4, 9.5.5, 9.5.6, 9.5.7 and 9.5.8 show a case of lower anterior tooth wear that has been treated using the process of injection moulding.

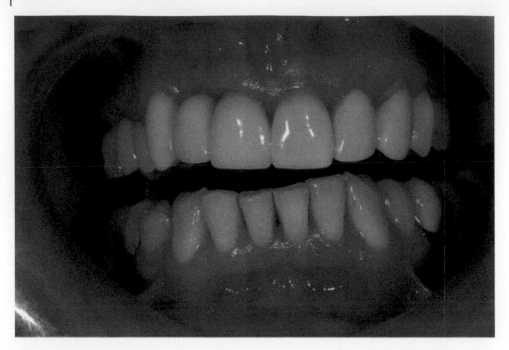

Figure 9.5.3 Pre-operative view showing the tooth wear present on the lower anterior teeth. *Source:* Courtesy of Dr Selar Francis.

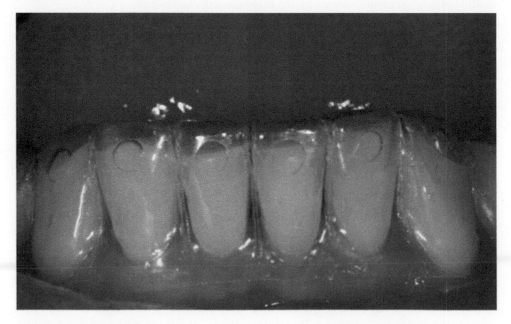

Figure 9.5.4 Stent try-in

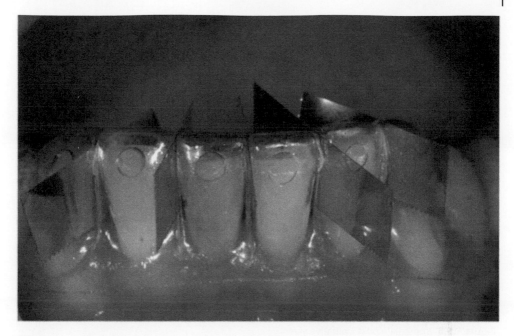

Figure 9.5.5  Matrices in situ

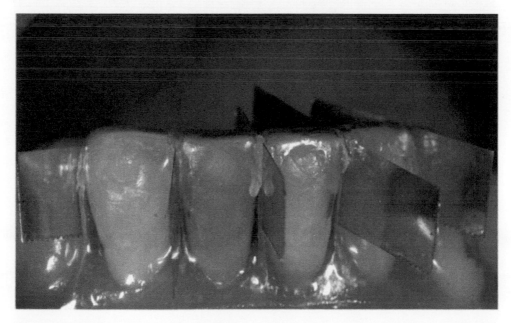

Figure 9.5.6  Warmed resin injected into stent

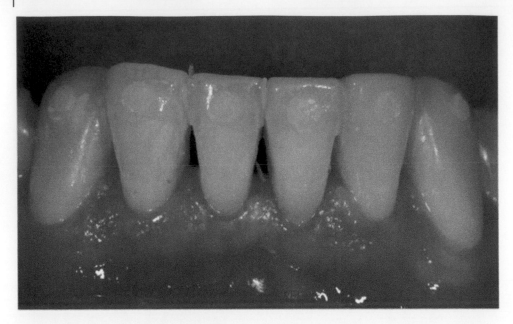

Figure 9.5.7 Immediate post-operative view

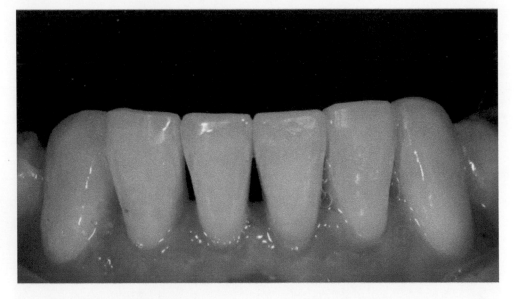

Figure 9.5.8 Post-operative view

## Tips

- A bespoke resin warmer is very helpful for this exercise.
- Spend time preparing the template before your patient arrives.

## Further Reading

Mehta SB, Banerji S, Millar BJ, Saures-Fieto JM. Current concepts in tooth wear managements. Part 1: Assessment, treatment planning and strategies for the prevention and passive monitoring of tooth wear. *Br Dent J.* 2012;212(1):17–27.

Mehta SB, Banerji S, Millar BJ, Saures-Feito JM. Current concepts in tooth wear management. Part 2 Active restorative care 1: the management of localised tooth wear. *Br Dent J.* 2012;212(2):73–82.

Mehta SB, Banerji S, Millar BJ, Saures-Fieto JM. Current concepts in tooth wear management. Part 3 Active restorative care 2: the management of generalised tooth wear. *Br Dent J.* 2012;212(3):121–7.

Mehta SB, Banerji S, Millar BJ, Saures-Fieto JM. Current concepts in tooth wear management. Part 4 An overview of the restorative techniques and materials commonly applied for the management of tooth wear. *Br Dent J.* 2012;212(4):169–77.

## 9.6

# Management of the Posterior Worn Dentition

*Subir Banerji and Shamir B. Mehta*

## Principles

For cases of early posterior tooth wear (TW), a **preventative approach** may be taken, including the prescription of a **riser restoration** (assuming that TW is present at the surfaces involved in mandibular guidance), as described in Chapter 9.2. Where the process of wear may have affected the **occlusal table** so as to lead to symptoms of pain, dysfunction or aesthetic concern (or where the rate of wear is deemed of notable concern to both the patient and the operator), there may be a need to restore this surface.

Restoration of the worn posterior occlusal anatomy may be undertaken using either a **direct** or **indirect approach**. Restorations may be placed to conform to the existing occlusion (which may involve further subtractive tooth preparation), or they may be placed in a supra-occlusal position or by planning an overall increase in the occlusal vertical dimension, as discussed in Chapter 9.7.

Where the placement of localised restorations is prescribed in the supra-occlusal position, there is a need to assess carefully the **eruptive potential** present as well to assess the effects of placing a restoration in supra-occlusion on the surrounding hard and soft tissues.

The direct application of resin composite overlays to attain the desired functional and morphological outcome can demand a high degree of operator skill. The prescription of direct resin onlays may prove highly valuable not only for the short-term protection of worn posterior surfaces such as **intermediate composite resin restorations**, so as to determine a patient's tolerance to a planned change in their occlusal scheme (with minimal intervention and optimal contingency planning), but also to provide protection to recently placed anterior restorations (which may otherwise be susceptible to failure from increased occlusal loading). However, advice on their longer-term use may be considered guarded.

Commonly prescribed indirect restorations used to manage worn posterior teeth include **full coverage crowns**, **partial coverage crowns** and **overlay restorations**. Full coverage crowns have the potential to offer desirable longer-term survival rates. Nevertheless, the risks of loss of tooth vitality and the need to remove further tooth tissue to permit successful crown placement are significant drawbacks.

Onlay and overlay restorations may be conventionally retained (by macro-mechanical retention form) or by a combination of chemical and micro-mechanical adhesion

*Practical Procedures in Aesthetic Dentistry*, First Edition. Edited by Subir Banerji, Shamir B. Mehta and Christopher C.K. Ho. © 2017 John Wiley & Sons, Ltd. Published 2017 by John Wiley & Sons, Ltd.
Companion website: www.wiley.com/go/banerji/aestheticdentistry

(adhesive onlay). The latter form of overlay restorations is particularly useful given the presence of a good quantity and quality of tooth enamel and the ability to attain effective moisture control, which is an essential prerequisite for effective resin bonding.

Indirect adhesive onlays may be fabricated from composite resin, metallic alloys or ceramic.

The advantages of indirect composite resin onlay restorations when used in the management of cases of TW include:

- Improved control over occlusal contour and vertical dimension, compared to direct restorations, particularly in the case of a large number of multiple restorations
- Potentially less time involved at the chair-side compared to direct techniques
- Can be added to and repaired relatively simply, intra-orally
- Aesthetically superior to cast metal restorations
- Less abrasive than indirect ceramic restorations
- Superior strength and wear resistance when compared to direct materials
- Polymerisation shrinkage negated intra-orally, other than at the level of the resin luting agent.[1]

The disadvantages include:

- Inferior marginal fit (versus metal and ceramic)
- Restorations may be bulky
- Multiple appointments required
- Laboratory costs
- May require the removal of hard-tissue undercuts
- Cementation line may require masking with direct materials
- Wear and leakage of the resin-based luting agent
- Possible inadequate wear resistance for posterior use.

Type III gold alloy and alloys based on nickel-chromium (Ni-Cr) are the most commonly used alloys for the fabrication of fixed metallic adhesive restorations. Ni-Cr alloys offer improved bond strengths to resin luting agents and a higher modulus of elasticity, thereby enabling application in thinner sections, in conjunction with more conservative tooth preparation(s) than Type III gold alloys. However, Type III gold alloys do offer easier working properties, superior polishability and desirable wear characteristics.

The advantages of adhesive cast restorations when applied to worn occluding surfaces include:

- They may be fabricated in thin sections (0.5 mm)
- A very accurate and predictable fit is attainable
- Minimal wear of antagonistic surfaces
- Protective of residual tooth structure
- Suitable for posterior restorations in parafunctional patients
- Placed supragingivally, therefore conducive to good periodontal health, and offer simplification of technique with regard to tooth preparation and impression making
- Minimal tooth preparation is required.[1]

Disadvantages include:

- May be cosmetically unacceptable due to the 'shine through' of metallic grey
- They do not offer the ease of repair, intra-orally

- There is a need for copious, good-quality enamel to create an acceptable bond interface
- Close proximal contacts with adjacent teeth among posterior teeth may pose a concern with the application of resin-bonded onlay restorations
- Difficulty with the placement of provisional restorations.

Type III gold restorations do require treatment to increase the surface energy to enhance bonding with resin cements. The combination of sandblasting and tin plating can be used to maximise resin retention to gold alloys.

Ceramic restorations when used in the management of cases of TW may provide the following:

- Superior aesthetics (although this will also depend on where the margin is located)
- Good abrasion resistance
- Lower relative surface free energy compared to resin composites, thus less susceptible to staining
- A higher level of gingival tissue tolerance.[1]

However, such restorations are:

- Brittle and prone to fracture unless applied in bulk, which may necessitate considerable tooth reduction, and associated potentially with higher failure rates in patients who display signs of wear by parafunctional tooth clenching and grinding habits
- Potentially abrasive to the opposing dentition (particularly in the case of feldspathic porcelains); glazed porcelain has been shown to be 40 times more abrasive to antagonistic surfaces than Type III gold[2]
- Difficult to repair intra-orally
- Difficult to adjust
- Susceptible to degradation wear in acidic environments
- Costly.

## Procedures

Where you are planning to provide a direct posterior resin onlay, there is a need to have 1.5–2.0 mm of interocclusal clearance in areas of loading. This may require some level of tooth preparation if the existing occlusal vertical dimension is to be maintained, or there may be a need to place the restoration in supra-occlusion. Following isolation with rubber dam, prepare the affected surface for resin bonding.

A diagnostic wax-up can be used to form a silicone key, which can be employed as a guide to the height of the occlusal table. Figure 9.6.1 shows a worn posterior surface, which is then restored by a direct resin onlay (Figure 9.6.2).

You may also choose to prescribe a direct resin onlay as an **intermediate restoration**, especially in an attempt to ascertain your patient's tolerance to a supra-occlusal restoration. Under such circumstances, the resin overlay should be finished to a 'flat' occlusal morphology, as shown in Figure 9.6.3. Once your patient has displayed acceptance, the resin onlay may be substituted with a more robust material with minimal further tooth reduction (as the required occlusal clearance will have been provided by the process of relative axial movement). When prescribing such restorations, you may choose to keep the restoration clear of occlusal contact during dynamic mandibular movements by the addition of a riser restoration, as described in Chapter 9.2. If the

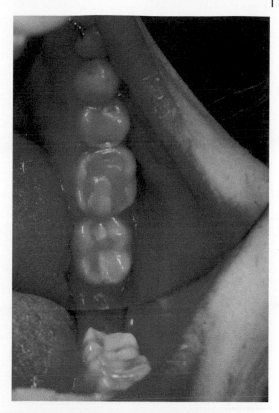

**Figure 9.6.1** A worn posterior occlusal surface that requires restorative intervention. A direct resin onlay has been provided, as seen in Figure 9.6.2

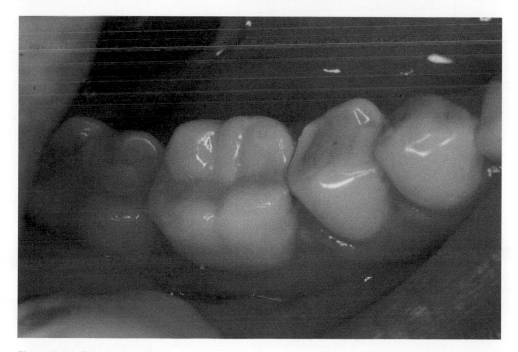

**Figure 9.6.2** Direct resin onlay

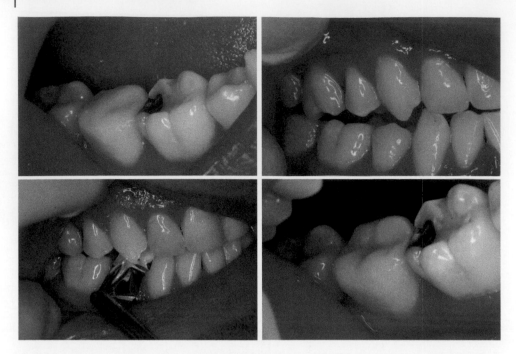

Figure 9.6.3 An intermediate direct resin onlay placed in supra-occlusion with a flat morphology on the lower right second molar tooth. On lateral excursion there is no contact on this tooth. Following re-establishment of the occlusal contacts, the restoration has been replaced with one presenting a more favourable anatomical form.

guiding tooth has signs of wear, a riser may be retained in the longer term. However, if there are no signs of wear present, the riser should be removed following the establishment of occlusal contacts.

For a Type III or IV cast gold alloy restoration, there will be a need to provide an inter-occlusal clearance of 1.0–1.5 mm; the preparation should be finished with a chamfer margin placed 1–2 mm circumferentially below the prepared occlusal surface. For ceramic restorations, there is a need to follow the manufacturer's instructions to avoid premature failure. For indirect resin onlays, an occlusal clearance of 1.5–2.0 mm is required.

The fabrication of a provisional restoration for an adhesive onlay restoration can prove challenging. If you have a diagnostic wax-up, this may be indexed and a custom direct provisional restoration formed using a bisacryl-based temporary crown and bridge material. Restorations may be cemented using zinc polycarboxylate cement. In the absence of a wax-up, isolate adjacent teeth using a circumferential matrix band. Acid etch (37% orthophosphoric acid, no more than 2 spots) can be placed on the buccal and palatal/lingual surfaces apical to the marginal finish line. You may wish to apply a dentine bonding agent, which will also help to immediately seal the dentine. Resin composite may then be applied and extended to the etched area.

The use of a putty and wash impression system is better avoided; putty will displace the wash material away from the marginal area, culminating in the critical marginal area being recorded in the less accurate material.

Instruct your dental technician to keep die spacer away from the margins when forming the die stone.

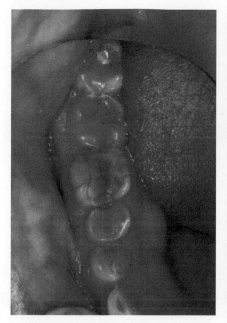 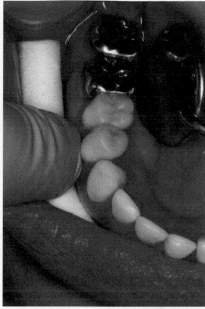

Figure 9.6.4 The use of adhesive ceramic and Type III adhesive gold onlays to treat a worn posterior dentition

Cementation should take place under rubber dam isolation. It is prudent also to isolate the adjacent teeth when preparing teeth for resin bonding, to avoid inadvertent adhesion with resin lute during the cementation space.

Figure 9.6.4 provides an example of a worn posterior dentition, restored using a combination of adhesive ceramic and Type III gold onlay restorations.

## Tips

- Develop familiarity with posterior tooth occlusal anatomy.
- Pay close attention to the process of precision tooth preparation, making sure to follow the recommended guidelines.

## References

1 Kilpatrick N, Mahoney E. Dental erosion: part 2. The management of dental erosion. *NZ Dent J.* 2004;100:42–7.
2 Wada T. Development of new adhesive material and its properties. *Proceedings of the International Symposium on Adhesive Prosthodontics.* 1986;9–19.

## Further Reading

Banerji S, Mehta SB, Millar BJ. Cracked tooth syndrome. Part Restorative options for the management of cracked tooth syndrome. *Br Dent J.* 2010 Jun;208(11):503–14.
Mehta SB, Banerji S, Millar BJ, Saures-Fieto JM. Current concepts in tooth wear management. Part An overview of the restorative techniques and materials commonly applied for the management of tooth wear. *Br Dent J.* 2012;212(4):169–77.

## 9.7

## Evaluation and Management of the Occlusal Vertical Dimension: Generalised Tooth Wear

*Subir Banerji and Shamir B. Mehta*

*Video: Evaluation and Management of the Occlusal Vertical Dimension*
*Presented by Subir Banerji and Shamir B. Mehta*

## Principles

For cases of generalised tooth wear (TW), active restorative intervention will invariably result in an increase in the patient's occlusal vertical dimension (OVD).

It is generally accepted that a freeway space (FWS) of 2–4 mm is considered to be 'physiological'. While the process of TW will usually culminate in a reduction in the vertical height of the tooth tissues, compensatory mechanisms have evolved (dento-alveolar compensation) to preserve the OVD, permitting masticatory function to continue at a physiological vertical dimension. The placement of dental restorations (which can have the effect of increasing the height of the clinical crown) may therefore result in a reduced or indeed obliterated FWS and manifest in an array of symptoms.

It is thus critical to assess the FWS when planning treatment provision.

For descriptive purposes, the restorative management of generalised TW patients may be considered according to the three categories described by Turner and Missirilian.[1] These are:

- **Category 1** – Excessive wear with loss of vertical dimension of occlusion.
- **Category 2** – Excessive wear without loss of vertical dimension, but with space available.
- **Category 3** – Excessive wear without loss of vertical dimension, but with limited space.

Regardless of the category, for any case of generalised TW where active intervention is being sought, a set of diagnostic casts mounted in centric relation (CR) is strongly advised. A semi-adjustable articulator with an arbitrary facebow may be considered acceptable, although a kinematic transverse horizontal axis facebow enables a more accurate transfer of the terminal hinge axis, helping to plan

*Practical Procedures in Aesthetic Dentistry,* First Edition. Edited by Subir Banerji, Shamir B. Mehta and Christopher C.K. Ho. © 2017 John Wiley & Sons, Ltd. Published 2017 by John Wiley & Sons, Ltd.
Companion website: www.wiley.com/go/banerji/aestheticdentistry

an increase in the OVD without introducing many errors in the horizontal jaw relationship. [2]

The desired increase in OVD will primarily be determined by what is necessary to produce functionally stable, aesthetic dental restorations and adequate FWS. Once this has been established, the planned increase may be programmed into the articulator (by raising the pin) and a diagnostic wax-up fabricated accordingly.

**Category 1** patients may be considered the most straightforward of all three categories to manage, as the resultant interocclusal clearance created through the process of TW will provide most, if not all, of the required space for the restorative material, while maintaining a physiological FWS. [3]

A full coverage, hard acrylic stabilisation splint such as a Michigan splint or Tanner appliance can be used to evaluate the patient's tolerance/adaptability to the planned occlusal changes.

In **Category 2** patients there is 'excessive wear without loss of OVD, but with limited space available'; in such cases a discrepancy will usually exist between centric occlusion (CO) and CR. CR may provide space to accommodate restorative materials; however, it might not always be fully adequate and there may be a need to plan an increase in the OVD. The patient should be provided with a full coverage, hard acrylic occlusal splint that will provide an increase in the OVD to the required range, while the mandible is manipulated into its retrusive arc of closure.[3]

The occlusal prescription of the splint should aim to provide a removable, mutually protective scheme. The patient should be instructed to wear the splint continually for a period of one month (at all times other than when eating) to evaluate the tolerance of the increase in OVD.

Unpredictable compliance with splint therapy has prompted an alternative approach, as described by Vialati and Belser.[4] This suggests that a more realistic approach would involve the placement of indirect provisional resin composite onlay and/or palatal resin veneers at the same occlusal prescription as would be provided by a full coverage, hard occlusal splint.

**Category 3** cases are usually the most difficult to restore, because space is not readily available due to tooth repositioning brought about by alveolar compensatory growth. For such cases, every effort should be made to obtain space by means other than an increase in the OVD.[1] Only if such methods fail to provide enough space would an increase in the OVD be advocated. This would be accomplished by programmed modification of the OVD through the careful use of occlusal splints.

Other methods that may be used to create space include the following:

- **Surgical crown lengthening** with osseous re-contouring to increase the quantity of coronal tooth tissue.
- **Elective endodontics** to permit the application of a post and core system to augment the available core material or, in the case of a grossly over-erupted tooth, to correct the occlusal plane discrepancy (where occlusal reduction would otherwise result in iatrogenic pulpal exposure). However, post and core restorations, particularly when placed in dentitions where there are signs of wear as a result of parafunctional tooth clenching or grinding habits, may be associated with a very bleak outlook. [5]
- **Orthodontic tooth** movement can also be used to permit the intrusion of grossly over-erupted teeth or the extrusion of teeth with short clinical crowns (where there is a copious quantity of alveolar bone support).

## Procedures

Your comprehensive patient assessment should include an evaluation of the space available in both the horizontal and vertical dimensions. This can be estimated by measurement of the existing OVD of the worn dentition and the face height with the mandible at rest and adequate lip seal, using a set of callipers or a Willis gauge.

In order to determine the aesthetic prescription, carry out a smile analysis, including an intra-oral mock-up. The information gathered from the aesthetic evaluation should be forwarded to the dental technician, with a detailed occlusal prescription. The final occlusal scheme should provide a mutually protected occlusal scheme, as described in Chapter 3.1.

Ideally, when planning the wax-up half the increase in OVD should be incorporated into each arch, but this depends on the pattern of wear and the desired aesthetic outcome. Where the increase in OVD is shared equally between the dental arches, it will not only allow for a better distribution of the increase in crown to root ratio, but also make the increase in OVD less abrupt, thereby improving the chances of successful adaptation. [3]

Having appraised the wax-up as described in Chapter 9.4, the transfer of the prescribed increase in OVD to the patient's dentition should initially be done by the use of fully reversible and adjustable materials, so as to determine the patient's tolerance and the aesthetic outcome of the proposed changes. For this purpose, you may choose to prescribe a full coverage, acrylic occlusal appliance or direct resin composite.

The decision on whether to restore the anterior or posterior dentition first may vary from patient to patient. However, the authors advocate initial restoration of the anterior dentition at the new vertical dimension, so as to determine the patient's acceptance of their anterior occlusion (with shared occlusal contacts during mandibular protrusion) and a canine-guided occlusion (on the assumption that the canine teeth are suitable for this purpose).

Anterior teeth may be built up using the techniques described in Chapters 9.4 and 9.5.

The posterior teeth may be restored shortly thereafter. Posterior 'occlusal stops' may be placed using direct resin composite, to provide function, protect the anterior restorations from excessive loading and avoid over-eruption of posterior teeth that will otherwise require restorative intervention.

Alternatively, where it may be decided to sequence the placement of restorations, such that either the anterior or posterior segments are restored in separate visits, the use of a stabilisation splint (which may be sectioned to accommodate the new restorations) can prove vital to ensure short-term longevity of the new restorations, by providing some level of protection from excessive occlusal loads.

As discussed in Chapter 9.6, direct resin occlusal stops do not offer a superior long-term prognosis, with bulk fracture being a primary concern. Therefore, once you are satisfied that your patient has accepted the planned aesthetic and occlusal changes, posterior teeth may be restored with indirect restorations, such as overlays or crowns.

Where a rehabilitation of the patient's occlusion is planned using conventional restorations (where adhesive techniques may not be suitable), preliminary tooth preparations (of at least one arch) can be carried out in a single visit. This will allow for fabrication of the provisional restorations for all the teeth at the planned OVD. The choice of which arch to prepare first will depend on the occlusal plane discrepancy (usually the arch with the greatest discrepancy will be prepared first). Acrylic or silicone indices formed from the diagnostic wax-up can be used to assist the operator with the level of occlusal reduction required.

The patient should be maintained in indirectly formed provisional restorations for a period of 6–8 weeks.[1] This time will allow for an evaluation of the aesthetics and function. The provisional restorations may require adjustments, however. Once deemed acceptable, the provisional restorations may be used as an occlusal and aesthetic guide for the fabrication of the definitive restorations. The construction of a customised anterior guidance table can prove to be very beneficial.

Where metallo-ceramic crowns are being prescribed, it may be worth undertaking either metal and or biscuit try-in stages, to minimise the risk of errors propagating during the undertaking of restorative care.

It is good practice to provide your patient with a full coverage, hard acrylic splint to protect their newly placed restorations.

Figures 9.7.1, 9.7.2, 9.7.3, 9.7.4 and 9.7.5 show an example of a patient who presented with generalised TW.

## Tips

- Where possible, try to adopt a fully reversible, adjustable approach.
- Do not hesitate to consider referral for specialist care or for advice.
- Make sure that your patient understands the limitations and risks as well as the benefits of treatment.

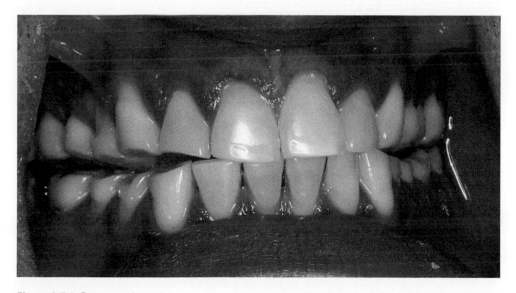

Figure 9.7.1 Pre-operative view

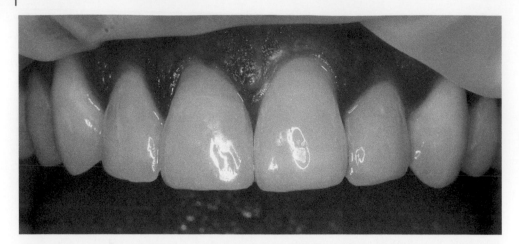

Figure 9.7.2 Restored anterior maxillary dentition, using direct resin composite

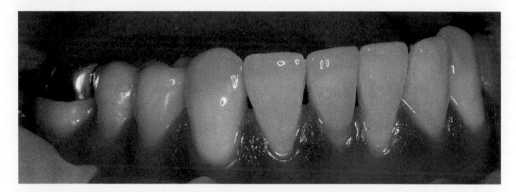

Figure 9.7.3 The lower anterior dentition restored in resin composite, with posterior adhesive onlays provided at the new OVD

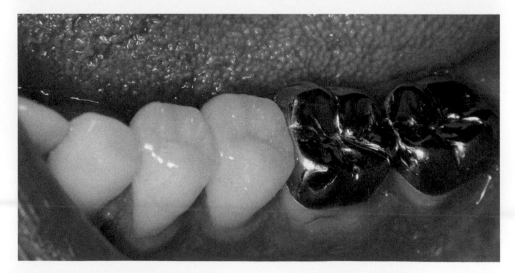

Figure 9.7.4 Adhesive onlay restorations (left posterior quadrant)

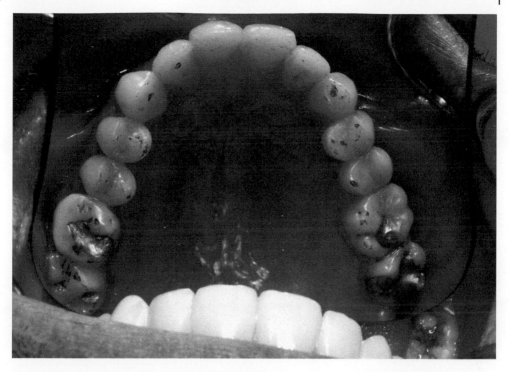

Figure 9.7.5 Restored dentition with mutual protection

## References

1 Turner K, Missirilian D. Restoration of the exteremely worn dentition. *J Prosthet Dent.* 1984;52:467–74.
2 Mehta SB, Banerji S, Millar BJ, Saures-Fieto JM. Current concepts in tooth wear management. Part 3 Active restorative care 2: The management of generalised tooth wear. *Br Dent J.* 2012;212(3):121–7.
3 Rivera-Morales W, Mohl N. Restoration of the vertical dimension of the occlusion in the severely worn dentition. *Dent Clin North Am.* 1993;36:651–63.
4 Vialati F, Belser C. Full mouth adhesive rehabilitation of a severely eroded dentition: the three step technique. Part 2. *Eur Jour Esthet Dent.* 2008;3:128–38.
5 Mehta SB, Millar BJ. A comparison of the survival of fibre posts cemented with two different resin systems. *Br Dent J.* 2008;13(11):1–7.

Part X

Tooth Whitening

# 10.1

## Assessment of the Discoloured Tooth

*Kyle D. Hogg*

Video: Assessment of the Discoloured Tooth
Presented by Kyle D. Hogg

## Principles

With the increased emphasis and importance placed on dento-facial aesthetics in today's society, it comes as no surprise that many patients are seeking to change or improve the colour of their teeth. In a recent survey conducted in the UK asking 3215 subjects to self-assess their dentition, 50% of the population studied perceived that they had some type of tooth discoloration.[1] This trend for patients desiring aesthetic improvement is not limited to young individuals. As people are maintaining more teeth longer into life, older individuals are also seeking out tooth whitening as a minimally invasive and safe way to improve their dental appearance.[2]

Performing a thorough pre-operative assessment of patients seeking tooth whitening is paramount to successfully identifying and treating patients who are suitable candidates. It is important to bear in mind that tooth colour is determined by both intrinsic qualities, such as the way in which enamel and dentine absorb and reflect light, and extrinsic qualities, such as external stains caused by smoking, diets rich in tannin-containing items or consumption of metal salts. There are also changes in the colour of teeth associated with the ageing process, as well as iatrogenic changes due to the patient's restorative dental history. In fact, tooth discoloration may manifest itself differently on individual teeth within the same arch (Figure 10.1.1). A thorough investigation of the patient's individual history and an understanding of the ways in which teeth become discoloured will allow the clinician to form a diagnosis for the type of discoloration and prescribe, where indicated, appropriate treatment protocols.

Perhaps the most frequent cause of tooth discoloration is via the process of cumulative extrinsic staining. This staining occurs when the organic material present in the interprismatic spaces located between enamel rods wicks pigments and dyes from the oral environment via capillary action. The organic material in these spaces is more susceptible to discoloration. Pigments present in the oral environment consist of a colour-bearing group (chromophore) in addition to another molecule(s). Pigments may or may not enter into the interprismatic space and adhere to the organic material located there. This is slightly different than a dye, which is a type of pigment that contains

*Practical Procedures in Aesthetic Dentistry*, First Edition. Edited by Subir Banerji, Shamir B. Mehta and Christopher C.K. Ho. © 2017 John Wiley & Sons, Ltd. Published 2017 by John Wiley & Sons, Ltd.
Companion website: www.wiley.com/go/banerji/aestheticdentistry

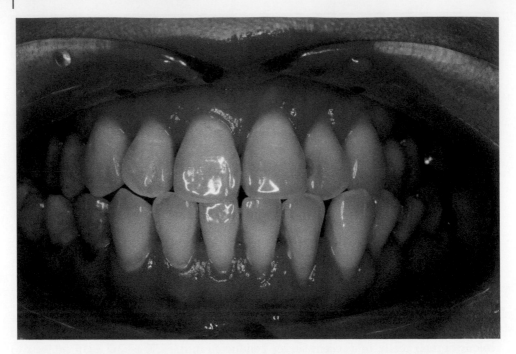

Figure 10.1.1 Intrinsic, extrinsic and iatrogenic discoloration. *Source*: Christopher C.K. Ho, BDS MClinDent Prosthodontics. Reproduced with permission from Christopher C.K. Ho.

reactive hydroxyl or amine groups that more readily adhere to the inorganic material in these spaces.[3] Dyes are ubiquitous and can be found in many commonly consumed food items such as tea, coffee, cola, berries and red wine, among many others. Figure 10.1.2 depicts how metal compounds can interact with dyes and pigments to form larger compounds and discolour the teeth.

Many sources of tooth discoloration can alternatively be considered intrinsic in origin. Non-vital or 'dead teeth' can become discoloured due to the presence of by-products from pulpal haemorrhage and death in a process similar to bruising. The breakdown of these by-products can penetrate the dentin proximal to the pulp chamber and result in a discoloration located deep within the tooth.

A process of calcific metamorphosis (Figure 10.1.3) can affect teeth with a history of trauma to the pulpal tissues and cause a 'yellowing' of the clinical crown due to calcification or deposition of hard tissue within the pulp chamber and canal spaces. In these instances the pulpal tissues are more frequently found to be vital.

Teeth may present with fluorotic brown, yellow or white discoloration of the enamel, focused in localised spots or expressed as a band. Fluorosis can range from minor superficial flecking to a more significant surface porosity or pitting that is also prone to external staining.

Another commonly observed condition is tetracycline discoloration, caused in part by the binding of tetracycline with both calcium and iron during development of the adult dentition. The tetracycline–calcium complex becomes incorporated into the hydroxyapatite within the dentine. On eruption and exposure to ambient light, the ultraviolet wavelength component brings about a photo-oxidation of the yellow or brown fluorescence present. The reaction results in a further darkening of the discoloured

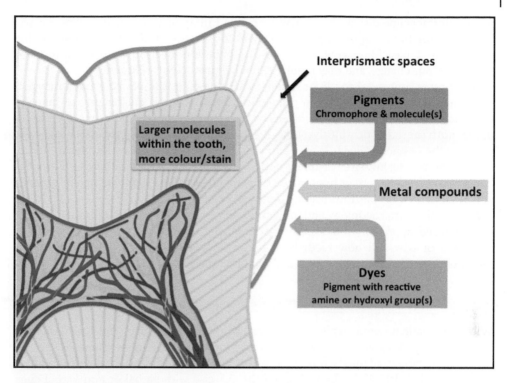

Figure 10.1.2 Process of extrinsic staining

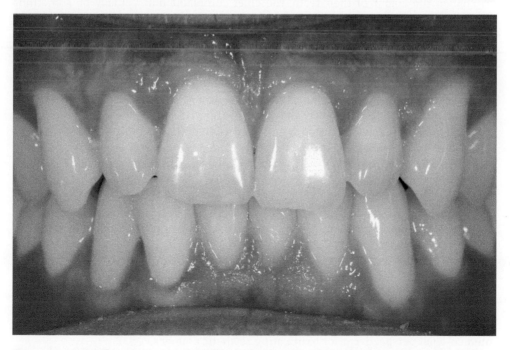

Figure 10.1.3 Calcific metamorphosis leading to discoloration of the UR 1. *Source*: Photo from the author's clinical practice.

tooth.[3] Tetracycline discoloration may be banded in appearance, with yellow, brown, blue and grey hues frequently present. Due to localisation of the discoloration within the dentine, a bleaching agent would have to penetrate deep into the tooth to bring about a colour change, and may require extended protocols for bleaching.

Other rarer congenital conditions, such as dentinogenesis imperfecta and amelogenesis imperfecta, can also result in discoloured teeth that are challenging to manage. Dentinogenesis imperfecta is characterised by a translucent or opalescent appearance of the tooth caused by dentine dysplasia. Bleaching over long periods has been shown to improve the aesthetic appearance of patients presenting with the condition while providing a minimally invasive treatment option.[3] Amelogenesis imperfecta can present as hypoplastic, hypomature or hypocalcified enamel that can be easily stained or abraded and is caries susceptible, thus leading to discoloration.

The multifactorial aetiology and individual expression of tooth discoloration require an organised approach to assess the patient comprehensively, develop an accurate diagnosis of why and how teeth have become discoloured, render treatment in a predictable and appropriate fashion and maintain the results over time.

## Procedures

With your patient comfortably seated upright in the dental chair, give them a mirror and ask them: 'What is it about your teeth that you would like to see changed?' Be sure to give the patient adequate time to respond and actively listen to what the patient says rather than lead the patient through the exercise with verbal or non-verbal cues. Bear in mind that while a patient initially says and even believes that they would like to change the colour of their teeth, the chief complaint may actually be something quite different. Often patients who state concerns about the colour of their teeth are in fact dissatisfied with other components of their smile, such as tooth form, contour, positioning, shape or embrasures. While a variety of aesthetic dental treatments are available to correct these concerns, tooth whitening alone will not address the patient's underlying complaint. Establishing and understanding the patient's chief complaint are paramount to assessing and treating the patient successfully.

Investigate the patient's medical and social history thoroughly to determine whether certain conditions, medications or habits have contributed to the discoloration of the dentition. In particular, social habits such as smoking, chewing tobacco or frequent consumption of red wine, coffee, tea or cola may contribute to extrinsic staining. Alteration of a patient's habits may be required for long-term treatment success and should be discussed before embarking on treatment.

A complete radiographic series that is both diagnostic and current must be reviewed and a photographic record, including pertinent intra-oral and extra-oral photos, should be taken at the consultation visit. The clinician is encouraged to capture an intra-oral image with a shade tab displaying the current shade as determined by conventional or digital shade-taking methods. These records provide important information, allowing the clinician to better establish a diagnosis of the underlying cause of the discoloration. Any active disease process must be diagnosed and stabilised prior to initiating elective treatment. It is also advisable to document the pre-existing conditions from a medico-legal perspective prior to initiating aesthetic changes.

**Table 10.1.1** Tooth whitening assessment form used to record patient assessment

| Tooth Whitening Assessment & Diagnosis Worksheet | | | | | | | | | | | | | | | | |
|---|---|---|---|---|---|---|---|---|---|---|---|---|---|---|---|---|
| **Patient Details** | | | | | | | | | | | | | | | | |
| Patient name: | | | | | | | | | | Date: | | | | | | |
| Address: | | | | | | | | | | | | | | | | |
| Contact No.: | | | | | | Email: | | | | | | | | | | |
| Date of birth: | | | | | | Sex (M/F) | | | | | | | | | | |
| **Medical & Social History** | | | | | | | | | | | | | | | | |
| Pertinent Medical Hx: | | | | | | | | | | | | | | | | |
| Medications: | | | | | | | | | | | | | | | | |
| Social habits: | Smoker (Y/N) | | | | | Chewing tobacco (Y/N) | | | | Tea (Y/N) | | | | | | |
| | Coffee (Y/N) | | | | | Red wine (Y/N) | | | | Cola (Y/N) | | | | | | |
| **Patient's Chief Complaint** | | | | | | | | | | | | | | | | |
| CC: | | | | | | | | | | | | | | | | |
| **Radiographic & Photographic Record** | | | | | | | | | | | | | | | | |
| Date of Radiographs | | | | | | Full Mouth Series | | | | | | | | | | |
| Bite Wings | | | | | | Periapicals | | | | | | | | | | |
| Panoramic | | | | | | CBCT | | | | | | | | | | |
| Date of Photographs | | | | | | Intra-oral Photos | | | | | | | | | | |
| Extra-oral Photos | | | | | | Other | | | | | | | | | | |
| **Intra-oral Examination** | | | | | | | | | | | | | | | | |
| Vitality Testing | | | | | | | | | | | | | | | | |
| Recession | | | | | | | | | | | | | | | | |
| Tx Required | | | | | | | | | | | | | | | | |
| Existing Rest. | | | | | | | | | | | | | | | | |
| Tooth Number | 8 | 7 | 6 | 5 | 4 | 3 | 2 | 1 | 1 | 2 | 3 | 4 | 5 | 6 | 7 | 8 |
| Existing Rest. | | | | | | | | | | | | | | | | |
| Tx Required | | | | | | | | | | | | | | | | |
| Recession | | | | | | | | | | | | | | | | |
| Vitality Testing | | | | | | | | | | | | | | | | |
| Restorative/Perio Treatment Needs | | | | | | | | | | | | | | | | |
| **Diagnosis of Discoloration:** | | | | | | | | | | | | | | | | |
| Current Shade | | | | | | Anticipated Shade | | | | | | | | | | |
| Tetracycline | | | | | | Fluorosis | | | | | | | | | | |
| White Spots | | | | | | Brown Spots | | | | | | | | | | |
| Enamel Defects | | | | | | Dentine Defects | | | | | | | | | | |
| Devital Teeth | | | | | | Other | | | | | | | | | | |
| **Whitening Prescription** | | | | | | | | | | | | | | | | |
| Technique | | | | | | | | | | | | | | | | |
| Product Name | | | | | | | | | | | | | | | | |
| Concentration | | | | | | | | | | | | | | | | |
| Desensitising Tx | | | | | | | | | | | | | | | | |
| **Informed Consent** | | | | | | | | | | | | | | | | |
| Advantages of Treatment | | | | | | | | | | | | | | | | |
| Disadvantages of Treatment | | | | | | | | | | | | | | | | |
| Maintenance Requirements | | | | | | | | | | | | | | | | |
| Alternative Treatments | | | | | | | | | | | | | | | | |
| Signature of Patient or Guardian | | | | | | | | | | Date | | | | | | |
| Signature of Provider | | | | | | | | | | Date | | | | | | |

*Source*: Adapted from Greenwall 2001[4]

The clinician should undertake a comprehensive intra-oral examination, noting the presence of existing restorations, treatment needs, presence of recession and confirmation of vitality of each tooth individually. Any treatment needs should be discussed with the patient, and a determination of the treatment sequence with respect to the timing of the tooth whitening agreed.

After the comprehensive assessment has been completed, a diagnosis of the discoloration should be made. In some instances the diagnosis will be homogeneous, or generalised to the majority or entirety of the dentition, while in other instances there will be more heterogeneity in the presentation and underlying causes of the discoloration. It may be important to note specific teeth that have certain types of discoloration such as tetracycline staining, white or brown spots, fluorosis, enamel or dentine defects or discoloration due to loss of vitality. Treatment of these teeth may require special techniques and planning to arrive at the desired result.

A whitening prescription should be selected based on the individual clinical presentation of the patient. The specific whitening technique, product name, active ingredient concentration and anticipated duration of the treatment would be included in the whitening prescription. Additionally, the need for any adjunctive desensitising treatment should be discussed.

Finally, the patient must be fully informed of the advantages and anticipated outcome of the whitening treatment, as well as any disadvantages or risks involved in the treatment. The patient must be aware of the maintenance requirements associated with the whitening treatment and have alternative treatment options discussed in order to give their informed consent to commence whitening treatment.

## Tips

- Make sure that you fully understand the nature of the patient's chief complaint with respect to their desire for aesthetic improvement.
- Establish the correct underlying diagnosis or diagnoses for the patient's tooth discoloration only after performing a thorough assessment (Table 10.1.1).
- Incorporate high-quality photography into your aesthetic dental practice as a means of recording baseline conditions, monitoring treatment progress and evaluating outcomes.

## References

1 Alkhatib M, Holt R, Bedi R. Prevalence of self-assessed tooth discolouration in the United Kingdom. *J Dent.* 2004;32:561–6.
2 Haywood V. History, safety, and effectiveness of current bleaching techniques and applications of the nightguard vital bleaching technique. *Quintessence Int.* 1992;23:471–88.
3 Kelleher M. *Dental bleaching.* London: Quintessence; 2008.
4 Greenwall L. *Bleaching techniques in restorative dentistry.* London: Martin Dunitz, Taylor & Francis; 2001.

# 10.2

## Vital Bleaching

*Kyle D. Hogg*

*Video: Vital Bleacing*
*Presented by Kyle D. Hogg*

## Principles

Noticeable tooth discoloration, particularly that which affects the teeth located within the aesthetic zone, can be a physical and emotional impairment to many individuals. Discoloured teeth can have a negative impact on an individual's self-esteem, self-confidence, physical appearance, attractiveness and social interactions. Vital bleaching, as described by Haywood and Heymann, utilising a viscous 10% carbamide peroxide gel in a close-fitting customised mouthguard or tray, has provided a predictable and non-invasive treatment modality to improve the shade of discoloured teeth (Figure 10.2.1).[1] Vital tooth bleaching is very safe, with no significant long-term oral or systemic health risks linked to the supervised use of 10% carbamide peroxide.[2] Additionally, 10% carbamide peroxide vital bleaching techniques have shown no adverse effects on enamel micro-hardness or on the surface morphology of treated teeth.[3] When appropriately utilised, vital bleaching can be a successful, predictable, minimally invasive and safe way to improve the overall aesthetics of an individual's smile.

Carbamide peroxide bleaching gel breaks down into hydrogen peroxide and urea, with hydrogen peroxide being the active bleaching agent. A bleaching gel containing 10% carbamide peroxide yields approximately 3.5% hydrogen peroxide. The hydrogen peroxide is able to penetrate enamel and dentine, where an oxidation/reduction reaction occurs (Figure 10.2.2). Hydrogen peroxide produces free radicals with unpaired electrons that interact with the larger molecules within the teeth that are responsible for the discoloration or stain. These larger molecules become oxidised and are broken down into smaller molecules, either leaving the tooth structure entirely or reducing discoloration.

The most commonly observed side effects with these peroxide-based bleaching agents are tooth sensitivity and occasional irritation of soft tissues in the mouth (oral mucosa), particularly the gums. Tooth sensitivity often occurs during the early stages of bleaching treatment. Tissue irritation may result from an ill-fitting tray used to contain the bleaching product. Both tooth sensitivity and tissue irritation are usually temporary and stop after the treatment.

*Practical Procedures in Aesthetic Dentistry*, First Edition. Edited by Subir Banerji, Shamir B. Mehta and Christopher C.K. Ho. © 2017 John Wiley & Sons, Ltd. Published 2017 by John Wiley & Sons, Ltd.
Companion website: www.wiley.com/go/banerji/aestheticdentistry

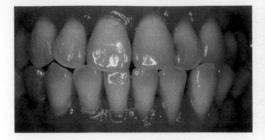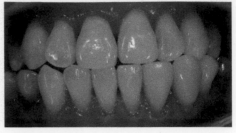

Figure 10.2.1 Initial presentation and after vital tooth bleaching. *Source*: Christopher C.K. Ho, BDS MClinDent Prosthodontics. Reproduced with permission from Christopher C.K. Ho.

## Procedures

With your patient comfortably seated upright in the dental chair, utilise lip retractors to aid in taking a separate baseline clinical photograph of each arch that the patient desires to bleach. It is advisable to place a shade tab adjacent to the teeth to be bleached to record the initial or baseline shade. This should ideally be completed before making impressions so as to avoid any shade distortion due to dehydration of the teeth.

Good-quality alginate impressions should be made, accurately capturing the details of each arch to be bleached. Precisely recording the details of the dentition with minimal incorporation of air bubbles will allow for the fabrication of suitable models. One

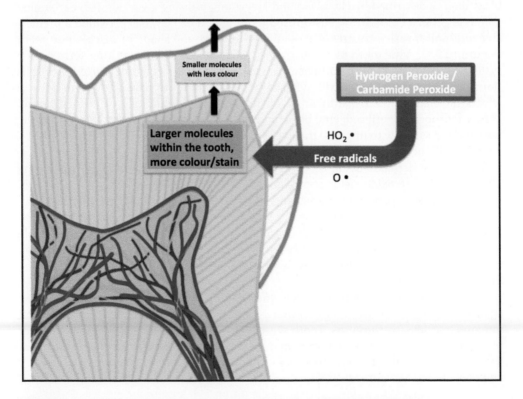

Figure 10.2.2 Bleaching producing oxidation and breakdown of complex molecules

method to minimise air bubble entrapment while making alginate impressions is to wipe alginate with a gloved finger across the occlusal and labial surfaces of the teeth prior to seating a properly loaded and well-fitting impression tray. This prevents air bubbles, which are negatives in the impression, from being incorporated as positives in the stone models. Fabricating bleaching trays on models with positives results in wells being incorporated in the vacuform bleaching tray, potentially allowing bleaching gel to accumulate unfavourably. It is imperative for predictable results that the bleaching material is held in close contact with the tooth surfaces to be bleached.

Teeth that are to be bleached should be noted clearly on the laboratory prescription, as well as the desired thickness and material to be utilised in the fabrication of the bleaching tray. There are a wide variety of material thicknesses and rigidities available in vacuform sheets. Typical tray thickness is 0.8–1.2 mm, while patients who exhibit signs and symptoms of parafunctional activity may benefit from a thicker, more rigid tray (1.5–2 mm).

The bleaching trays may be designed in a number of different ways, but should serve to hold the bleaching gel in close contact with the tooth surface (Figure 10.2.3). Trays may be scalloped to follow the gingival margin or finished in a straight line on the buccal aspect of the teeth, extending approximately 2 mm beyond the gingival margin. Trays constructed with a straight finish line on the buccal may be more effective at bleaching the cervical portion of teeth by maintaining an effective amount of bleaching material in that area, while reducing the potential for salivary peroxidases and catalases from neutralising the bleaching activity. This design may also cause higher incidences of transient and minor gingival irritation. Lingually the trays are routinely finished in a straight line, as this design is often less irritating to the tongue.

Reservoirs are often incorporated into the bleaching trays by placing a block-out resin or composite on the tooth surfaces intended for bleaching. The bleaching gel will flow, rather than compress, when the loaded tray is seated. The reservoirs allow for a sufficient volume of bleaching gel to be maintained over the tooth while the tray is worn, rather than being displaced outside of the tray or preventing the tray from fully seating.

Trays should be checked by the clinician to ensure proper fit and seating. The soft tissue should be evaluated to ensure that the trays do not cause any blanching. Any objectionable or sharp edges of the tray extensions should be modified for patient comfort.

There are a number of formulations of bleaching gel commercially available. The most documented and well-researched bleaching gel is 10% carbamide peroxide (Figure 10.2.4).[4] Carbamide peroxide contains a thickening agent, carbapol, which allows for extended activity of the bleaching gel by slowly releasing hydrogen peroxide. Thus patients should be advised to wear the bleaching tray for at least two hours, and

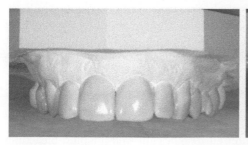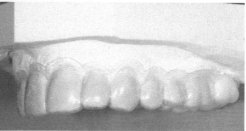

Figure 10.2.3 Tray fabrication with block-out resin utilised to create reservoirs. *Source*: Photo from the author's clinical practice.

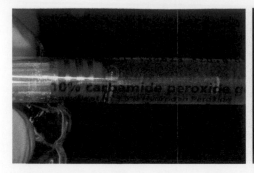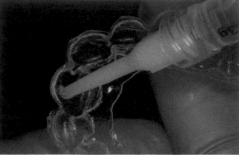

Figure 10.2.4 Application of 10% carbamide peroxide into tray reservoirs. *Source*: Subir Banerji, BDS MClinDent PhD Prosthodontics, London. Reproduced with permission from Subir Banerji.

even overnight if the patient desires. Be sure to check with the manufacturer's guidelines on other bleaching gel formulations for the recommended length of time for which the bleaching gel should be applied.

Patients should be instructed on how much gel to apply in the tray and where it should be applied, which will vary depending on the teeth and surfaces intended for bleaching. Frequently only a small amount of gel is required per tooth and should be applied halfway down the facial aspect of the reservoir. Advise the patient to wipe off any excess gel after seating the tray, as it may cause unnecessary gingival irritation. After the tray has been worn for the prescribed time, the patient should be instructed to brush both their teeth and the tray to remove any residual gel that may be present. The trays should be stored dry between uses.

The patient should be scheduled for a re-evaluation appointment at approximately two weeks following initiation of the bleaching treatment to check the progress of the shade change and monitor any soft or hard tissue sensitivity. It is strongly advised to take photographs documenting the shade changes as treatment progresses. Patients should monitor shade changes at home as well and discontinue bleaching if the teeth become lighter than adjacent restorations. Conversely, if teeth seem refractory to bleaching, additional treatment time and bleaching material may be required. It is important to discuss the responsibility for the burden of cost should a longer course of bleaching be required prior to initiating treatment.

Nearly 70% of patients encounter some hypersensitivity while bleaching.[4] It is important to advise patients that the sensitivity is quite common and most frequently transient. Strategies can be implemented utilising toothpaste containing 5% potassium nitrate, a desensitising agent, either applied in the tray and worn like the bleaching gel for 30 minutes prior to bleaching, used as a dentifrice for two weeks prior to initiating bleaching, or both.

Patients should also be advised that the shade change brought about by the course of bleaching may require topping up from time to time, depending on the individual dentition, habits and diet. Extrinsic stains should be minimised via meticulous home care and regular professional hygiene supportive care.

## Tips

- Accurate impressions and models are required to fabricate well-adapted bleaching trays. If the bleaching material is not held in close contact to the tooth surfaces to be bleached, then the treatment will be ineffective.

- Discuss with patients in advance of treatment that many individuals will encounter transient sensitivity while bleaching. Manage the sensitivity by utilising toothpaste containing 5% potassium nitrate for two weeks prior to treatment, or applied in the bleaching tray and worn for 30 minutes immediately prior to bleaching.
- Advise patients to discontinue bleaching in the unplanned event that the teeth become lighter than the restorations.

## References

1 Haywood V, Heymann H. Nightguard vital bleaching. *Quintessence Int.* 1989;20:173–6.
2 Ritter A, Leonard R, St Georges A, Caplan D, Haywood V. Safety and stability of nightguard vital bleaching: 9–12 years post-treatment. *J Esthet Rest Dent.* 2002;14:275–85.
3 Lopes G, Bonissoni L, Baratieri L, Vieira L, Montiero S. Effect of bleaching agents on the hardness and morphology of enamel. *J Esthet Rest Dent.* 2002;14(1):24–30.
4 Kelleher M. *Dental bleaching*. London: Quintessence; 2008.

## 10.3

## Non-vital Bleaching

*Kyle D. Hogg*

*Video: Non-vital Bleaching*
*Presented by Kyle D. Hogg*

## Principles

One of the more common causes of localised discoloration of a tooth or teeth is the presence of residual pulpal haemorrhage by-products in the pulp chamber, canal space and proximal dentine. Often there has been a history of trauma to the affected teeth, resulting in a disruption of the vascular supply to the pulpal tissues. This may be associated with a loss of pulpal tissue vitality, haemorrhage or both. It is important to note that not all localised discoloured teeth are non-vital, nor are all non-vital teeth discoloured. Thus a thorough and accurate assessment should be made regarding the history and vitality of the teeth in question prior to embarking on treatment.

It has been stated that nearly 10% of patients receiving root canal therapy are unhappy with the colour of the treated tooth on completion of the procedure.[1] Given the relative frequency of root canal therapy being performed in the aesthetic zone, it is important that the clinician be skilled in performing bleaching of non-vital teeth in order to conservatively manage the aesthetic demands of the patient.

A variety of techniques have been employed to bleach non-vital teeth following root canal therapy. Strategies for bleaching the external surface of teeth are also successful for bleaching the internal surface of a non-vital tooth, and form the basis of the 'inside/ outside' bleaching technique (Figure 10.3.1). A 10% carbamide peroxide gel is often utilised to bleach not only the outside of the tooth, with a conventional bleaching tray, but also the inside of the tooth via application of the gel directly into the pulp chamber through an access opening. This access opening is then effectively sealed off from the oral cavity by the close-fitting bleaching tray extending over the access on the palatal aspect. Other bleaching agents such as sodium perborate added to water, sodium perborate added to various concentrations of hydrogen peroxide, and high concentrations of hydrogen peroxide and heat have all been shown to bleach the internal aspect of the discoloured non-vital tooth effectively.

In contrast with vital tooth bleaching, the duration of treatment in non-vital tooth bleaching is abbreviated, typically lasting only 2–5 days. The bleaching tray is worn

*Practical Procedures in Aesthetic Dentistry*, First Edition. Edited by Subir Banerji, Shamir B. Mehta and Christopher C.K. Ho. © 2017 John Wiley & Sons, Ltd. Published 2017 by John Wiley & Sons, Ltd.
Companion website: www.wiley.com/go/banerji/aestheticdentistry

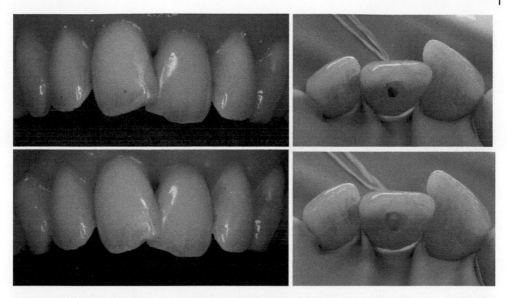

Figure 10.3.1 Initial presentation and after non-vital tooth bleaching using 10% carbamide peroxide and an inside/outside technique. *Source*: Subir Banerji, BDS MClinDent PhD Prosthodontics, London. Reproduced with permission from Subir Banerji.

constantly, except during eating, and the bleaching gel is changed approximately every two hours. Unlike in vital tooth bleaching, there is no concern for pulpal hypersensitivity during treatment due to the root canal therapy performed on the tooth. Soft-tissue irritation can be a concern if the tray is sharp or ill fitting, or if excess bleaching gel is left in contact with the soft tissues. The higher concentrations of hydrogen peroxide and heat application utilised in some chairside bleaching techniques seem to result in more frequent occurrences of cervical resorption than the other bleaching strategies, without showing significantly better aesthetic results.[2] It is hypothesised that the higher-concentration hydrogen peroxide may leach out of a defect present in the cemento-enamel junction (CEJ) in a small percentage of teeth, damaging the periodontal ligament in this area and increasing the risk of cervical resorption.[1]

Effective non-vital tooth bleaching can help preserve the discoloured tooth by allowing the aesthetic challenge to be treated using less invasive methods. Instead of managing the discoloured non-vital tooth with a full coverage restoration with or without a post, further reducing precious remaining tooth structure on the already compromised endodontically treated tooth, clinicians may elect for simple bleaching, direct or indirect composite veneers or indirect porcelain veneers as viable alternatives.

## Procedures

The quality of the endodontic treatment should be evaluated to ensure that the tooth is well sealed and asymptomatic. Any revision of the endodontic treatment should be carried out prior to initiating non-vital tooth bleaching. Treatment on teeth with questionable healing should be delayed until a more definitive condition of health is achieved.

It is necessary to remove the restoration sealing the access opening and to reduce the gutta percha obturation material to a level of approximately 2–3 mm below the CEJ. A glass ionomer cement (GIC) should be applied using a Dycal instrument (Dentsply Sirona, Salzburg, Austria) precisely over the gutta percha and allowed to cure. Care should be taken not to cover any of the stained dentinal walls, as this would prevent the bleaching gel from penetrating the exposed dentinal tubules and reaching the stain, and may result in unsatisfactory bleaching or uneven colour changes. Appropriately placed GIC should maintain the seal of the radicular canal system and allow for adequate bleaching to occur, without compromising the integrity of the obturation or having a negative impact on endodontic success rates.

The access opening and pulp chamber should be thoroughly inspected with magnification for any residual debris or haemorrhage by-products. Ultrasonic scaling with small tips can prove particularly useful in removing unwanted debris while maintaining better visualisation of the residual dentine. Composite restorations present in the non-vital tooth may have to be removed, as the resin serves to block the infiltration of the dentinal tubules with hydrogen peroxide and prevent the bleaching gel from working in that area.

Bleaching trays should be fabricated and cared for in the same manner as in vital tooth bleaching, outlined in Chapter 10.2. It is important to ensure that the bleaching tray has a close but comfortable fit, with a reasonable seal over the access opening of the discoloured tooth.

A high-quality diagnostic photo should be taken with a baseline shade tab adjacent to the teeth to be bleached at the initiation of treatment. Patients should be instructed on how best to perform the inside/outside technique by demonstrating where and how much 10% carbamide peroxide should be applied. It is often helpful to utilise a patient mirror to show clearly how the bleaching gel syringe tip can be introduced into the access opening. Confirm that the patient can perform the necessary procedure of introducing bleaching gel into the access opening on their own, as well as how to load the bleaching tray appropriately and seat it fully into place. Patients who lack the dexterity to perform the necessary procedures may require sealing of bleaching gel or a sodium perborate/water mix into the access opening. Often this modified technique is not as effective, as the bleaching agent cannot be changed as frequently as the ideal inside/outside technique dictates.

Once the loaded tray is seated, excess bleaching gel should be wiped away to avoid minor gingival irritation. The tray should remain in place at all times, except during eating or drinking. The bleaching gel should be replaced every two hours and again just before the patient sleeps during the 2–5 days of bleaching treatment to maintain the optimum effect of the bleaching gel. During the course of treatment the patient should refrain from consuming food or beverages that have the potential to stain, such as red wine, coffee or tea, while the endodontic access is open.

Sealing the access opening should be conducted in a biomimetic fashion with composite resin for optimum aesthetic outcomes. Studies show a transient bond strength reduction following bleaching with a number of agents, including 10% carbamide peroxide. Thus it may be beneficial to allow 1–3 weeks to transpire between cessation of inside/outside bleaching and placing the definitive composite restoration (Figure 10.3.2).[3]

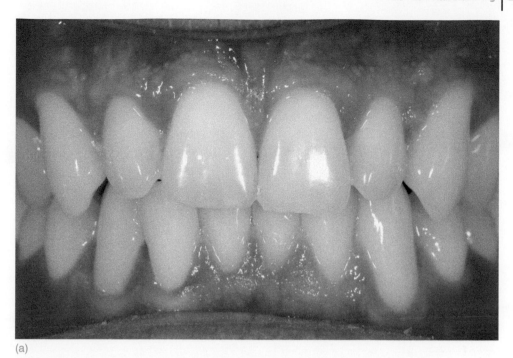

(a)

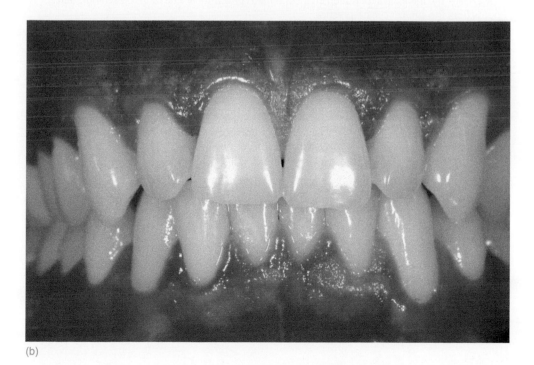

(b)

**Figure 10.3.2** Inside/outside non-vital tooth bleaching using 10% carbamide peroxide.
(a) Pre-operative condition of the discoloured non-vital UR 1. (b) UR 1 after inside/outside bleaching.

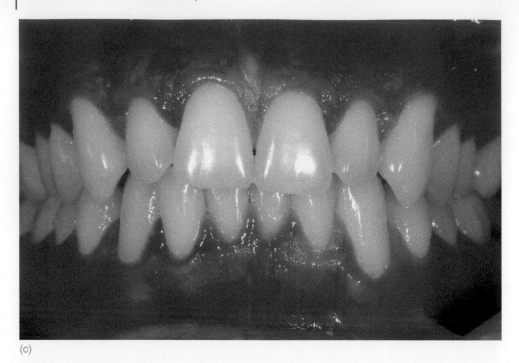

(c)

**Figure 10.3.2** (continued)
(c) Maxillary and mandibular dentition after continued conventional vital tooth bleaching. *Source:* Photos from the author's clinical practice.

## Tips

- Assess the quality of the endodontic therapy and the healing response before initiating non-vital tooth bleaching with an inside/outside technique.
- Teach patients how much and where bleaching gel should be applied and have them demonstrate the process back to you to ensure that they understand the technique and possess the dexterity to administer the bleaching gel appropriately.
- Patients should wear the bleaching tray at all times except when eating or drinking, and change the bleaching gel every two hours for optimum results.

## References

1 Kelleher M. *Dental bleaching*. London: Quintessence; 2008.
2 Dahl J, Pallesen U. Tooth bleaching: a critical review of the biological aspects. *Crit Rev Oral Biol Med*. 2003;14(4):292–304.
3 Attin T, Hannig C, Wiegand A, Attin R. Effect of bleaching on restorative materials and restorations: a systematic review. *Dent Materials*. 2004;20:852–61.

# Part XI

# Implants in the Aesthetic Zone

# 11.1

# Pre-operative Evaluation

*Kyle D. Hogg*

*Video: Pre-operative Evaluation*
*Presented by Kyle D. Hogg*

## Principles

Planning for the replacement of a missing tooth or missing teeth in the aesthetic zone requires a thorough pre-operative evaluation to facilitate a predictable treatment outcome, meeting the functional and aesthetic requirements as well as the expectations of both patient and provider. A number of treatment modalities can be selected to achieve these requirements, including:

- Orthodontic space closure
- Removable partial denture
- Adhesive or resin-bonded fixed partial denture
- Fixed partial denture
- Dental implant-supported restoration.

Successful prosthetic rehabilitation in the aesthetic zone hinges on selecting the most appropriate treatment option for the individual patient; within the confines of the specific localised clinical situation; and within the broader comprehensive restorative treatment plan.[1]

Recent systematic reviews have validated the use of dental implant-supported restorations as a means of reliably replacing single or multiple missing teeth, showing excellent survival rates.[2]

A thorough and meticulous patient assessment based on comprehensive evaluation of the patient is paramount for adequate diagnosis and treatment planning of any dental rehabilitation. A template flow diagram for undertaking a comprehensive patient assessment has been proposed by Mehta et al.[3] (Figure 11.1.1).

Dental implant rehabilitation is inherently interdisciplinary, with both surgical and prosthetic phases of treatment that require a coordinated assessment. The comprehensive pre-operative assessment for dental implant rehabilitation should begin with the establishment, from the perspective of the patient, of the chief complaint. A thorough medical history review must be undertaken to ensure that the patient is fit

*Practical Procedures in Aesthetic Dentistry*, First Edition. Edited by Subir Banerji, Shamir B. Mehta and Christopher C.K. Ho. © 2017 John Wiley & Sons, Ltd. Published 2017 by John Wiley & Sons, Ltd.
Companion website: www.wiley.com/go/banerji/aestheticdentistry

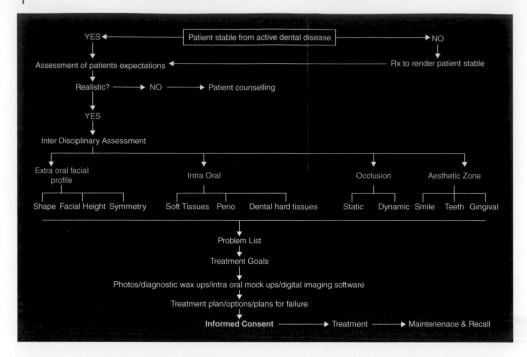

Figure 11.1.1 Flow diagram for undertaking a comprehensive patient assessment. *Source*: Mehta, Banerji, and Aulakh, 2015. Reproduced with permission from George Warman Publications UK Ltd.

to undergo the required surgical and prosthetic procedures. It is important to bear in mind that dental implant therapy is typically elective treatment. Therefore, the patient must not be placed at any undue risk in the pursuit of treatment. Specialist referral for medical consultations may be required or advisable in patients with more compromised conditions or with complex medical histories. The patient must also be satisfactorily stable from active dental disease and have reasonable treatment outcome expectations prior to embarking on a more focused interdisciplinary assessment of the prospective implant sites.

The interdisciplinary assessment includes an intra-oral and extra-oral examination of the patient with an evaluation of the facial aesthetics, temporomandibular joint, muscles of mastication, dental hard and soft tissues, occlusion and both the static and dynamic nature of the aesthetic zone. A thorough and detailed evaluation of the site to be restored with implants is imperative to achieve a successful, restoratively driven treatment outcome. Special diagnostic records, radiographic imaging and diagnostic wax-ups of the proposed restoration provide the surgical and restorative team with valuable information that enables appropriate planning and execution of treatment in a predictable fashion.

Patients must ultimately be educated on the risks, benefits and maintenance requirements of all treatment options that might be suitable for them. In addition to developing a treatment plan, the clinician must also discuss with the patient the steps involved in rendering care, the duration of the planned rehabilitation, the number of visits required, maintenance and the financial obligations of the selected treatment in order to achieve informed consent.

## Procedures

Refer to the procedures in Chapter 2.3, 'Evaluation of the Aesthetic Zone', for a review of how to perform a comprehensive aesthetic zone evaluation. Evaluating a patient for implant rehabilitation in the aesthetic zone is an extension of the comprehensive aesthetic zone evaluation, with additional patient factors and site-specific factors to be considered.

With your patient comfortably seated upright in the dental chair, and you seated at the same height facing them, ask the patient to describe in their own words what their dental problem is and what they would like to have done to correct the problem. Allow the patient to speak, listening carefully to the patient's description of both their condition and desired solution without interruption, and repeat it back to the patient in a paraphrased manner. This exercise, while seemingly simplistic, establishes the patient's chief complaint, provides valuable information on the patient's preferences, expectations for rehabilitation and level of dental knowledge, and develops trust and rapport between patient and provider.

In the same manner, perform a detailed review of the patient's medical and social history. Of particular note would be patients with a positive history of radiation therapy to the head and neck, history of taking bisphosphonate medications or who have had bisphosphonate-related osteonecrosis of the jaw (BRONJ), insulin-dependent diabetics, patients with unfinished cranio-facial growth and incomplete tooth eruption (females younger than 18–19 years, males slightly older), patients undergoing immunosuppressant therapy, patients undergoing chemotherapy and heavy smokers. Caution should be taken when considering treating patients with these conditions or others that might prevent or hinder the predictability of soft- or hard-tissue healing, and the long-term survival and success of dental implant rehabilitation. Specialist referral to appropriate medical colleagues for pre-operative evaluation and clearance is advisable for patients who have a complicated medical history or a high American Society of Anesthesiology (ASA) score.

Next, perform an extra-oral clinical examination, as outlined in detail in Chapter 2.3.

Continuing with the intra-oral examination, note the arrangement and condition of the patient's remaining dentition, occlusal scheme, temporomandibular joint function, presence of parafunctional activity, oral hygiene, periodontal status, caries rate and additional restorative, periodontal, endodontic and orthodontic needs. A complete radiographic survey and periodontal charting are necessary to determine fully whether the patient is stable from active disease, which should be a prerequisite before proceeding to implant rehabilitation.

As the examination progresses from global patient factors to site-specific factors, the focus narrows to the characteristics of the site requiring rehabilitation. In planning for an implant rehabilitation in the aesthetic zone, it is particularly important to assess both the tooth and gingival display at repose and at the maximum dynamic smile, or high 'E' smile. The amount of tooth display that a patient exhibits is variable over time, with younger individuals typically showing around 3 mm of maxillary central incisors and 0.5 mm of mandibular central incisors at repose. With age and decreased muscle tonicity and elasticity of the peri-oral tissues, patients typically show progressively more of the mandibular incisors and less of the maxillary incisors. The dynamic smile should be evaluated by observing the lip morphology and mobility from a frontal position when the patient says 'EEEEE' or laughs. The lip may appear thin, medium or full, in addition to being classified by length as short, medium or long. The relative mobility of the lips also influences the display of anterior teeth during dynamic movements.[4] The degree to which the proposed implant restoration and peri-implant tissues are visible in the aesthetic zone can greatly influence the aesthetic demands of the patient and the difficulty of the rehabilitation.

Attention should also be given to the presence or absence of keratinised gingival tissues in the area requiring rehabilitation. The gingival biotype (relative thickness or thinness of the tissue), the degree of scallop of the gingival tissues (low flat tissue or highly scalloped tissue), gingival symmetry and interdental papillae height should all be considered with respect to how the proposed rehabilitation can re-create the patient's naturally occurring appearance. In general, thick gingival biotypes with low flat tissue and shorter papillae are more predictably reproducible and stable than thin biotypes with highly scalloped tissue and tall papillae. A good starting point for discussing the anterior aesthetics and kinetics of tooth display is by photographing the maximum high 'E' smile and exploring the patient's chief complaint and your observations as you both view the photograph (Figure 11.1.2).

A thorough evaluation of the restorative requirements, endodontic health and periodontal health of the adjacent teeth must be undertaken to ensure that pathological conditions of these teeth will not negatively influence the predictable healing and function of the dental implant. Adjacent teeth should be healthy and stable before implant rehabilitation proceeds.

An assessment of the bone volume at the proposed surgical site is required to determine whether an implant can be placed in the appropriate three-dimensional location to allow for the ideal aesthetic and functional restoration. There must be sufficient inter-radicular space to permit placement of the dental implant between neighbouring teeth while leaving a zone of safety between the dental implant and adjacent tooth roots and pertinent neuro-vascular anatomy. A pre-operative evaluation of available bone volume, density and quality can be performed with the aid of cone-beam computed tomography (CBCT) or other three-dimensional imaging techniques (Figure 11.1.3). These detailed

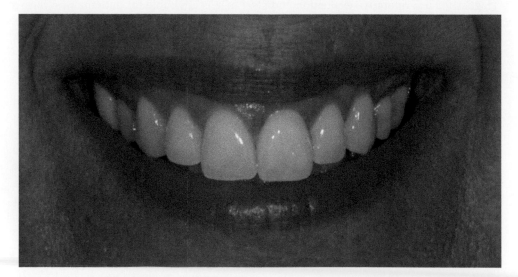

Figure 11.1.2 Evaluation of anterior tooth and gingival display. In this image, taken from the author's clinical practice, the UL 1 is failing and requires extraction. The patient exhibits a high lip line that exposes all of the maxillary anterior and posterior teeth in addition to several millimetres of thin and highly scalloped gingival tissues with tall papillae. The aesthetic demands of the patient will be high and the rehabilitation of the UL 1 with an implant will require complex treatment.

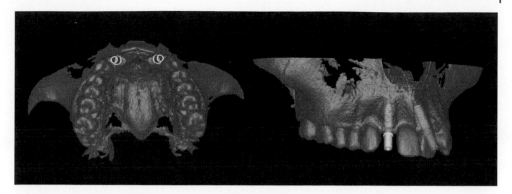

Figure 11.1.3 CBCT scan of the maxilla taken from the author's clinical practice, allowing for detailed surgical and prosthetic planning

images can allow the restorative dentist and surgeon to assess the hard and soft tissues in the proposed site and evaluate the need for any grafting or augmentation. These specialised images also allow for previously performed augmentations to be evaluated.

Good-quality alginate impressions and pre-operative photographs should be taken to facilitate planning of the proposed implant rehabilitation and further discussion with the patient. Diagnostic casts should be transferred to an articulator with a properly recorded facebow and mounted in centric relation. The shape and symmetry of adjacent teeth should be assessed and any planned corrections undertaken. A full-contour diagnostic wax-up or fabrication of an interim prosthesis should be performed to evaluate the availability of interocclusal, mesial-distal and bucco-lingual space. Utilisation of the articulator can better allow the dental technician to provide a prototype of the restoration that blends the aesthetic demands with the functional requirements of the patient's existing or planned static and dynamic occlusal scheme. This prototype can be incorporated into a scan guide for use with advanced imaging techniques such as CBCT, a surgical guide to direct implant placement or both. Working backwards from the intended restorative result prior to surgical intervention ensures that the process is prosthetically driven, with a greater degree of predictability in the final treatment outcome.

Discussion with the patient about their expectations for the proposed implant rehabilitation is vital. It is paramount that an open and honest conversation be held regarding the patient's aesthetic and functional expectations of the proposed implant treatment, as well as other alternative treatment options, with full explanations of the relative risks and benefits inherent in each option. Patients should be informed about the anticipated treatment time and costs of the treatment options. The future maintenance requirements of the rehabilitation and necessity for follow-up care should be established, as well as the financial obligations of the patient for any future repairs. These discussions are required to achieve informed consent from the patient and should be well documented in the treatment record.

## Tips

- Make the undertaking of an implant evaluation in the aesthetic zone a methodical and comprehensive process, progressing from global patient factors to site-specific factors. An evaluation form for this process is provided in Table 11.1.1.

Table 11.1.1 Implant case evaluation form

| Implant Case Evaluation | | | |
| --- | --- | --- | --- |
| | Characteristic | Favourable | Unfavourable |
| Patient factors | Medical health (ASA I/II/III/IV) | | |
| | Age/growth | | |
| | Smoking habit | | |
| | Occlusion | | |
| | Temporomandibular joint/muscles of mastication | | |
| | Parafunctional habits | | |
| | Oral hygiene | | |
| | Previous or current periodontal disease | | |
| | Caries rate | | |
| | Additional rest/perio/endo/ortho needs | | |
| | Ability to tolerate surgery (recline etc.) | | |
| | Previous radiation therapy/bisphosponates | | |
| | Sufficient oral opening for instrumentation | | |
| | Other | | |
| Site-specific factors | Tooth/gingival display at repose | | |
| | Tooth/gingival display at high 'E' smile | | |
| | Presence of keratinised gingiva | | |
| | Gingival biotype (thick/thin) | | |
| | Gingival scallop (low flat/high scallop) | | |
| | Gingival symmetry | | |
| | Papillae height | | |
| | Bone density/quality | | |
| | Bone volume | | |
| | Inter-radicular space (parallel/converge/diverge) | | |
| | Soft-tissue deficiency (vertical/horizontal) | | |
| | Hard-tissue deficiency (vertical/horizontal) | | |
| | Soft/hard-tissue grafting required | | |
| | Previous soft/hard-tissue graft suitability | | |
| | Adjacent teeth periodontal health | | |
| | Adjacent teeth endodontic health | | |
| | Adjacent teeth restorative requirements | | |
| | Adjacent teeth shape | | |
| | Adjacent teeth symmetry and proportion | | |
| | Interocclusal space availability | | |
| | Mesial-distal space availability | | |
| | Bucco-lingual space availability | | |
| Patient expectations | Aesthetic expectations | | |
| | Functional expectations | | |
| | Treatment time expectations | | |
| | Maintenance expectations | | |
| | Financial expectations | | |

*Source*: Developed by Cliff Starr DMD and Kyle D. Hogg DDS MClinDent Prosthodontics.

- Take appropriate records, including photographs, conventional radiographs, diagnostic casts and three-dimensional images where indicated. The fabrication of a diagnostic wax-up or diagnostic interim prosthesis is strongly recommended prior to embarking on definitive treatment.
- Discuss patient expectations of the proposed treatment with respect to aesthetics, function, treatment time, maintenance requirements and financial obligations. Make sure that the patient has reasonable expectations prior to giving treatment.

## References

1 Zitzmann N, Margolin M, Filippi A, Weiger R, Krastl G. Patient assessment and diagnosis in implant treatment. *Aust Dent J*. 2008;53 (Suppl 1):S3–10.

2 Pjetursson B, Asgeirsson A, Zwahlen M, Sailer I. Improvements in implant dentistry over the last decade: comparison of survival and complication rates in older and newer publications. *Int J Oral Maxillofac Implants*. 2014;29 (suppl):308–24.

3 Mehta S, Banerji S, Aulakh R. Patient assessment: preparing for a predictable aesthetic outcome. *Dent Update*. 2015;42:78–86.

4 Vig R, Brundo G. The kinetics of anterior tooth display. *J Prosth Dent*. 1978;39(5):502–4.

## 11.2

## Abutment Selection

*Christopher C.K. Ho*

## Principles

An abutment is an intermediary component inserted on the implant, with the restoration then seated over the abutment. An abutment screw normally retains the abutment in place. This abutment provides the retention, support and final position of the restoration.

The abutment can be constructed in a two-piece combination consisting of the abutment and the restoration, with the latter cemented into place or as a one-piece combination consisting of an abutment/restoration screwed into place as one unit. They are generally available as either prefabricated (stock) abutments from the implant manufacturer or customised for the patient through CAD/CAM or casting procedures via a dental laboratory. Prefabricated abutments (Figure 11.2.1) are less expensive and relatively easy to use, although they have limitations due to not being customised. A customised abutment is made to fit the implant position specifically, taking into consideration the adjacent teeth, soft tissues and general contours. Situations that may require a custom abutment include the following:

- Angle correction greater than 15 degrees – the abutment may be used to correct the implant angulation.
- Minimal interocclusal space – the abutment height should not exceed the space required for the restorative material.
- Splinted multiple unit cases to allow parallelism.
- Ability to replicate anatomical cross-sectional profile of teeth.
- Collar height needed more than 1 mm above the largest collar height of a stock abutment, to allow easier clearance of cement. Abutment margins should be supragingival in non-aesthetic zones and slightly subgingival in the aesthetic zone.
- Interproximal distance whereby the abutment width must be sufficient to support the crown, but possess adequate interproximal access for hygiene maintenance.

The final choice between a custom abutment and a prefabricated abutment depends on the clinical situation, practitioner's experience and preference. The various types are summarised in Figure 11.2.2.

**Custom abutments** are used in situations where stock abutments cannot be used to correct angulations, and also to provide an ideal anatomical profile and customised marginal position of a restoration.

*Practical Procedures in Aesthetic Dentistry*, First Edition. Edited by Subir Banerji, Shamir B. Mehta and Christopher C.K. Ho. © 2017 John Wiley & Sons, Ltd. Published 2017 by John Wiley & Sons, Ltd.
Companion website: www.wiley.com/go/banerji/aestheticdentistry

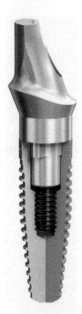

Figure 11.2.1 Implant and prefabricated titanium abutment (Esthetic abutment, Nobel Biocare Services AG, Zurich, Switzerland). Note that the margins are available with different collar heights and are made to simulate the typical marginal positioning

These are fabricated in two ways:

1) **Castable abutments** that are waxed by a dental technician to the required contours and customised for the restorative space. These techniques require waxing, investing and casting with alloys at high temperature. This can be more labour intensive and subsequently costly.

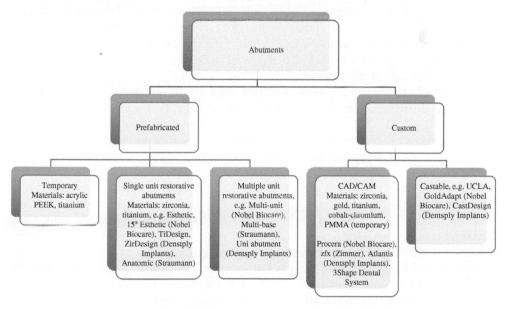

Figure 11.2.2 Implant abutments available

2) **Computer-generated abutments**, e.g. NobelProcera (Nobel Biocare), Atlantis (Dentsply, Dentsply Sirona, Salzburg, Austria). The use of CAD/CAM technology for this purpose was developed in the 1980s. Further developments are occurring with digital impression taking, scanning, milling abutments and restorations with great accuracy and precision. Conventional techniques rely on the accuracy of many steps including impression taking, investment materials, wax and casting, which can often lead to errors. CAD/CAM abutments have the potential to provide the most accurate fit due to minimal manipulation after milling. This is particularly useful in implant dentistry where precision is crucial for fit, longevity, distribution of stress, ease of insertion and long-term success.

**Prefabricated (stock) abutments** are available from implant manufacturers and either used intact or further modified by the dentist or dental technician. These are available with various anatomical cross-sections and alignments for common clinical scenarios. It is advised to place the marginal design of an abutment equigingival or in a position that can be accessed when cementing a restoration, due to the possibility of cement being left undetected when a margin is placed deep subgingivally. Linkevicius has reported that the amount of residual cement left increases as margins are located more subgingivally, and at 2–3 mm subgingival the residual cement is 10 times that of margins that are either equigingival or 1 mm subgingival.[1]

Available prefabricated abutments include the following:

- **Temporary abutments** made of plastic or titanium. These are often used to prosthetically guide soft-tissue healing for improved soft-tissue contours, progressive and immediate loading, or for assessing occlusion and phonetics in a more complex rehabilitation.
- **Multiple unit abutments**, e.g. Multi-unit abutments (Nobel Biocare), Uni abutments (Denstply Sirona), are used in partially or fully edentulous patients. These components may allow movement of the restorative platform to a location that is not so deep subgingivally, allowing simpler insertion and removal of a prosthesis as well as allowing for divergent alignment of implants. In addition, many of these multiple unit abutments have a taper that allows for divergent implant alignments, such as are seen in the fully edentulous maxilla where implants may be splayed buccally. Inserting and removing an implant without use of these more tapered abutments may be difficult due to the nature of the connections.
- **Angulated abutments** are used to correct angulations in cases where implants are inserted intentionally at an angle, as in All on Four Treatment Concepts (Nobel Biocare; Figure 11.2.3), where there is limited bone or to allow for screw access in multiple unit cases. They are available in a number of different angulations allowing for correction of the prosthetic screw access.

### Material Selection

The materials commonly used for abutments are zirconia, titanium and gold. Gold abutments are fabricated using casting procedures, while zirconia and titanium abutments are milled to the correct shape and contours. The success of these materials is dependent on correct handling and case selection. Sailer et al. found in a systematic review of 29 studies in single and fixed partial dentures that the estimated 5-year survival for ceramic and metal abutments is 99.1% and 97.4%, respectively.[2] A study by Abrahamson et al. found that abutments made of CP (commercially pure) titanium or

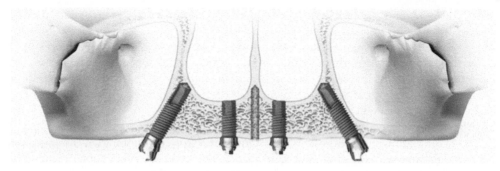

Figure 11.2.3 All on Four® Treatment Concept (Nobel Biocare) – anterior implants have straight multi-unit abutments, while posterior implants have angulated abutments correcting the access for the prosthetic screws

ceramic allowed the formation of a mucosal attachment that included one epithelial and one connective tissue portion, which were about 2 mm and 1–1.5 mm high, respectively.[3] At sites where abutments were made of gold alloy or dental porcelain, no proper attachment formed at the abutment level, but the soft-tissue margin receded and bone resorption occurred. The abutment fixture junction was thereby occasionally exposed and the mucosal barrier became established to the fixture portion of the implant. This was confirmed by Welander et al., who demonstrated that the soft-tissue dimensions at titanium and zirconia abutments remained stable between 2 and 5 months of healing.[4] At gold/platinum-alloy abutment sites, however, an apical shift of the barrier epithelium and the marginal bone occurred between 2 and 5 months of healing.

Reviews of selected articles[2,5] suggest that zirconia abutments are reliable in the anterior region from both biological and mechanical points of view. Furthermore, zirconia abutments may represent a material surface that is less attractive to early plaque retention compared to titanium.

## Procedures

After the impression is taken, a model is constructed within the laboratory, or if a digital impression is taken the file is exported for a model to be fabricated.

The dentist and dental technician must arrive at a decision on whether to use a custom or a prefabricated abutment. The use of a prefabricated abutment requires information on the size of the implant platform and also a decision on the profile of the abutment. Many different-shaped profiles are offered by manufacturers to allow for different emergence profiles. These abutments may also have different angulations to allow for different alignments of implant positions. Additionally, many of these abutments have different collar heights, situating the margin in a more appropriate position for cementation.

Preparation of prefabricated abutments can be performed for the most part extra-orally, although some clinicians will prefer to place the prefabricated abutment and prepare the abutment intra-orally, placing retraction cord and then taking an impression like a conventional crown preparation (i.e. abutment-level impression).

Insertion of the abutment or a screw-retained one-piece abutment/crown requires removal of the healing abutment and irrigation of the connection of the implant. The author advises the use of a chlorhexidine gel to disinfect the connection before placing the abutment onto the implant. It is prudent to warn the patient that there may be some pressure on the soft tissues as the restoration is inserted, especially if there has been no grooming of the tissues with a provisional restoration. This is the result of tissue compression from the transition from a circular healing abutment to a correctly profiled restoration. This discomfort will gradually resolve over a few minutes, although if there is too much tissue impingement then the subgingival profile of the abutment may require adjustment, as it could be over-contoured.

After the abutment has been hand tightened, it is customary to take a radiograph to ensure complete seating of the abutment. Once there is confirmation that the abutment is completely seated, the abutment is torqued to the correct level as recommended by the implant manufacturer with the appropriate instrumentation.

## Tips

- In the aesthetic zone where the tissue is a thin biotype or the implant is superficially placed, it may be advisable to use a zirconia abutment to allow improved aesthetics, especially if there is any tissue recession.[6]
- The insertion of abutments for a cemented restoration may be simpler with the use of an insertion jig, which orientates the correct position of the abutment in relation to the adjacent teeth (Figure 11.2.4).
- Over-contouring of an abutment has the effect of putting pressure on the soft tissues, leading to compressive forces that can often result in recession. Special caution should be undertaken in the design of the labial region of anterior abutments to ensure that there are no deleterious consequences.

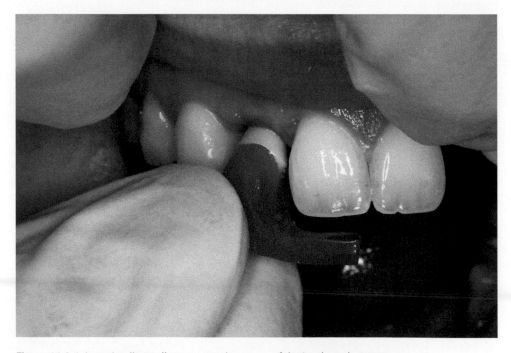

Figure 11.2.4  Location jig to allow correct placement of the implant abutment

# References

1 Linkevicius T, Vindasiute E, Puisys A, Peciuliene V. The influence of margin location on the amount of undetected cement excess after delivery of cement-retained implant restorations. *Clin Oral Implants Res.* 2011;22(12):1379–84.
2 Sailer I, Philipp A, Zembic A, Pjetursson BE, Hämmerle CH, Zwahlen M. A systematic review of the performance of ceramic and metal implant abutments supporting fixed implant reconstructions. *Clin Oral Implants Res.* 2009 Sep;20 Suppl 4:4–31.
3 Abrahamsson I, Berglundh T, Glantz PO, Lindhe J. The mucosal attachment at different abutments. An experimental study in dogs. *J Clin Periodontol.* 1998;25(9):721–7.
4 Welander M, Abrahamsson I, Berglundh T. The mucosal barrier at implant abutments of different materials. *Clin Oral Implants Res.* 2008;19(7):635–41.
5 Zembic A, Philipp AO, Hämmerle CH, Wohlwend A, Sailer I. Eleven-year follow-up of a prospective study of zirconia implant abutments supporting single all-ceramic crowns in anterior and premolar regions. *Clin Implant Dent Relat Res.* 2015 Oct;17 Suppl 2:e417–26.
6 Jung RE, Sailer I, Hämmerle CH, Attin T, Schmidlin P. In vitro color changes of soft tissues caused by restorative materials. *Int J Periodontics Restorative Dent.* 2007;27(3):251–7.

## Further Reading

Giglio G. Abutment selection in implant supported fixed prosthodontics. *Int J Periodont Restorative Dent.* 1999;19:233–41.
Nakamura K, Kanno T, Milleding P, Ortengren U. Zirconia as a dental implant abutment material: a systematic review. *Int J Prosthodont.* 2010 Jul;23(4):299–309.
Scarano A, Piattelli M, Caputi S, Favero GA, Piattelli A. Bacterial adhesion on commercially pure titanium and zirconium oxide disks: an in vivo human study. *J Periodontol.* 2004;75(2):292–6.

## 11.3

# Impression Taking in Implant Dentistry

*Christopher C.K. Ho*

*Video: Impression Taking in Implant Dentistry*
*Presented by Christopher C.K. Ho*

## Principles

An impression is necessary to transfer the position and design of an implant or abutment to a master cast. Additionally, this captures the soft-tissue contours that frame the restoration, providing the pink aesthetic frame around the tooth. An impression is usually made at the implant level or abutment level with an elastomeric impression material such as polyether or polyvinyl siloxane. A poor impression may lead to an inaccurately fitting prosthesis or compromised result, which may add to the cost incurred as well as extend treatment times and inconvenience for the patient.

The implant impression will provide:

- Position
- Depth
- Axis/angulation
- Rotational position
- Soft-tissue contour (emergence profile).

The requirements of impression materials include:

- Accuracy
- Rigidity yet resilience
- Ability to be removed from undercuts
- Dimensional stability.

The use of polyether or additional polyvinyl siloxane has been recommended. Silicone impression materials have better biomechanical stability than polyether, which is susceptible to moisture and sunlight. Silicone tends to have a favourable modulus of elasticity that allows simpler removal from the mouth, especially in soft-tissue undercuts.

The fit of implant prostheses requires extreme accuracy due to the precise machine fit and the rigid connection to bone. Implants do not have a periodontal ligament that may allow for minor inaccuracies such as in teeth. Impressions for multiple implant

*Practical Procedures in Aesthetic Dentistry*, First Edition. Edited by Subir Banerji, Shamir B. Mehta and Christopher C.K. Ho. © 2017 John Wiley & Sons, Ltd. Published 2017 by John Wiley & Sons, Ltd.
Companion website: www.wiley.com/go/banerji/aestheticdentistry

Table 11.3.1 Comparison between open- and closed-tray implant impression taking

| Factors | Transfer (closed-tray) coping | Pick-up (open-tray) coping |
|---|---|---|
| **Ease of use** | Simpler, may be better for gagging patients | More steps involved |
| **Tray preparation** | None | Tray must be perforated where the impression coping is situated |
| **Interocclusal space** | Less space required and simpler in posterior region | More space is required to access screw to insert and remove coping |
| **Multiple unit splinting** | Not possible | Possible |
| **Precision of impression** | Possible inaccuracy due to having to reinsert the coping back into the impression | Less inaccuracy due to coping remaining in the impression |
| **Divergent implants** | Difficult to remove impression | Simpler to remove impression |
| **Depth of implants** | Deeper placement may preclude use of a closed-tray coping as it may not engage the impression material sufficiently | Impression coping is square and can engage impression material, and can be modified if required |

restorations are even more critical. A passive fit is the objective, as a misfit may lead to stress placed on the implants, resulting in bone loss and even loss of integration.

Impression techniques used in implant dentistry include abutment-level impressions, both direct and indirect; and implant-level impressions, both pick-up (open-tray) and transfer (closed-tray). See Table 11.3.1 for a comparison of the latter types.

### Abutment-Level Impression Copings

**Direct** abutment-level impressions require placement of the abutment and then preparation and impression, similar to a conventional crown preparation.

**Indirect** abutment-level impressions require the use of snap-on abutments such as Snappy abutments (Nobel Biocare Services AG, Zurich, Switzerland) or Solid abutments (Straumann AG, Basel, Switzerland), which involve placing a standard abutment with an impression cap that gets picked up within the impression. An analogue to fit this abutment is then inserted and a model made.

### Implant-Level Impression Techniques

A **transfer (closed-tray)** impression is where the impression coping remains in the mouth following removal of the set impression. An analogue is then placed on the impression coping and the coping replaced back into the impression. These copings are normally tapered to allow removal.

A **pick-up (open-tray)** impression (Figure 11.3.1) is where the coping is incorporated within the impression and unscrewed, then removed on setting of the impression. This requires the tray to be open to allow access to the retaining screw, enabling release and removal of the impression. These copings are normally square, allowing the coping to be locked within the impression.

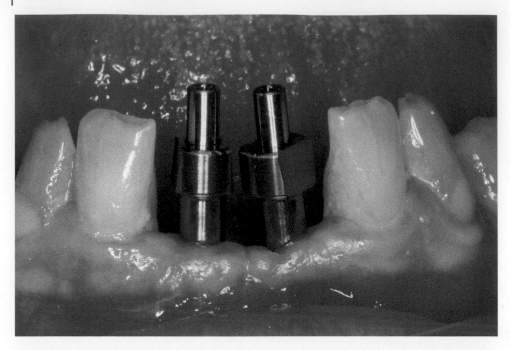

Figure 11.3.1 Open-tray impression copings – notice the square form of the coping, which is picked up in the impression

Digital impression techniques are now being developed with the use of scan markers that are inserted onto an implant and the patient scanned for a digital impression, with the registration of the implant carried out concurrently.

### Customised Impression Copings

Manufacturers' impression copings are standardised and do not take into account the varying soft-tissue profiles that may be formed by provisional restorations or contoured healing abutments. Impression copings may be customised to accurately record soft tissue by inserting an analogue into a provisional restoration and forming an impression of the provisional crown and analogue assembly by placing this into impression material, covering up to the submucosal portion of the provisional restoration (Figure 11.3.2). Once set the provisional restoration is removed, leaving the analogue within the impression material and the contours of the provisional crown left as a negative, for an impression coping then to be placed onto the analogue. The negative space can be filled with acrylic or flowable composite resin, giving a customised impression coping that can be used intra-orally, capturing the provisional crown contours.

### Multiple Unit Impressions

Due to the machine fit of implants, the objective is passive fit of a prosthesis or, put simply, to create as accurate a fit as is clinically possible to avoid bone strain resulting from uncontrolled loading of the implants through the superstructure.

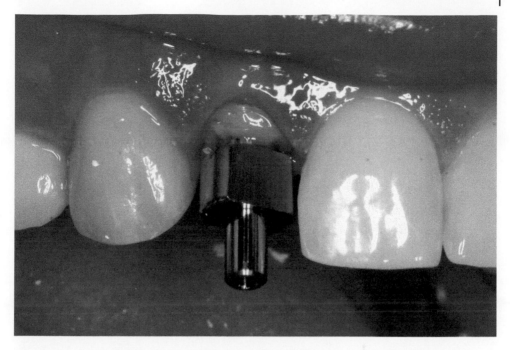

Figure 11.3.2 Customised impression coping in place, supporting and reproducing the gingival architecture developed by the provisional restoration

To increase the accuracy of multiple unit impressions, it has been suggested that there is improved precision of fit if impression copings are splinted with auto-polymerising resin prior to taking the impression.

A recent systematic review by Papaspyridakos et al. found that the splinted impression technique is more accurate for both partially and completely edentulous patients.[1] The open-tray technique is more accurate than closed-tray for completely edentulous patients, but for partially edentulous patients there seems to be no difference. If you have multiple implants but plan on restoring them as single units, you may choose closed-tray impression copings for ease of use.

## Procedures

The procedure for an implant-level impression is as follows:

- After removal of the healing abutment or provisional restoration, the impression coping should be inserted without delay, as the soft tissue can collapse inwards, making it more difficult to insert the coping.
- Insert either an open- or closed-tray impression coping. If taking a multiple unit impression, consider splinting of the impressions with wire, resin or other framework with an open-tray technique (Figure 11.3.3).
- Take a periapical radiograph. A paralleling technique is utilised so as to visualise the complete seating of the copings (Figure 11.3.4). The use of a film holder is encouraged.
- Try-in the tray and prepare it by perforating it in the region of the impression coping if utilising an open-tray technique.

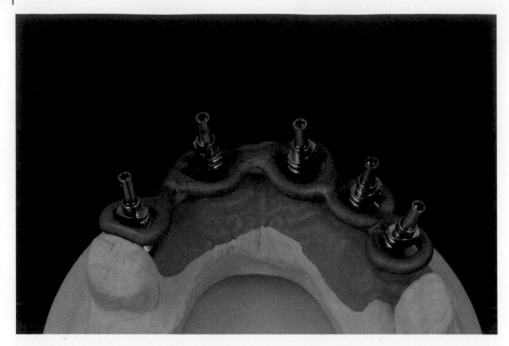

Figure 11.3.3 Jig constructed in the laboratory for pick-up intra-orally by splinting of copings to the jig

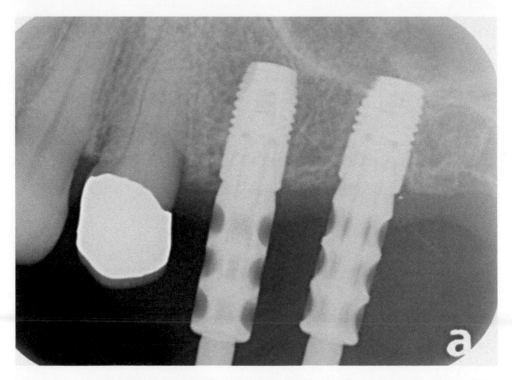

Figure 11.3.4 Paralleling technique used to take radiograph of implant and impression coping – note that there has been complete seating of the impression coping

- Proceed to take the impression. Inspect to see that the impression is accurate and extends to all the teeth required. Additional attention should be made to assess that the coping fits into the impression if a closed-tray technique is used, and if an open-tray technique is used ensure that the coping is sitting firmly within the material with no chance of dislodgement.
- Reinsert the healing abutment or provisional restoration.

## Tips

- Take a periapical radiograph to check the fit and seating of copings that are below the mucosa and not visible.
- If implants are in close proximity to each other, it may be impossible to place the impression copings together. If this happens, you may wish to modify the impression copings with a bur to allow complete seating. Another solution may be to employ an engaging temporary cylinder or other abutment that can be used like a pick-up coping.
- In splinting of multiple unit impressions when implants are spaced some distance apart, there may be more inaccuracy due to the polymerisation contraction that resins undergo, and hence stiff wire and resin may be substituted to minimise the volume of resin contraction.

## Reference

1 Papaspyridakos P, Chen CJ, Gallucci GO, Doukoudakis A, Weber HP, Chronopoulos V. Accuracy of implant impressions for partially and completely edentulous patients: a systematic review. *Int J Oral Maxillofac Implants*. 2014;29(4):836–45.

## Further Reading

Buskin R, Salinas T. Transferring emergence profile created from provisional to definitive restoration. *Pract Perio Aest Dent*. 1998;10:1171–9.

Chee W, Jivraj S. Impression techniques for implant dentistry. *Br Dent J*. 2006 Oct 7;201(7): 429–32.

Karunagaran S, Paprocki GJ, Wicks R, Markose S. A review of implant abutments – abutment classification to aid prosthetic selection. *J Tenn Dent Assoc*. 2013;93(2): 18–23.

## 11.4

## Screw versus Cemented Implant-Supported Restorations

*Christopher C.K. Ho*

## Principles

An implant-supported restoration can be inserted onto an implant by either attaching it to the implants with screws or cementing it onto abutments that have been secured by screws. There are advantages and disadvantages to each procedure, and the decision of whether to screw retain or cement a restoration is often dependent on the implant position and clinician preference.

The factors that determine the decision are outlined in the following sections.

### Retrievability

Screw retention allows the ability to remove a restoration for repair, prosthetic modification or soft-tissue inspection, and creates access for hygiene if required. Many clinicians prefer to treat implant restorations similarly to conventional crowns and bridgework, cementing the final restoration and, if there is any maintenance required such as screw loosening, then destroying the restoration and replacing it accordingly. The incidence of screw loosening has diminished with improved screw-joint mechanics and connections, although it may still occur. When abutment screws loosen, cement-retained restorations are not always predictably removed from abutments to allow screws to be re-tightened, and hence the restoration may need to be removed. This would often destroy the restoration and render it unusable. Thus it would be prudent and simpler to manage if the restorations were planned for screw retention where, if a problem did occur, the restoration could be accessed through the screw hole, removed and tightened. Additionally, as the complexity of the restoration and the number of units increase, the expense of re-making an extensive restoration becomes untenable for the patient, so retrievability is paramount. Alternatively temporary soft cement can be used to cement the final restoration, this will require an accurate fit of the restoration to minmise the risk of inadvertent decementaion and preserve retrievability.

### Aesthetics

Screw retention requires a screw-access hole to be made through the restoration that is normally restored with composite resin once the restoration is in place. In the anterior

*Practical Procedures in Aesthetic Dentistry*, First Edition. Edited by Subir Banerji, Shamir B. Mehta and Christopher C.K. Ho. © 2017 John Wiley & Sons, Ltd. Published 2017 by John Wiley & Sons, Ltd.
Companion website: www.wiley.com/go/banerji/aestheticdentistry

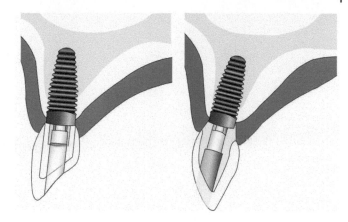

Figure 11.4.1  Screw-retained crowns require an access hole on the cingulum area to enable access to the screw. The image on the right demonstrates the alignment of the implant, with the access to the screw leading to a hole on the labial surface of the crown, which would not be acceptable and necessitates a cement-on crown

region of the mouth screw retention may not be possible due to implant position, as having a screw access in a visible area, such as the labial face of a maxillary incisor, is unacceptable (Figure 11.4.1). When screw access to the implants is in aesthetic areas, the screw access can be re-aligned with the use of angulated abutments, or the restoration should be retained with custom abutments and cemented. Screw-retained restorations can only be used when the trajectory of the implant allows the screw access to be in a non-aesthetic area. There are also clinicians who object to having a hole in the restoration that is restored with composite resin, as this may wear and discolour over time. Additionally, to achieve screw retention in the anterior region often involves aligning the implant slightly more palatally in the anterior maxilla to allow screw access in the cingulum area, which may leave a ridge lap or unaesthetic crown.

### Passivity

A passive fit is desirable for implant restorations, as stress to an implant may overload the prosthesis, causing a technical complication, or lead to strain between the bone interface and implants, resulting in peri-implant bony changes. It has been advocated that one of the advantages of cement-retained restorations is that frameworks are more passive, as the abutments are individually retained to the implants by screws and the restoration is cemented over the abutments. This cement space allows for passivity, on the assumption that the cement acts as a shock absorber and reduces stress to the bone and implant interface. There is very little evidence to support this theory, however. Impression taking and handling of the casts are crucial to minimise errors and the advent of CAD/CAM milling has eliminated many of the errors from casting and metal work. Due to the passive fit, there is a belief that there is less fatigue and fracture of componentry, and that should there be overloading forces to the restoration, the cement layer would fail first, thereby saving the implant and restoration from failure.

### Hygiene (Emergence Profile)

To achieve screw access in maxillary anterior implant restorations, it may be necessary to align an implant in a more palatal trajectory, which may leave the implant more palatally placed, especially in a resorbed alveolar ridge. The final restoration may thus possess a ridge lap and subsequently be more difficult to clean effectively, or there may be an unaesthetic appearance (Figure 11.4.2).

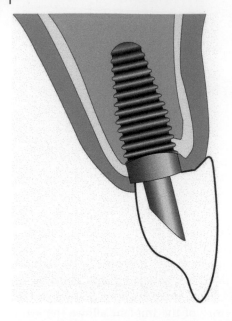

Figure 11.4.2 Achieving screw retention in the anterior region may involve aligning the implant slightly more palatally in the anterior maxilla to allow screw access in the cingulum area, which may leave a ridge lap or unaesthetic crown

### Reduced Occlusal Material Fracture

A screw-retained restoration will have a screw-access hole, which disrupts the structural continuity of porcelain, leaving some unsupported porcelain at the hole. Cemented restorations are one piece without any weakening of the structure of the crown. However, it should be noted that if veneering porcelain chips or fractures off an implant restoration in a screw-retained restoration, it would be a relatively simple procedure to remove and carry out an indirect repair on the implant restoration.

### Interarch Space

A cemented restoration requires sufficient axial wall height to allow for retention form, hence in those situations where there is limited interarch space it may not be possible to achieve adequate retention for a cemented restoration. However, screw-retained restorations can be secured to implants with as little as 4 mm of space from the platform of the implant to the opposing teeth.

### Occlusion

In a cement-retained restoration there is no screw-access hole that may interfere with occlusal stops or excursive movements. Often composite resin is used to cover access channels and these materials are susceptible to wear under functional forces, so the occlusal contacts are preserved with cement-retained restorations.

### Health of Peri-implant Tissue

Incomplete removal of cement may result in peri-implant inflammation, soft-tissue swelling, bleeding and/or suppuration and eventual resorption of peri-implant bone. It has been demonstrated that even in experienced practitioners a surprising amount of cement remnants and scratching of abutments are observed when removing cement from subgingival margins around implants.[1] The use of screw retention or a customised abutment with the margins placed supragingivally or equigingivally is recommended to minimise trapping of cement. Linkevicius et al. have highlighted that the deeper the position of the margin, the greater the amount of undetected cement in a cemented restoration. They also reported that dental radiographs should not be considered a reliable method for cement.[2,3]

### Provisionalisation

Provisional restorations may be used for immediate loading, as well as achieving better aesthetics by developing a proper emergence profile with guiding of soft-tissue contours during healing. A screw-retained is preferred over a cement-retained restoration, as the screw can be used to seat the provisional restoration and expand the peri-implant mucosa. It can also be very difficult to remove excess cement and manage bleeding while seating a cemented provisional crown during implant surgery.

### Clinical Performance

Sailer et al. conducted a systematic review on the 5-year survival and complication rates of cemented and screw-retained implant reconstructions, and found that cement-retained reconstructions exhibited more serious biological complications.[4] They also found that 2.8% of patients had a marginal bone level of >2 mm in cement-retained crowns as compared with 0% for screw-retained crowns. Comparatively, however, the screw-retained reconstructions exhibited more technical problems, with an estimated 5-year incidence of technical complications of 24.4% as compared with 11.9% for cement-retained crowns. They concluded that cemented reconstructions exhibited more serious biological complications (implant loss, bone loss >2 mm), while screw-retained reconstructions exhibited more technical problems. Screw-retained reconstructions are more easily retrievable than cemented reconstructions and, therefore, technical and eventually biological complications can be treated more easily.

Wittneben et al., in a longer systematic review over 12 years, found that there was no statistical difference between cement and screw-retained reconstructions for survival or failure rates; however, screw-retained reconstructions exhibited fewer technical and biological complications overall.[5]

An overall comparison of cement and screw-retained restorations is presented in Table 11.4.1.

Table 11.4.1 A comparison between cement-on and screw-retained restorations

|  | Cement | Screw |
| --- | --- | --- |
| Retrievability | + | +++ |
| Aesthetics | + |  |
| Passive casting | + |  |
| Hygiene (emergence profile in anterior) | + |  |
| Reduced occlusal material fracture | + |  |
| Decreased fatigue/fracture of components | + |  |
| Limited interarch space: low profile retention |  | + |
| No cement in sulcus |  | + |

## Procedures

### Screw-Retained Restoration

- Remove the one-piece abutment and crown from the model and disinfect the restoration prior to insertion.
- Remove the healing abutment or provisional restoration from the mouth and clean the implant platform with disinfectant/water spray.
- Try-in the restoration by hand tightening it until the screw fully seats. The restoration may not seat fully because of:
  - Tight interproximal contacts
  - Not seating into internal/external connection
  - Soft-tissue impingement.

In the latter case, ensure that no soft-tissue tags are caught within the connection. If there is too much tissue blanching where the emergence profile of the subgingival contours is over-contoured, then this may be adjusted. Usually within 5 minutes the tissue blanching should disappear, but if there is still blanching then this will require adjustment. This principle also applies to pontic spaces for implant-supported bridgework.

- Check the functional occlusion and confirm with the patient that they are happy with the aesthetics of the restoration.
- Once the screw is hand tightened, take a paralleling periapical radiograph to inspect whether the restoration is fully seated onto the implant platform.
- Torque the restoration to the manufacturer's instructions to the appropriate amount, using a torque wrench or other device.
- In the screw-access hole, a cotton wool pellet, gutta percha or Teflon tape can be used on top of the head of the screw to ensure that access can be made through the crown in the future without damage to the head of the screw.
- Seal off the access hole with a restorative material; in most cases this will be composite resin.
- Check the final occlusion and function.

### Cement-Retained Restoration

- Remove the separate abutment and crown from the model and disinfect the restoration prior to insertion.
- Remove the healing abutment or provisional restoration from the mouth and clean the implant platform with disinfectant/water spray.
- Seat the abutment by ensuring that the orientation is correct. If the restoration does not seat fully, which may be due to not engaging the connection (often a hex) correctly, loosen the abutment, carry out a slight rotation to seat it and hand tighten the screw. If there is too much tissue blanching that does not dissipate over 5 minutes, adjust the contours of the abutment accordingly
- Once the abutment is fully seated, a radiograph should be taken to ensure that there is complete seating.
- Torque the abutment to the manufacturer's instructions to the appropriate amount using a torque wrench or other device.

- Ensure that the restoration is seated completely around the margins. If a restoration does not seat completely, this is often due to tight interproximal contacts or soft-tissue impingement.
- Check the functional occlusion and confirm with the patient that they are happy with the aesthetics of the restoration.
- Cover the access hole in the abutment with a cotton wool pellet, gutta percha or Teflon tape, so that when cementing the restoration no cement is inadvertently trapped in the screw.
- Cement the restoration. It is extremely important not to allow cement to be trapped in the peri-implant sulcus. Ensuring that there are no remnants is crucial, as this may predispose the implant to a biological problem. Techniques to minimise this from happening include the use of retraction cords, use of minimal cement and vent holes in the lingual of the restoration. It may also be difficult to seat a restoration if margins are subgingival, due to the hydraulic pressure that builds up, with the cement not being able to escape.

### Lateral Set-Screw (Cross-Pinning)

Lateral set-screws are an attempt to overcome the problems of unpredictable retention and retrievability of implant restorations. The screw engages threads in the restoration, normally perpendicular to the long axis of the abutment by the set-screw located in a non-aesthetic region (usually the lingual surface). This technique allows relatively easy retrieval of the restoration, with screw-hole access in a non-aesthetic and/or functional area (Figure 11.4.3).

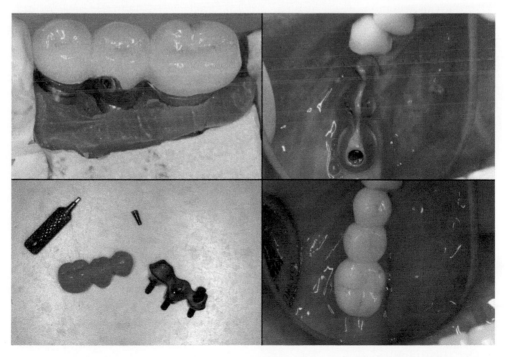

Figure 11.4.3 Use of a lateral set-screw to allow a bridge to be temporarily cemented, enabling retrievability if required

There can be difficulty using this technique in some patients due to the angulation of the long axis of the tooth, such as lingual inclination, which may present a challenging access to the set-screw. Additionally the lingual walls of restorations are often thin, resulting in an insufficient number of screw threads to house the screw. This insufficient bulk in the restoration can also lead to distortion of the restoration or stripping of the screw threads when the set-screw is tightened.

## Tips

- A technique to minimise entrapped cement remnants in a cemented restoration is to use a **chairside copy abutment**. This involves duplicating an abutment by copying it with an impression material. Seating the restoration can be then carried out extra-orally on the duplicate abutment, removing all excess except a thin film that coats the internal surface of the restoration and then seating intra-orally. This ensures that there is only the exact amount of cement on the restoration, leaving minimal excess to clean up.
- It has been shown that resin cements are the hardest to remove. If a restoration has sufficient retention, it may be best to use cement that is easier to remove.[1]
- Seating a restoration that may be more anatomically correct than a healing abutment often flares the emergence profile, making insertion of the restoration uncomfortable for the patient. It is prudent to warn the patient on seating a restoration that there may be pressure pain on insertion, and to reassure them that this disappears over a few moments. It would be good practice to seat it gently and slowly over a few moments to lessen the discomfort to patients.

## References

1 Agar JR, Cameron SM, Hughbanks JC, Parker MH. Cement removal from restorations luted to titanium abutments with simulated subgingival margins. *J Prosthet Dent.* 1997 Jul;78(1):43–7.
2 Linkevicius T, Puisys A, Vindasiute E, Linkeviciene L, Apse P. Does residual cement around implant-supported restorations cause peri-implant disease? A retrospective case analysis. *Clin Oral Implants Res.* 2013 Nov;24(11):1179–84.
3 Linkevicius T, Vindasiute E, Puisys A, Linkeviciene L, Maslova N, Puriene A. The influence of the cementation margin position on the amount of undetected cement. A prospective clinical study. *Clin Oral Implants Res.* 2013 Jan;24(1):71–6.
4 Sailer I, Muhlemann S, Zwahlen M, Hammerle CH, Schneider D. Cemented and screw-retained implant reconstructions: a systematic review of the survival and complication rates. *Clin Oral Implant Res.* 2012;23(Suppl 6):163–201.
5 Wittneben JG, Millen C, Brägger U. Clinical performance of screw- versus cement-retained fixed implant-supported reconstructions: a systematic review. *Int J Oral Maxillofac Implants.* 2014;29 Suppl:84–98.

## Further Reading

Chee W, Jivraj S. Screw versus cemented implant supported restorations. *Br Dent J.* 2006 Oct 21;201(8):501–7.
Chee W, Torbati A, Albozy JP. Retrievable cemented implant restorations. *J Prosthodont.* 1998;7:120–25.

## 11.5

# Implant Provisionalisation

*Kyle D. Hogg*

*Video: Implant Provisionalisation*
*Presented by Kyle D. Hogg*

## Principles

The success of dental implant rehabilitation cannot be entirely measured by implant and prosthesis survival, but rather must incorporate additional elements such as dento-gingival aesthetics, prosthesis aesthetics, functionality, phonetics, maintenance of the soft- and hard-tissue health of the surrounding dentition, rate of mechanical complications, rate of biological complications and overall patient satisfaction. This is of particular importance when providing treatment in the aesthetic zone, where the demand for a harmonious and visually pleasing replacement for missing teeth is at a premium. Numerous surgical protocols, implant designs, abutment designs and restoration designs have been developed to provide treatment outcomes that satisfy the aesthetic and functional requirements of replacing missing maxillary and mandibular anterior teeth.

An important element in performing predictable and aesthetic implant restorations in the aesthetic zone is provisionalisation. Provisional restorations have a variety of purposes in relation to implant dentistry. These restorations allow for acceptable patient comfort, aesthetics and function during the treatment process, while maintaining occlusal stability and the position of adjacent or opposing teeth. Provisional restorations provide a template for peri-implant soft-tissue contouring and development of an ideal emergence profile, critical factors in the overall appearance of the final restoration. These restorations allow for a trial of the proposed restorative prototype, providing an opportunity for critical appraisal and alteration of the aesthetics and function of the provisional restoration intra-orally. Once approved by both patient and clinician, provisional restorations can be utilised to transfer important design information to the dental technician for use in fabrication of the definitive restoration.

Providing appropriate provisional restorations during the course of implant rehabilitation can be a challenging and time-consuming aspect of clinical treatment. Provisionalisation can be divided into three phases: provisionalisation prior to implant placement; provisionalisation after implant placement but before placement of an implant-supported provisional restoration; and implant-supported provisional restoration.[1] Some patients may not require all three phases of provisionalisation,

*Practical Procedures in Aesthetic Dentistry*, First Edition. Edited by Subir Banerji, Shamir B. Mehta and Christopher C.K. Ho. © 2017 John Wiley & Sons, Ltd. Published 2017 by John Wiley & Sons, Ltd.
Companion website: www.wiley.com/go/banerji/aestheticdentistry

depending on the timing of implant placement relative to the loss or agenesis of the tooth to be replaced, the preferences of the individual patient and the loading protocol chosen for that implant. Selecting the appropriate provisionalisation strategy for the patient should be based on the specific clinical presentation and preferences of that individual.[2] It is important to have a clear understanding between the patient and clinician regarding the cost, limitations and duration of the provisional restorations, as well as the therapeutic benefits of the process.

There are three broad categories of provisional restorations available for use during the course of treatment: removable prostheses; fixed tooth–supported prostheses; and implant-supported prostheses.[3] Refer to Table 11.5.1 for a review of the relative advantages and disadvantages of each provisionalisation strategy.

There are a variety of methods for replacing missing teeth in the early phases of provisionalisation. The final phase, namely the implant-supported provisional restoration, is a critical step in achieving a predictable aesthetic result. This phase of treatment is designed to develop the perimucosal emergence profile and gingival margin contours to be copied in the final restoration/abutment complex, confirm the position of the incisal edge, facilitate the development of interproximal papillae, determine the location of the proximal contacts and establish the overall restoration length, width and contour.

Table 11.5.1 Provisionalisation strategies for implants in the aesthetic zone

| Restoration type | Removable | | | Fixed (tooth supported) | | | Implant supported |
| --- | --- | --- | --- | --- | --- | --- | --- |
| Criteria | Interim RPD | Essix retainer | Bonded tooth | Resin-bonded bridge (metal wing) | Reinforced provisional FPD (metal, fibre) | Acrylic resin provisional FPD | Implant-retained provisional restoration |
| Durability | Good | Poor | Fair | Good | Good | Fair | Excellent |
| Modifiability | Easy | Moderate | Moderate | Moderate | Moderate | Easy | Easy |
| Aesthetics | Good | Fair | Fair | Good | Good | Good | Excellent |
| Comfort | Poor | Fair | Good | Good | Good | Good | Excellent |
| Hygiene | Easy | Easy | Difficult | Moderate | Difficult | Difficult | Easy |
| Function | Poor | Poor | Fair | Good | Excellent | Good | Excellent |
| Phonetics | Fair | Fair | Excellent | Good | Good | Good | Excellent |
| Patient satisfaction | Poor | Poor | Good | Good | Excellent | Excellent | Excellent |
| Transmucosal loading | Poor | Excellent | Excellent | Excellent | Excellent | Excellent | Excellent |
| Soft-tissue contouring | Poor | Poor | Good | Good | Good | Good | Excellent |
| Occlusal clearance | Significant | None | None | Moderate | Significant | Moderate | Moderate |
| Cost of fabrication | Medium | Low | Low | High | High | Low | Variable |
| Access to surgical site | Easy | Easy | Difficult | Difficult | Moderate | Moderate | Moderate |

*Notes*: FPD = fixed partial denture; RPD = removable partial denture

## Procedures

Selection of a provisionalisation option that can fulfil the aesthetic and functional demands of the patient for an implant placed in the anterior region should start at the patient assessment and case-planning level. The assessment should include some form of restorative prototype from which the surgeon, restorative dentist and dental technician can work backwards in a prosthetically driven workflow. The implant placement and provisionalisation should be made with a clear restorative endpoint in mind (Figure 11.5.1). The following clinical procedures will help the clinician predictably choose or prescribe appropriate provisionalisation strategies.

With the patient comfortably seated in the dental chair, perform a thorough intra-oral examination, with particular attention paid to the edentulous site or site where the tooth will be removed. Evaluate the hard- and soft-tissue contours of the proposed implant site, determining whether any soft- or hard-tissue augmentation will be necessary. The restorative and periodontal needs of the adjacent teeth should be ascertained. Pre-operative diagnostic photos are recommended for treatment planning and

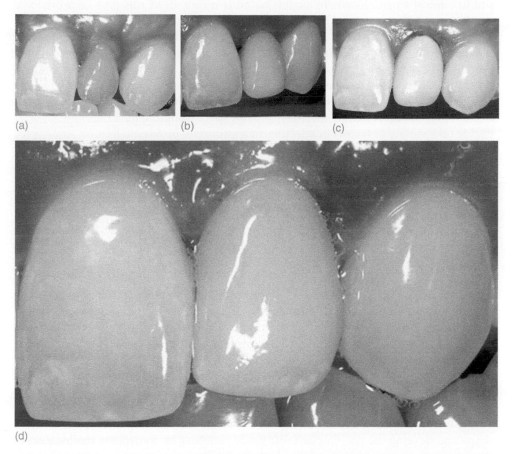

(a)  (b)  (c)

(d)

Figure 11.5.1 Progression from pre-operative condition to final implant restoration. Failing retained primary lateral incisor (a); resin-bonded bridge with single metal wing placed over immediate implant (b); implant-supported provisional restoration (c); definitive custom zirconia abutment and lithium disilicate crown (d)

documentation purposes. Good-quality alginate impressions of the maxillary and mandibular arches are often very helpful in developing a provisionalisation strategy. It is important that these impressions fully record pertinent anatomy accurately for either removable or fixed provisional restoration fabrication. Additionally, capturing a bite registration and utilising a facebow record allow diagnostic casts to be mounted accurately on a semi-adjustable articulator. Using an articulator in this manner can aid the clinician in planning for removable or fixed provisionalisation strategies by allowing an unimpeded view of the dentition, static and dynamic occlusion, interocclusal space availability, and potential for adjacent teeth to support adhesively or conventionally fixed partial dentures.

In the event that the patient presents with a provisional restoration already in place prior to implant placement, evaluate the suitability for purpose of the restoration during the initial stages of treatment. If there is a need for soft- or hard-tissue augmentation resulting in a change in contour at the edentulous site, select a provisionalisation strategy that allows for easy modification to accommodate these changes. It is prudent to avoid interim removable partial dentures that place pressure on the edentulous site in clinical situations where augmentation is required, as this type of provisional can frequently result in transmucosal loading, which can be deleterious to soft-tissue and bone-graft healing as well as implant survival.[2] Care should be taken to prevent pressure from being placed on the grafted sites or implants by relieving the overlying pontics. This may have a negative effect on the aesthetics of the provisional restoration. Figure 11.5.2 gives an example of pontic relief.

In the event that the patient does not have a provisional restoration in place prior to implant placement, or has an unsuitable provisional restoration, then the clinician must decide on a variety of factors in selecting an appropriate provisionalisation strategy for that individual. When providing a provisional restoration prior to implant placement, consider incorporating a radiopaque marker, such as barium sulfate, into the restoration to allow the prototype to appear on radiographs and cone-beam computed tomography (CBCT) scans. This may aid the surgeon greatly in placing the implant in the ideal three-dimensional location.

While immediate loading of dental implants can be a predictable treatment modality following appropriate protocols, not all implants placed are candidates for immediate loading. When a period of healing is required before progressing to an implant-supported provisional restoration, consideration must be given to allowing access to the surgical site. Being able to access the implant site easily allows for fabrication of the implant-supported provisional restoration indirectly, either by the clinician or the dental technician, and may save valuable chair time (Figure 11.5.3). In the event that conditions are favourable for immediate loading protocols, a provisional implant-supported restoration may be fabricated chairside at the time of surgery (Figure 11.5.4). Care should be taken to minimise the occlusion and eliminate excursive contacts on the implant-supported provisional restorations when immediate or delayed loading protocols are implemented.

Implant-supported provisional restorations allow the clinician the opportunity to shape and develop the peri-implant soft-tissue contours by controlling the location of the proximal contact points and facial convexity. By imparting a particular shape to the provisional restoration/abutment complex, the gingival margins and interproximal papillae can be optimised (Table 11.5.2).

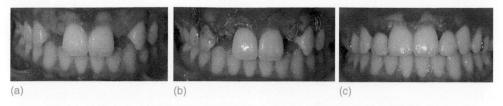

(a)                                    (b)                                    (c)

Figure 11.5.2 Modification of interim removable partial denture pontics to prevent transmucosal loading. Pre-operative condition with congenitally missing UR 2, UL 2 and deficient soft- and hard-tissue contours (a); implant placement into the edentulous sites with simultaneous hard- and soft-tissue grafting (b); interim partial denture with modified pontics to eliminate contact with implants or grafted sites (c)

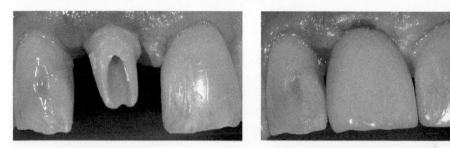

Figure 11.5.3 Laboratory-fabricated implant-supported provisional crown on definitive custom zirconia abutment

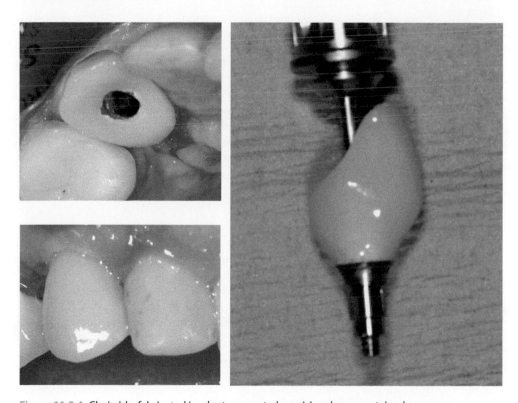

Figure 11.5.4 Chairside-fabricated implant-supported provisional screw-retained crown on temporary titanium cylinder

Table 11.5.2  Modification of provisional restoration contours to optimise the peri-implant soft-tissue profile

| Peri-implant soft-tissue profile | Provisional restoration contour |
| --- | --- |
| To position papilla apically | Decrease proximal contours, position proximal contact apically |
| To position papilla coronally | Increase proximal contours, position proximal contact coronally |
| To position facial margin apically | Increase facial convexity |
| To position facial margin coronally | Decrease facial convexity |

*Source*: Adapted from Priest 2006[3]

When osseo-integration and soft-tissue maturation have occurred, and both the patient and clinician approve of the intra-oral prototype, high-quality digital photographs of the provisional restoration in place should be taken to convey important information to the dental technician regarding the prescription of the definitive restoration. It is also good practice to take an impression of the seated provisional restoration to provide the technician with a tangible model of the restorative contours and dimensions that have been tested and approved over the healing phase.

## Tips

- Select a provisionalisation plan that is based on the objective clinical findings and preferences specific to the individual patient, rather than applying one strategy for all patients.
- While a variety of provisionalisation strategies may be employed in the early phases of treatment, the final phase of provisionalisation should consist of an implant-supported provisional crown (either screw retained or cemented).
- Utilise the implant-supported provisional crown to communicate important design features in your prescription for the definitive restoration to the dental technician by taking photos and capturing an impression of the implant-supported provisional crown in place.

## References

1 Weber H, Sing T. Provisional restorations in implant dentistry. *Inside Dent.* 2014;10(11).
2 Cho S, Shetty S, Froum S, Elian N, Tarnow D. Fixed and removable provisional options for patients undergoing implant treatment. *Compendium.* 2007;28(11):604–9.
3 Priest G. Esthetic potential of single-implant provisional restorations: selection criteria of available alternatives. *J Esthet Restor Dent.* 2006;18:326–39.

## 11.6

## Pink Aesthetics

*Brian Chee*

## Principles

To achieve a natural appearance, the peri-implant soft tissues should closely mimic those of the adjacent dentition. Several key features have been highlighted, including papilla height and the position of the mucosal margin, as well as the texture, colour and contour of the peri-implant mucosa.[1–3]

### Gingival Biotype

Gingival thickness can be broadly categorised into either thin or thick biotype. The thin gingival biotype has been associated with long-narrow teeth and a highly scalloped gingival margin, whereas the thick biotype is associated with short-wide teeth and a flat, low-scalloped gingival margin.[4]

Appreciation of the gingival biotype is important, since it can influence the aesthetic risk and complexity of treatment. The thick gingival biotype represents robust tissues with a lower risk of mucosal recession. In contrast, a thin gingival biotype is more susceptible to surgical trauma due to reduced vascularisation. This can lead to a greater risk of recession and aesthetic failure.[5–7]

### Papilla

The re-creation of papilla-like tissue is one of the most challenging goals of implant therapy in the aesthetic zone. The principal factor determining the presence of a papilla is the distance of the bone crest to the proximal contact point. A seminal study by Tarnow et al.[8] found that when the distance from the contact point to the crestal bone was 5 mm or less, the papilla between teeth was present nearly 100% of the time. However, when this distance was increased to 6 mm and 7 mm, the papilla was only present 56% and 27% of the time, respectively. Similarly, the regeneration of papillae adjacent to single implants is not predictable when the distance from bone crest to contact point is above 5 mm.[9] Moreover, the papilla level associated with single-implant restorations is related to the bone crest at the adjacent teeth and is independent of the bone level at the implant.[9,10] A minimum safe lateral distance of 1.5 mm has been suggested to preserve

*Practical Procedures in Aesthetic Dentistry*, First Edition. Edited by Subir Banerji, Shamir B. Mehta and Christopher C.K. Ho. © 2017 John Wiley & Sons, Ltd. Published 2017 by John Wiley & Sons, Ltd.
Companion website: www.wiley.com/go/banerji/aestheticdentistry

the papilla, as positioning the implant too close to the adjacent tooth can result in loss of the proximal bone.[11] Recent studies suggest that a greater potential for complete papilla fill may be achieved if the distance from the adjacent teeth is increased to 3 mm or more.[12–14] However, this minimum distance may be less important when using implants with a platform-switched design.[15]

Even though spontaneous improvement in papilla fill has been observed adjacent to single-implant restorations,[1,14] this is rarely achieved between multiple adjacent implants. Findings by Tarnow et al.[16] suggest that a mean soft-tissue height of 3.4 mm can be expected to cover the crestal bone between two implants. Due to this deficiency in papilla height, it may be necessary to modify the shape of the teeth to provide a longer contact areas and smaller embrasure space.[17] With severe deficiencies, the papilla can be re-created prosthetically with pink porcelain (Figure 11.6.1), acrylic or composite resin.

### Implant Position

Incorrect implant position is a major cause of aesthetic failure due to peri-implant soft-tissue defects.[18]

### Apico-coronal Position

Observations in histological studies have confirmed that a consistent soft-tissue dimension occurs at implants similar to the biologic width associated with teeth.[19,20] Furthermore, the bone resorption associated with development of the biologic width is greater if the implant–abutment interface is placed below the bone crest.[21,22] This will

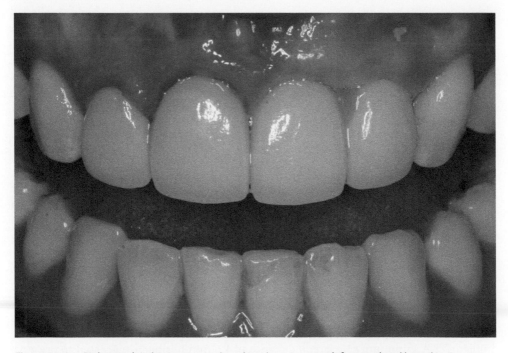

**Figure 11.6.1** Pink porcelain between two dental implants in upper left central and lateral incisor to simulate missing papilla. Meticulous attention to oral hygiene is required to maintain the gingival health for this area. *Source:* Christopher C.K. Ho, BDS MClinDent Prosthodontics. Reproduced with permission from Christopher C.K. Ho.

also be influenced by the type of connection between the implant and the abutment. Deeper placement can lead to excessive bone remodelling with subsequent recession, short papillae and long clinical crowns, particularly when there is a compromise in the bacterial seal between the implant and abutment connection. The ideal shoulder position for implants in the aesthetic zone should be approximately 3 mm apical to the planned restoration margin.

### Mesio-distal Position

Placement of the implant too close to the adjacent tooth can also result in loss of crestal bone to the level of the implant.[11] Additionally, the horizontal component of the biologic width means that a minimum distance of 3 mm is required between implants to prevent additional interproximal bone loss.[23]

### Bucco-lingual Position

Buser et al.[18] recommend that the implant shoulder is positioned 1–2 mm lingual to the emergence of the adjacent teeth. Implants positioned too buccally are associated with mid-buccal recession and aesthetic failure (Figure 11.6.2).[7]

## Procedures

Papilla reconstruction and recession coverage procedures for implants are currently unpredictable.[24] A strong emphasis should therefore be placed on the prevention of soft-tissue defects at implants in the aesthetic zone. Several key principles can be applied in order to reduce the risk of these complications:

- Appropriate flap design, atraumatic handling of the soft tissues and tension-free primary wound closure

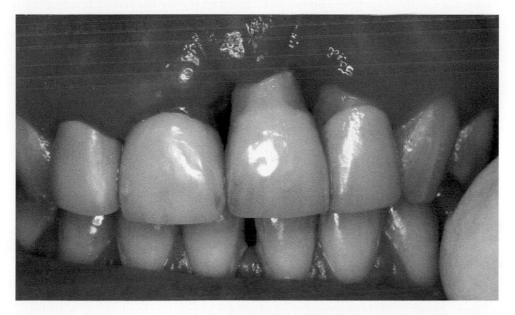

Figure 11.6.2 Implant placed in extreme buccal position leading to severe recession and an aesthetic disaster

- Selection of an appropriate post-extraction timing protocol according to individual aesthetic risk
- Implant placement in the correct prosthetically driven position
- Buccal bone augmentation for long-term tissue stability and prevention of mid-buccal recession
- Consider soft tissue augmentation for patients with a thin biotype
- Support and conditioning of the peri-implant soft tissues prior to definitive restorations.

### Flap Design and Wound Closure

Selection of an appropriate flap design and careful handling of the soft tissues are essential in achieving aesthetic wound healing. Flap design should allow good visualisation and access to the bony architecture, while keeping disruption of the blood supply and visible scarring to a minimum.[25] Additionally, there should be adequate mobilisation of the flap to allow passive closure over augmented sites. The following principles can be applied to flap design and manipulation:

- Most implant cases in the aesthetic zone can be managed using a combination of Intrasulcular and mid-crestal incisions. Clinical experience has shown that this approach provides good access with minimal risk of recession, if the flap is well adapted with a tension-free primary closure. Disruption of the papilla at adjacent teeth can be avoided using papilla-base incisions.[26]
- A single relieving incision at the distal line angle of the canines or premolars provides good access to the alveolar bone while maintaining blood supply to the flap. The relieving incision should be at 90° to the gingival margin to facilitate flap approximation. Cutting across the papilla or at the mid-facial aspect of the teeth should be avoided.
- Papilla-sparing flaps have also been advocated to reduce the risk of proximal bone loss and papilla deficiency.[27,28] While papilla-sparing incisions are routinely used for second-stage surgery, the main disadvantages for implant placement are impaired access and closure in cases with large bone defects requiring augmentation. Papilla-sparing flaps involving alveolar mucosa are also associated with significantly more scarring compared with intrasulcular and papilla-base incisions.[29]
- Incisions should be perpendicular to the surface of the tissues to maximise thickness and blood supply at the flap margin, reducing the risk of necrosis and wound dehiscence.
- A periosteal incision at the base of the flap promotes mobilisation and advancement over grafted sites.
- Use of microsurgical techniques (i.e. magnification, small elevators, microsurgical needle holders) can improve soft-tissue healing by promoting less tissue trauma, precise flap adaptation and wound closure without tension.
- Clinical experience has shown that 5-0 and 6-0 monofilament suture materials (e.g. expanded polytetrafluoroethylene, nylon and polypropylene) are suitable for implant therapy in the aesthetic zone. Thinner suture (6-0 and smaller) leads to thread breakage rather than tissue tearing under excessive tension, with the potential to reduce wound dehiscence.[30] Finer suture diameters can therefore achieve passive wound closure more predictably, although the selection of thicker suture (such as 5-0) is still necessary for repositioned flaps and when interproximal suturing dictates a larger needle size.

- Flapless surgery has many advantages, including reduced bone resorption and surgical trauma, as well as improved wound stability. However, there is significantly impaired visualisation and access for implant placement and grafting. For this reason, computer-assisted guided surgery is recommended with a flapless approach.

### Bone Augmentation

The thickness of the buccal alveolar bone is critical for optimal pink aesthetics, since the stability of the soft tissues is largely determined by the underlying bone support. A minimum buccal bone thickness of 2 mm has been suggested to reduce the incidence of future bone loss.[31] However, a recent study suggests that most sites at the anterior maxilla have less than this 'critical' thickness, with the majority (71%) of cases demonstrating a buccal bone thickness of only 0.5–1 mm.[32] This suggests that most implants in the aesthetic zone will require contour augmentation for optimal aesthetics in the long term. Simultaneous guided bone regeneration (GBR), combining autogenous bone chips, a low substitute graft material (such as demineralised bovine bone mineral, Bio-Oss, Geistlich Pharma AG, Wohlhusen, Switzerland) and collagen membrane, is a predictable and well-documented technique.[33,34]

### Timing of Implant Placement

Immediate implant placement or early placement 6–8 weeks after extraction may be indicated if the implant can be placed in the correct three-dimensional position with adequate primary stability. The soft-tissue healing that has occurred with an early placement protocol facilitates simultaneous ridge augmentation and primary closure.

The immediate placement of implants at the time of tooth extraction is an attractive approach due to the significantly reduced number of procedures and treatment time. However, immediate implant placement is unable to prevent dimensional changes in the socket wall caused by loss of the periodontal ligament-associated bundle bone.[35] Clinical studies indicate an increased risk of recession with an immediate protocol, and the technique is not recommended for high-risk cases with a thin biotype or buccal bone defect.[36]

Staged bone grafting followed by delayed implant placement may be indicated if there is inadequate bone volume. The placement of an implant in a grafted, fully healed ridge is less complex and technique sensitive than early or immediate placement. Although ridge preservation can partially compensate for post-extraction bone resorption, there is considerably greater treatment time and cost.

### Second-Stage Surgery and Soft-Tissue Augmentation

Waiting until second-stage surgery to assess the need for soft-tissue augmentation has several advantages. Many cases will not require additional soft-tissue grafting if the horizontal deficiency has been corrected by simultaneous bone augmentation at the time of implant placement. This approach also facilitates passive wound closure at the time of placement, since the flap does not have to accommodate the increased volume of both hard- and soft-tissue grafts. Delayed soft-tissue augmentation also increases the surface area for plasmatic diffusion compared with placement of the connective tissue graft (CTG) in contact with avascular bone graft materials.

If a small to moderate buccal deficiency remains following implant placement with simultaneous GBR, this can be addressed using a modified roll flap at the time of second-stage surgery.[37] This technique is straightforward and avoids the donor-site morbidity associated with a conventional CTG. Larger ridge deficiencies can be managed with a CTG harvested from the hard palate or tuberosity. The collagen-rich and dense connective tissue harvested from the tuberosity area is well suited for augmentation at implants.[38]

## Tips

- Gingival biotype can be assessed by the transparency of a periodontal probe through the gingival margin when probing.
- Simultaneous contour augmentation using the principles of GBR is often indicated in the aesthetic zone to provide long-term tissue stability and reduce the risk of recession.
- The use of a submerged (two-stage) protocol should be considered if a residual ridge deficiency in the aesthetic zone is anticipated. This allows further opportunities for soft-tissue augmentation at the time of implant exposure.
- Small soft-tissue deficiencies can be corrected by exposing the implant with a crestal incision towards the palatal aspect, displacing the soft tissue in a buccal direction after insertion of the abutment.
- The tissue-punch technique reduces the amount of keratinised tissue and should therefore be avoided in the aesthetic zone unless there is an excess of soft tissue.
- A connective tissue graft with a tunnel approach has the advantage of minimal disruption of the papilla, lower risk of scarring, as well as good wound stability and blood supply.

## References

1 Jemt T. Regeneration of gingival papillae after single-implant treatment. *Int J Periodont Restorative Dent.* 1997;17:326–33.
2 Fürhauser R, Florescu D, Benesch T, Haas R, Mailath G, Watzek G. Evaluation of soft tissue around single-tooth implant crowns: the pink esthetic score. *Clin Oral Implants Res.* 2005;16:639–44.
3 Belser UC, Grütter L, Vailati F, Bornstein MM, Weber H-P, Buser D. Outcome evaluation of early placed maxillary anterior single-tooth implants using objective esthetic criteria: a cross-sectional, retrospective study in 45 patients with a 2- to 4-year follow-up using pink and white esthetic scores. *J Periodontol.* 2008;80:140–51.
4 Olsson M, Lindhe J. Periodontal characteristics in individuals with varying form of the upper central incisors. *J Clin Periodontol.* 1991;18:78–82.
5 Bengazi F. Recession of the soft tissue margin at oral implants. A 2-year longitudinal prospective study. *Clin Oral Implants Res.* 1996;7:303–10.
6 Kan JYK, Rungcharassaeng K, Lozada J. Immediate placement and provisionalization of maxillary anterior single implants: 1-year prospective study. *Int J Oral Maxillofac Implants.* 2003;18:31–9.
7 Evans CDJ, Chen ST. Esthetic outcomes of immediate implant placements. *Clin Oral Implants Res.* 2008;19:73–80.

8  Tarnow DP, Magner AW, Fletcher P. The effect of the distance from the contact point to the crest of bone on the presence or absence of the interproximal dental papilla. *J Periodontol.* 1992;63:995–6.

9  Choquet V, Hermans M, Adriaenssens P, Daelemans P, Tarnow DP, Malevez C. Clinical and radiographic evaluation of the papilla level adjacent to single-tooth dental implants. A retrospective study in the maxillary anterior region. *J Periodontol.* 2001;72:1364–71.

10  Kan JYK, Rungcharassaeng K, Umezu K, Kois JC. Dimensions of peri-implant mucosa: an evaluation of maxillary anterior single implants in humans. *J Periodontol.* 2003;74:557–62.

11  Esposito M, Ekestubbe A, Gröndahl K. Radiological evaluation of marginal bone loss at tooth surfaces facing single Brånemark implants. *Clin Oral Implants Res.* 1993;4:151–7.

12  Gastaldo JF, Cury PR, Sendyk WR. Effect of the vertical and horizontal distances between adjacent implants and between a tooth and an implant on the incidence of interproximal papilla. *J Periodontol.* 2004;75:1242–6.

13  Cosyn J, Sabzevar MM, De Bruyn H. Predictors of inter-proximal and midfacial recession following single implant treatment in the anterior maxilla: a multivariate analysis. *J Clin Periodontol.* 2012;39:895–903.

14  Schropp L, Isidor F. Papilla dimension and soft tissue level after early vs. delayed placement of single-tooth implants: 10-year results from a randomized controlled clinical trial. *Clin Oral Implants Res.* 2015;26:278–86.

15  Vela X, Mendez V, Rodriguez X, Segala M, Tarnow DP. Crestal bone changes on platform-switched implants and adjacent teeth when the tooth-implant distance is less than 1.5 mm. *Int J Oral Maxillofac Implants.* 2012;32:149–55.

16  Tarnow D, Elian N, Fletcher P et al. Vertical distance from the crest of bone to the height of the interproximal papilla between adjacent implants. *J Periodontol.* 2003;74:1785–8.

17  Kois JC. Predictable single-tooth peri-implant esthetics: five diagnostic keys. *Compend Contin Educ Dent.* 2004;25:895–902.

18  Buser D, Martin W, Belser UC. Optimizing esthetics for implant restorations in the anterior maxilla: anatomic and surgical considerations. *Int J Oral Maxillofac Implants.* 2004;19:43–61.

19  Berglundh T. Dimension of the periimplant mucosa. Biological width revisited. *J Clin Periodontol.* 1996;23:971–3.

20  Cochran DL, Hermann JS, Schenk RK, Higginbottom FL, Buser D. Biologic width around titanium implants. A histometric analysis of the implanto-gingival junction around unloaded and loaded nonsubmerged implants in the canine mandible. *J Periodontol.* 1997;68:186–98.

21  Hämmerle CHF, Brägger U, Bürgin W, Lang NP. The effect of subcrestal placement of the polished surface of ITI® implants on marginal soft and hard tissues. *Clin Oral Implants Res.* 1996;7:111–19.

22  Hermann JS, Cochran DL, Hermann JS, Buser D, Schenk RK, Schoolfield JD. Biologic width around one- and two-piece titanium implants. *Clin Oral Implants Res.* 2001;12:559–71.

23  Tarnow DP, Cho SC, Wallace SS. The effect of inter-implant distance on the height of inter-implant bone crest. *J Periodontol* 2000;71:546–9.

24 Levine RA, Huynh-Ba G, Cochran DL. Soft tissue augmentation procedures for mucogingival defects in esthetic sites. *Int J Oral Maxillofac Implants.* 2014;29 Suppl:155–85.

25 Kleinheinz J, Buchter A, Kruse-Losler B, Weingart D, Joos U. Incision design in implant dentistry based on vascularization of the mucosa. *Clin Oral Implants Res.* 2005;16:518–23.

26 Velvart P, Ebner-Zimmermann U, Ebner JP. Comparison of long-term papilla healing following sulcular full thickness flap and papilla base flap in endodontic surgery. *Int Endod J.* 2004;37:687–93.

27 Gomez-Roman G. Influence of flap design on peri-implant interproximal crestal bone loss around single-tooth implants. *Int J Oral Maxillofac Implants.* 2001;16:61–7.

28 Greenstein G, Tarnow D. Using papillae-sparing incisions in the esthetic zone to restore form and function. *Compend Contin Educ Dent.* 2014;35:315–22.

29 Von Arx T, Salvi GE, Janner S, Jensen SS. (2008) Scarring of gingiva and alveolar mucosa following apical surgery: visual assessment after one year. *Oral Surg.* 2008;1:178–89.

30 Burkhardt R, Preiss A, Joss A, Lang NP. Influence of suture tension to the tearing characteristics of the soft tissues: an in vitro experiment. *Clin Oral Implants Res.* 2008;19:314–19.

31 Spray JR, Black CG, Morris HF, Ochi S. The influence of bone thickness on facial marginal bone response: stage 1 placement through stage 2 uncovering. *Ann Periodontol.* 2000;5:119–28.

32 Huynh-Ba G, Pjetursson BE, Sanz M et al. Analysis of the socket bone wall dimensions in the upper maxilla in relation to immediate implant placement. *Clin Oral Implants Res.* 2010;21:37–42.

33 Buser D, Chappuis V, Bornstein MM, Wittneben J-G, Frei M, Belser UC. Long-term stability of contour augmentation with early implant placement following single tooth extraction in the esthetic zone: a prospective, cross-sectional study in 41 patients with a 5- to 9-year follow-up. *J Periodontol.* 2013;84:1517–27.

34 Jensen SS, Bosshardt DD, Gruber R, Buser D. Long-term stability of contour augmentation in the esthetic zone: histologic and histomorphometric evaluation of 12 human biopsies 14 to 80 months after augmentation. *J Periodontol.* 2014;85:1549–56.

35 Araújo MG, Wennström JL, Lindhe J. Modeling of the buccal and lingual bone walls of fresh extraction sites following implant installation. *Clin Oral Implants Res.* 2006;17:606–14.

36 Chen ST, Buser D. Esthetic outcomes following immediate and early implant placement in the anterior maxilla: a systematic review. *Int J Oral Maxillofac Implants.* 2014;29:186–215.

37 Scharf DR, Tarnow DP. Modified roll technique for localized alveolar ridge augmentation. *Int J Periodontics Restorative Dent.* 1992;12:415–25.

38 Zuhr O, Baumer D, Hurzeler M. The addition of soft tissue replacement grafts in plastic periodontal and implant surgery: critical elements in design and execution. *J Clin Periodontol.* 2014;41 Suppl 15:S123–42.

## 11.7

## Implant Maintenance and Review

*Kyle D. Hogg*

*Video: Implant Maintenance and Review*
*Presented by Kyle D. Hogg*

## Principles

Dental implants can be an aesthetic and predictable method of replacing missing teeth. While dental implants are not subject to caries or endodontic pathology like natural teeth, they can develop peri-mucositis and peri-implantitis, similar to the natural dentition exhibiting gingivitis and periodontitis. Long-term studies show that both biological and technical complications can arise for both implants and implant-supported restorations.[1] Despite very high survival rates over long periods of time, the need does exist for maintenance and revision procedures related to dental implants and their restorations. This can result in significant amounts of time and financial resources allocated to keep the implants healthy and functioning appropriately. The need for continual maintenance, a defined individualised maintenance plan consisting of both at-home and professional care, as well as the cost of ownership of the implant rehabilitation should be discussed and documented as part of the process of achieving informed consent prior to treatment. Furthermore, surgical and prosthetic planning should be conducted in such a way as to minimise avoidable biological and technical complications.

The most common biological complications that occur with dental implant treatment are peri-mucositis and peri-implantitis. Peri-mucositis is the plaque-induced reversible inflammatory response of the marginal peri-implant soft tissues (Figure 11.7.1). It does not present with appreciable bone loss. While it is also plaque induced, peri-implantitis features progressive marginal bone loss and clinical signs of infection of the peri-implant soft tissues. Central to the disease process of both conditions is the accumulation or presence of bacterial plaque. A causative relationship has been shown between plaque accumulation and inflammatory changes in the peri-implant soft tissues.[2] It is generally thought that untreated peri-mucositis can progress into peri-implantitis, which can lead to implant failure. This is of importance because the incidence of peri-mucositis is fairly common and is likely to be under-diagnosed.

Different maintenance regimens as well as surgical and non-surgical interventions have been proposed for treatment of peri-mucositis and peri-implantitis (Table 11.7.1). Prevention strategies should be aimed at eliminating the accumulation of bacterial plaque

*Practical Procedures in Aesthetic Dentistry*, First Edition. Edited by Subir Banerji, Shamir B. Mehta and Christopher C.K. Ho. © 2017 John Wiley & Sons, Ltd. Published 2017 by John Wiley & Sons, Ltd.
Companion website: www.wiley.com/go/banerji/aestheticdentistry

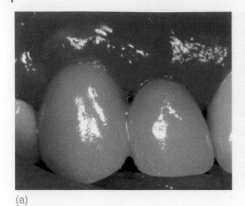
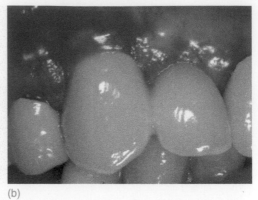

(a)                                          (b)

Figure 11.7.1 Comparison of peri-mucositis and healthy peri-implant. Gingival inflammation, soft-tissue swelling and tissue that bleeds easily on gentle probing (a). The patient was reluctant to perform basic hygiene around the cantilevered provisional fixed partial denture (FPD) UR 2–3 on the implant in the UR 3 position. Healthy peri-implant environment on the same individual around the final cantilevered FPD UR 2–3 after non-surgical supportive therapy and patient education (b). Note the lack of swelling, inflammation and bleeding

on restorations, abutments and any susceptible surface of the implant itself via patient education on home care and hygiene instruction, professional in-office supportive therapy on a recall that matches the individual's risk assessment, and provision of restorations that facilitate cleaning. At this time there is no definitive regimen or intervention that has

Table 11.7.1 Treatment strategies for maintaining or re-establishing peri-implant tissue health

| Maintaining soft-tissue health | Treatment of peri-mucositis | Treatment of peri-implantitis |
|---|---|---|
| • Patient education<br>• At-home mechanical debridement<br>• Professional in-office mechanical debridement<br>• Chlorhexidine mouthwash/gel<br>• Antiseptic mouthwash<br>• Subgingival irrigation (WaterPik) | • Patient education<br>• At-home mechanical debridement<br>• Professional in-office mechanical debridement<br>• Chlorhexidine mouthwash/gel<br>• Antiseptic mouthwash<br>• Subgingival irrigation (WaterPik)<br>• Submucosal placement of chemotherapeutic agents<br>• Ultrasonic debridement | • Patient education<br>• At-home mechanical debridement<br>• Professional in-office mechanical debridement<br>• Chlorhexidine mouthwash/gel<br>• Antiseptic mouthwash<br>• Subgingival irrigation (WaterPik)<br>• Submucosal placement of chemotherapeutic agents<br>• Ultrasonic debridement<br>• Air-abrasion debridement<br>• Er:YAG laser therapy<br>• Flap surgery with:<br>  ○ Degranulation<br>  ○ Direct mechanical debridement<br>  ○ Direct chemical debridement<br>  ○ Direct chemotherapeutic application to implant surface<br>  ○ Er:YAG laser therapy of implant surface<br>  ○ Implantoplasty to remove roughened surface of implant<br>  ○ Hard-tissue grafting and barrier membrane placement |

Table 11.7.2 Commonly occurring technical complications in implants restored with single crowns

| Complication | Cumulative incidence after 5 years of observation |
| --- | --- |
| Abutment screw loosening | 8.8% |
| Loss of retention of restoration | 4.1% |
| Fracture of veneering material | 3.5% |
| Fracture of framework material | 3.5% |
| Implant fracture | 0.18% |
| Abutment or abutment screw fracture | 0.18% |

*Source*: Adapted from Jung et al. 2012[1]

been shown to be the most effective in management of peri-mucositis or peri-implantitis.[3] When the diagnosis of peri-implant pathology has been made, an interventive treatment should be initiated promptly to avoid disease progression. As peri-mucositis and peri-implantitis have high rates of recurrence, repeated interventions and close monitoring of patients with a past history of the conditions should be considered.

Technical complications can arise over the the lifetime of the implant rehabilitation, sometimes necessitating repair or replacement of the implant restoration. Steps should be taken in the selection of appropriate patients, treatment planning and execution of treatment to minimise the risks of the most commonly occurring technical complications. These complications are listed in Table 11.7.2.

It is essential to plan for contingencies and complications when carrying out implant rehabilitations, particularly if the restorative planning is extensive or involves multiple splinted restorations. Retrievability of the restoration allows for easier periodical access and evaluation of the peri-implant soft tissues and restorative components. Being able to retrieve the restoration can also make it easier to clean the prosthesis and perform repairs if necessary. Consideration should be given to segmented treatment, breaking the rehabilitation into smaller units so that technical complications that arise may have a more limited effect. Special attention should be paid to the occlusion on the implant restoration, as well as the surrounding dentition. While controversy exists about the effect that occlusion can have on bone loss around dental implants and osseointegration, it is generally agreed that pathological occlusion and parafunctional activity can cause an increase in the frequency of technical complications. Occlusion and tooth movement are dynamic, and change throughout a patient's life (Figure 11.7.2).

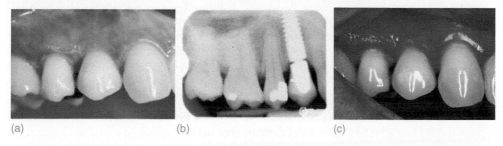

(a)  (b)  (c)

Figure 11.7.2 Changes in tooth position over 12 years of observation. Implant restoration of the UR 4 soon after it was delivered (a); clinical presentation 12 years after initial placement of the implant restoration (b and c). Note that while the peri-implant soft and hard tissues have remained healthy around the UR 4, the contact between the UR 3 and UR 4 has opened. *Source*: Subir Banerji, BDS MClinDent PhD Prosthodontics. Reproduced by permission of Subir Banerji.

It is important periodically to evaluate the occlusal demands placed on the implant restoration, as teeth move, wear and are changed iatrogenically.

## Procedures

Developing an individualised maintenance programme for patients receiving a dental implant restoration with a structured schedule of review will help to prevent biological and technical complications from occurring, or allow the clinician to recognise the need for intervention and potentially limit the extent of the complication. To be effective, the maintenance programme must collect clinical and, when appropriate, radiographic data in an organised and repeatable fashion. The plan must be frequently evaluated to determine its effectiveness, and altered as conditions change. A good maintenance programme allows for the patient, dental auxiliaries and clinician to work together to maintain the health, function and aesthetics of the implant restoration. The discussion of clinical procedures will commence with delivery of the definitive implant restoration.

With the patient comfortably seated in the dental chair, prepare to deliver the definitive implant restoration. It is good practice to show the patient the component restorative parts prior to delivery to help them better understand how to clean around the restoration adequately. A trial fitting of the restoration should then be conducted to permit the clinician to evaluate, among other things, the contours, proximal contacts, gingival embrasures and both static and dynamic occlusion. The contours of the restoration should allow for cleansing and prevent stagnation or plaque accumulation. The proximal contacts should be sufficiently loose to allow floss to access, but not so open as to allow food to impact. The gingival embrasure design should permit the insertion of cleaning aids or floss threaders. Generally speaking, the static occlusion of a single implant restoration should be light enough that a ribbon of shim stock is not held by the implant restoration and the antagonistic tooth is under light to moderate pressure, but under increasing occlusal force the shim stock is held by the pair. Additionally, excursive contacts on the implant restorations should be eliminated or kept to a minimum when possible.

With the trial fitting completed to the satisfaction of the clinician, the implant restoration may be definitively delivered. When providing implant abutments with cemented crowns, great care must be taken not to introduce excess cement into the peri-implant sulcus. Excess cement in this area is often hard to detect, can be even more challenging to remove and can lead to peri-implant pathology. On delivery of the restoration a baseline radiograph should be taken. The film or sensor should be oriented parallel to the long axis of the implant. The baseline radiograph establishes a reference point of where the hard-tissue contours were in relation to the implant at the time of restoration. It is important to note that while the radiograph may pick up excess radiopaque cement present on the image, it is not very sensitive and not a reliable means of establishing that all cement has been removed from the peri-implant sulcus (Figure 11.7.3). Steps taken to minimise excess cement being loaded in the crown and a thorough tactile and visual examination of the sulcus are more appropriate means to avoid cementation-related complications. Time should be taken to instruct and demonstrate to the patient how to clean around the delivered restoration adequately. The patient should then repeat back and perform the cleaning exercise, allowing for remediation of the hygiene techniques and establishing that the patient is equipped to perform the at-home care required proficiently.

A recall interval of between 3 and 6 months should be established based on the patient's individual risk factors. The factors to be considered in determination of the recall interval include oral hygiene and effectiveness of plaque control, previous history of peri-mucositis

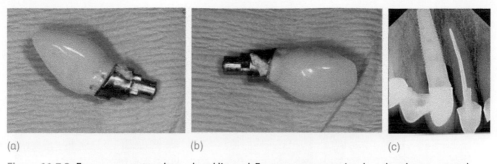

(a)       (b)       (c)

**Figure 11.7.3** Excess cement on buccal and lingual. Excess cement retained on the abutment and crown of the implant in the UR 3 site (a and b); radiograph showing recurrent decay of the UR 2 and peri-implant bone loss around the UR 3 (c). The patient presented clinically with pain, swelling and suppuration from the implant sulcus consistent with peri-implantitis

or peri-implantitis, peri-implant bleeding or suppuration, tobacco use and the needs of the remaining dentition. When examined by the clinician or dental hygienist at a recall visit, the patient should be asked whether they are having any trouble with the implant rehabilitation, along with the rest of the dentition. Prior to any instrumentation of the implant the site should be visually inspected, the clinician noting the appearance of the peri-implant soft tissues and checking for any signs of oedema or tissue recession. The soft tissues around the implant should be gently compressed to check for any signs of suppuration from the sulcus, which would indicate pathology. Following this, gentle periodontal probing can be conducted. Because of the differences in the attachment of natural teeth and implants and the prosthetic transition from implant to clinical crown, the absolute probing depth around implants is not comparable to that of teeth. What is more important is the presence or absence of bleeding on probing and the relative changes in probing depths over time associated with the implant. The implant can be percussed to check for mobility or pain. The static and dynamic occlusion should also be re-evaluated with thin articulating paper and a ribbon of shim stock to ensure its stability and fidelity to the prescribed occlusal scheme. The patient should also be screened for parafunctional activity.

Professional mechanical debridement with gold or titanium scalers, and/or ultrasonic or piezoelectric scalers with plastic or carbon tips, is suitable for debridement of the restored implant. While some standard metal scalers may be too hard or abrasive for debridement of the implant, many plastic hand scalers are not sufficiently rigid to remove plaque or calculus effectively.

A second pre-scripted radiograph, taken in the same fashion as the baseline radiograph, should be conducted 1 year following restoration of the implant (Figure 11.7.4). The capture of a similar high-quality image allows the clinician to evaluate the stability of the bone levels visible on the radiograph when compared to the baseline. In the absence of clinical and radiographic signs of peri-mucositis or peri-implantitis, the radiographic interval can be extended to match that of the remaining dentition. If those conditions are not met, then an interventive treatment should be initiated promptly or the patient referred to a specialist colleague for further management.

## Tips

- Discuss with the patient the expectations for maintenance and review prior to initiating treatment. Be sure that the patient understands the potential for biological and technical complications associated with implant rehabilitation, the importance

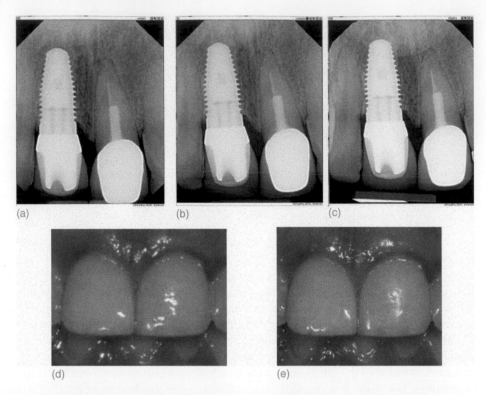

**Figure 11.7.4** Series of radiographs and photographs from the author's clinical practice permitting evaluation of peri-implant hard and soft tissues. High-quality repeatable radiographs demonstrating the stability of the crestal bone relative to the implant over time: baseline (a), 1-year follow-up (b) and 6-year follow-up (c). Subsequent photographs depict the stability and health of the peri-implant soft tissues over the same 6-year interval (d and e).

of at-home and professional debridement, and the responsibility for the cost of future maintenance.
- Develop an individualised maintenance plan for the patient focusing on disease prevention and review the effectiveness of and compliance with the plan frequently.
- Recognise the clinical and radiographic signs and symptoms of peri-mucositis or peri-implantitis early and intervene or refer to a specialist colleague for further care.
- Re-assess occlusion on implant restorations frequently, particularly if there have been changes to the dentition.

## References

1 Jung R, Zembic A, Pjetursson B, Zwahlen M, Thoma D. Systematic review of the survival rate and the incidence of biological, technical, and aesthetic complications of single crowns on implants reported in longitudinal studies with a mean follow-up of 5 years. *Clin Oral Implants Res.* 2012;23 (Suppl. 6):2–21.
2 Pontoriero R, Tonelli M, Carnvale G, Mombelli A, Nyman S, Lang N. Experimentally induced peri-implant mucositis: a clinical study in humans. *Clin Oral Impl Res.* 1994;5:254–9.
3 Esposito M, Grusovin M, Worthington H. Treatment of peri-implantitis: what interventions are effective? A Cochrane systematic review. *Euro J Oral Implant.* 2012;5 (Suppl):S21–41.

# Index

*Practical Procedures in Aesthetic Dentistry*, First Edition. Edited by Subir Banerji, Shamir B. Mehta and
Christopher C.K. Ho. © 2017 John Wiley & Sons, Ltd. Published 2017 by John Wiley & Sons, Ltd.
Companion website: www.wiley.com/go/banerji/aestheticdentistry